PHARMACOPOEIAS, DRUG REGULATION, AND EMPIRES

INTOXICATING HISTORIES

Series editors: Virginia Berridge and Erika Dyck

Whether on the street, off the shelf, or over the pharmacy counter, interactions with drugs and alcohol are shaped by contested ideas about addiction, healing, pleasure, and vice and their social dimensions. Books in this series explore how people around the world have consumed, created, traded, and regulated psychoactive substances throughout history. The series connects research on legal and illegal drugs and alcohol with diverse areas of historical inquiry, including the histories of medicine, pharmacy, consumption, trade, law, social policy, and popular culture. Its reach is global and includes scholarship on all periods. Intoxicating Histories aims to link these different pasts as well as to inform the present by providing a firmer grasp on contemporary debates and policy issues. We welcome books, whether scholarly monographs or shorter texts for a broad audience focusing on a particular phenomenon or substance, that alter the state of knowledge.

1 Taming Cannabis
Drugs and Empire in Nineteenth-Century France
David A. Guba, Jr

2 Cigarette Nation
Business, Health, and Canadian Smokers, 1930–1975
Daniel J. Robinson

3 Remedicalising Cannabis
Science, Industry, and Drug Policy
Suzanne Taylor

4 Mixing Medicines
The Global Drug Trade and Early Modern Russia
Clare Griffin

5 Drugging France
Mind-Altering Medicine in the Long Nineteenth Century
Sara E. Black

6 Psychedelic New York
A History of LSD in the City
Chris Elcock

7 Disparate Remedies
Making Medicines in Modern India
Nandini Bhattacharya

8 Art, Medicine, and Femininity
Visualising the Morphine Addict in Paris, 1870–1914
Hannah Halliwell

9 A Thirst for Wine and War
The Intoxication of French Soldiers on the Western Front
Adam D. Zientek

10 Pharmacopoeias, Drug Regulation, and Empires
Making Medicines Official in Britain's Imperial World, 1618–1968
Stuart Anderson

Pharmacopoeias, Drug Regulation, and Empires

*Making Medicines Official
in Britain's Imperial World,
1618–1968*

STUART ANDERSON

McGill-Queen's University Press
Montreal & Kingston • London • Chicago

© McGill-Queen's University Press 2024

ISBN 978-0-2280-2104-9 (cloth)
ISBN 978-0-2280-2105-6 (paper)
ISBN 978-0-2280-2158-2 (ePDF)
ISBN 978-0-2280-2159-9 (ePUB)

Legal deposit second quarter 2024
Bibliothèque nationale du Québec

Printed in Canada on acid-free paper that is 100% ancient forest free (100% post-consumer recycled), processed chlorine free

 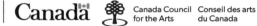

We acknowledge the support of the Canada Council for the Arts.

Nous remercions le Conseil des arts du Canada de son soutien.

McGill-Queen's University Press in Montreal is on land which long served as a site of meeting and exchange amongst Indigenous Peoples, including the Haudenosaunee and Anishinabeg nations. In Kingston it is situated on the territory of the Haudenosaunee and Anishinaabek. We acknowledge and thank the diverse Indigenous Peoples whose footsteps have marked these territories on which peoples of the world now gather.

Library and Archives Canada Cataloguing in Publication

Title: Pharmacopoeias, drug regulation, and empires : making medicines official in Britain's imperial world, 1618–1968 / Stuart Anderson.
Names: Anderson, Stuart, 1946– author.
Series: Intoxicating histories ; 10.
Description: Series statement: Intoxicating histories ; 10 | Includes bibliographical references and index.
Identifiers: Canadiana (print) 2024030604x | Canadiana (ebook) 20240306058 | ISBN 9780228021049 (cloth) | ISBN 9780228021056 (paper) | ISBN 9780228021582 (ePDF) | ISBN 9780228021599 (ePUB)
Subjects: LCSH: Pharmacopoeias—Great Britain—History.
Classification: LCC RS141.3 .A53 2024 | DDC 615.1/141—dc23

This book was typeset by True to Type in 10½/13 Sabon

For Liz

Contents

Figures and Tables ix
Acknowledgements xi
Abbreviations xiii

Introduction: Medicines, Trade, and Pharmacopoieas 3

1 The Many Meanings of 'Pharmacopoiea' 24

2 Pharmacopoeias and Drug Regulation 44

3 Pharmacopoeias in European Colonial Empires 64

4 Pharmacopoeias for England, Scotland, and Ireland 84

5 The Emergence of Colonial Pharmacopoeias 108

6 One Empire, One Pharmacopoeia 130

7 Towards an Imperial Pharmacopoeia 150

8 From Colonial Addendum to Imperial Pharmacopoeia 176

9 A Committee of Inquiry 198

10 Decolonizing the Pharmacopoeia 218

Conclusion 240

Notes 257
Index 325

Figures and Tables

FIGURES

0.1 Expeditions to the New World, 1494–1788. Source: adapted from Francisco Guerra, "Medical Colonization of the New World," *Medical History* 7, no. 2 (1963): 154-1. 9

2.1 An unscrupulous chemist selling a child arsenic and laudanum. Wood engraving after J. Leech. Source: Wellcome Collection, https://wellcomecollection.org/works/hcw9dhst. 49

3.1 Codex Medicamentarius seu Pharmacopoeia Parisiensis, 1732 Cum Privilegio Regis. Source: Wellcome Collection, https://wellcomecollection.org/works/kepk9yye. 72

4.1 Frontispiece from the second issue of first edition of the *Pharmacopoeia Londinensis*, December 1618. Source: *Moments in Medicine*, Bodleian Libraries, Oxford University, https://visit.bodleian.ox.ac .uk/sites/default/files/bodwhatson/documents/media/mim-pharma-copoeia-londinensis.pdf. 88

5.1 William Brooke O'Shaughnessy (1809–1889) around 1844. Source: Wikipedia, s.v. "William Brooke O'Shaughnessy," last modified 23 November 2023, 04:20, https://en.wikipedia.org/wiki/William _Brooke_O%27Shaughnessy#/media/File:William_Brooke_O%E2 %80%99Shaughnessy_1.jpg. 118

5.2 *Bengal Pharmacopoeia* 1844. Source: author's photograph. 121

6.1 *Pharmacopoeia of India* 1868. Source: Wikisource, https://en.wiki source.org/wiki/Index:Pharmacopoeia_of_India_%281868%29 .djvu. 141

6.2 Robert Bentley (1821–1893), John Attfield (1835–1911), and Theophilus Redwood (1806–1892), ca 1881–87. Source: Julia Martín, Purificación Sáez-Plaza, and Agustín García Asuero, "Theophilus Redwood, Hero of the British Pharmacy, First President of 'The Society of Public Analysts.' Part 1," *Anales de la Real Academia Nacional de Farmacia* 84, no. 4 (2018), https://idus.us.es/bitstream/handle/11441/96375/ARANF_garcia-asuero_2018_theophilus-I.pdf?sequence=1&isAllowed=y.   147

7.1 John Wodehouse, 1st Earl of Kimberley (1826–1902), ca 1897. Source: National Portrait Gallery, https://www.npg.org.uk /collections/search/portrait/mw138539/John-Wodehouse-1st-Earl-of-Kimberley.   157

7.2 *Indian and Colonial Addendum to the British Pharmacopoeia* 1898. Source: Wellcome Collection, https://wellcomecollection .org/works/bxsp5gv7.   170

8.1 Orange quinine wine, prepared according to the *British Pharmacopoeia* 1898. Source: Wellcome Collection, https://wellcome collection.org/works/h9dz64et.   183

8.2 '"Wellcome" brand chloroform fulfils all B.P. requirements', 1916. Source: Wikimedia Commons, https://commons.wikimedia.org /wiki/File:Wellcome_chloroform.jpg.   191

9.1 Hugh Pattison Macmillan, KC (1873–1952) in 1924. Source: National Portrait Gallery, https://www.npg.org.uk/collections /search/person/mp52845/hugh-pattison-macmillan-baron-macmillan.   202

10.1 The *Indian Pharmacopoeial List* 1946. Source: Internet Archive, https://archive.org/details/dli.ernet.16223/page/n5/mode/2up.   229

TABLES

0.1 British dependencies and colonies, 1914   20
2.1 Models of drug regulation   51
3.1 European colonial powers and pharmacopoeias, 1550–1920   82
4.1 Drug imports into England by region of origin, 1567–1774   90
4.2 Drug imports and inclusion in official pharmacopoeias, 1618–1775   92
6.1 Plant medicines included in the BP 1885 by continent of origin   149
7.1 Drugs in the *Indian and Colonial Addendum* official in colonies besides India and Eastern Division   172
8.1 Alternatives to products of German origin in BP 1914   190
10.1 Year of independence of selected British Dominions and colonies   234

Acknowledgements

The origins of this book lie in insights and reflections gained through several strands of previous research. Firstly, work for the International Society for the History of Pharmacy's (ISHP) Working Group on the History of Pharmacopoeias drew attention to differences in approaches to the compilation and use of pharmacopoeias both in the metropoles and colonies of European colonial powers. Secondly, a workshop on pharmacopoeias and healing knowledge in the early modern Atlantic world held at the University of Wisconsin in April 2016 brought together scholars from a wide range of backgrounds. Whilst illustrating the depth and range of scholarship then taking place on pharmacopoeias, it also raised many questions about definition, status, compilation, content, and use in colonies. Thirdly, a subsequent study of British pharmacy and professionalization in the colonial context highlighted differences in the role and use of pharmacopoeias across the empire. Together, these strands exposed a very wide range of meanings and functions attached to the word.

In writing this book I have received help from many colleagues across the world, and especially those on the ISHP Working Group; they include Bruno Bonnemain, Antonio Isacio Gonzalez Bueno, Giovanni Cipriani, Axel Helmstädter, Paul Kruse, Francois Lederman, Joao Rui Pita, and Stefan Wulle. Tony Cartwright and the late Harkishan Singh gave much support and advice over several years, including directing me to many important references, and readily providing copies of material that was otherwise difficult to access.

Others who have provided valuable assistance or information at various times include Ben Breen, Patrick Chiu, Joanne Collin, Matthew Crawford, John Crellin, Greg Higby, Wouter Klein, Toine Pieters, André Schön, and Paula de Vos. I am indebted to the advice and help

xii Acknowledgements

of staff at archives and libraries in London and elsewhere, especially those at the National Archives, the British Library, and the Wellcome Collection. Particular thanks are due to librarians Jane Trodd and Karen Horn and museum manager Catherine Walker at the Royal Pharmaceutical Society, Katie Birkwood at the Royal College of Physicians, and Nick Wood at the Society of Apothecaries. Lee Williams helped in the adaptation of maps.

My thanks are due to the series editors, Virginia Berridge and Erika Dyck, for their continued support and encouragement, to the anonymous referees for much helpful feedback, to Richard Baggeley at McGill-Queen's University Press for his support and guidance, and to Ryan Perks, copy editor, and Alyssa Favreau, production editor at McGill-Queen's, for turning a manuscript into a book.

As always, my greatest debt is to my wife, Liz, for her continued patience and support for my researching and writing activities.

Stuart Anderson

Abbreviations

APF	*Australian Pharmaceutical Formulary*
BMA	British Medical Association
BP	*British Pharmacopoeia*
BPC	*British Pharmaceutical Codex*
BW	Burroughs Wellcome & Co.
CIDC	Central Indigenous Drugs Committee (India)
CMA	Canadian Medical Association
CPA	Canadian Pharmaceutical Association
DP	*Dublin Pharmacopoeia*
EIC	English East India Company
EP	*Edinburgh Pharmacopoeia*
GMC	General Medical Council
ICA	*Indian and Colonial Addendum*
IPL	*Indian Pharmacopoeial List*
IOR	India Office Records
ISHP	International Society for the History of Pharmacy
LP	*London Pharmacopoeia*
MRC	Medical Research Council
NAI	National Archives of India
OCP	Ontario College of Pharmacy
PA	*Pharmacopoeia Amstelredamensis*
PI	*Pharmacopoeia of India*
PSGB	Pharmaceutical Society of Great Britain
PSI	Pharmaceutical Society of Ireland
RCP	Royal College of Physicians
TNA	The National Archives, Kew, London
USP	*United States Pharmacopoeia*

PHARMACOPOEIAS, DRUG REGULATION, AND EMPIRES

INTRODUCTION

Medicines, Trade, and Pharmacopoeias

This book problematizes use of the term 'pharmacopoeia' in scholarly writing. In recent years it has come to have many different meanings: sometimes it refers to an official publication that has been authorized by an appropriate body; more often it refers to something that has not. Scholarly writing on pharmacopoeias is now to be found across a very broad range of academic disciplines, from history and economics to ethnopharmacology and geography. It encompasses both 'official' and 'unofficial' pharmacopoeias, but the distinction between the two is not always clear. Even when one is made, a simple binary division between traditional and official pharmacopoeias is no longer sufficiently informative.

Much scholarly writing on pharmacopoeias now relates to the use of natural materials by Indigenous communities for medicinal purposes. 'Pharmacopoeia' in this context may not even refer to a written text; the term is also used to describe knowledge passed on across time and space through oral testimony. It may point to materials of animal, vegetable, and mineral origin, or only those sourced from plants. The word is now used to describe, for example, the medicines used by an Indigenous group (the Kallawaya pharmacopoeia), in a country (the Mexican pharmacopoeia), in a region of the world (the European pharmacopoeia), within a system of medicine (the Western pharmacopoeia), or those used for a specific disease (the syphilitic pharmacopoeia). But a range of other terms – including antidotaria, dispensatories, and formularies – are also used to describe written texts that may or may not have been produced under official authority.

If non-official pharmacopoeias are problematic, the difficulties are even greater when discussing official pharmacopoeias. There have been many definitions for such volumes, but many pharmacopoeias usually recognized as official did not meet many or even most of the criteria listed. They could be 'official' by virtue of being published by a monarch, a college of physicians, a church authority, or a government. Yet they were not necessarily 'statutory' by being incorporated into parliamentary legislation, and many – including the London and Edinburgh pharmacopoeias – were not. The extent of their statutory nature also varied enormously; it might extend to the strict enforcement of their use and harsh penalties for infringements, but it might equally relate only to their production, to the use of one named pharmacopoeia, or to restricting the supply of medicines to preparations included in them.

Even when pharmacopoeias had statutory recognition their use in practice might be negligible as a result of weak or no enforcement, lack of inspection, rare prosecutions, and limited sanctions. Their scope varied greatly; whilst some official pharmacopoeias included all the medicines that doctors could prescribe and that pharmacists supplied, others were lists only of those in most common use, and even then their use might be voluntary. Countering fraudulent activities such as adulteration and counterfeiting and the supply of substandard drugs required not just standards for drugs specified in a pharmacopoeia, but the application of a drug regulatory framework underpinned by legislation.

The relationship between official pharmacopoeias and drug regulation systems is a convoluted one. They could and did operate independently of each other. The use of pharmacopoeias could be incorporated into the same legislation as drug regulation. More commonly pharmacopoeias were referenced in a patchwork of medical, pharmacy and poisons, food and drugs, customs and excise, and other legislation. It was also possible for pharmacopoeial requirements to be undermined by other legislation. But if these were problems in the metropole for European colonial powers they were even more so in colonies, since the list of functions assigned to pharmacopoeias grew as empires expanded.

THIS BOOK'S APPROACH

This book explores issues resulting from use of the term 'pharmacopoeia' in scholarly writing by considering them from several perspectives. A cross-disciplinary perspective examines how scholars from a wide range of disciplines use the term in different ways and with differing meanings. A cross-imperial power perspective enables the iden-

Introduction 5

tification of ways in which the British approach to the use of pharmacopoeias in its empire differed from that of other European colonial powers. The book also takes a cross-colony perspective in identifying ways in which the use of official metropolitan pharmacopoeias differed between British colonies. Finally, it takes a cross-temporal perspective, exploring how the meaning and function, legal status, content, and use of pharmacopoeias changed over both space and time.

These issues are important since lack of clarity about the definition, status, and function of pharmacopoeias has significant consequences. It can result in confusion, uncertainty, and misunderstanding, or another word might be more inappropriate. 'The *British Pharmacopoeia*' is very different to 'the British pharmacopoeia', which refers solely to medicines native to the British Isles. Yet this kind of confusion is common across the literature. As a result, opportunities have been missed for cross-disciplinary learning between disciplines such as ethnopharmacology and history. Lack of distinction between the official and statutory status of pharmacopoeias often results in their role and use not being located within a broad regulatory framework as relates to drugs. Finally, insufficient acknowledgement of changing meanings and functions of pharmacopoeias over time has meant that important historical features and opportunities for new avenues of research have been missed.

The study of pharmacopoeias still has much to reveal about the complex relationship between medicines, regulation, trade, and empire. This book offers new insights on scholarly work in this field. It calls on all those engaged in research on pharmacopoeias, from whatever discipline, to be more explicit in their use of the term, to explore what lessons and insights might be learned from other disciplines, and to locate findings in a context that embraces not only medicine and trade but also pharmacy professionalization and drug regulation. It advocates clearer explanation of meaning when using the word; it urges greater cross-disciplinary collaboration between scholars researching pharmacopoeias; and it seeks to promote further historical studies of pharmacopoeias.

PHARMACOPOEIAS AND EMPIRES

At its most fundamental the word 'pharmacopoeia' is used to describe a list of materials used for medicinal purposes in communities, either in general or as determined by some authority. What items are included in such lists is determined by many factors: the transmission of knowledge between communities; the search for useful products in distant lands; the professionalization of medicine and pharmacy; and attempts to control the use and quality of certain items, among other issues. Bioprospecting for drugs and international trade played central roles in determining the content, purpose, and use of pharmacopoeias, both Indigenous and metropolitan, in the colonial context.

The role of official pharmacopoeias in the colonies of European powers has received little attention to date from historians. This book considers that role in the British Empire. In choosing to 'imperialize the pharmacopoeia' Britain took a rather different approach to the role of metropolitan pharmacopoeias in its empire than did other European colonial powers. The role they played was the result of complex interrelationships between medicines and trade, science and belief, politics and warfare, authority and power, and between professionalization and drug regulation. Three main themes run through most of the book: the international drugs trade and its expansion from the sixteenth century; the professionalization and institutionalization of apothecaries and their transition into pharmacists in Britain and its colonies; and the interaction between physicians and apothecaries with regard to drug regulation and standardization. The aim of this introduction therefore is to set the scene for what follows by exploring the relationships between medicines, regulation, trade, and empire, and their connections with pharmacopoeias.

These disparate factors coalesced to create a need for the standardization and regulation of medicines and a space for pharmacopoeias. Their complexity multiplies when discussion is extended over several centuries, particularly following Christopher Columbus's arrival in the 'New World' in 1492. The *Receptario Florentino*, considered to be the first official pharmacopoeia in Europe, was published in Florence just six years later, under the authority of the Florentine College of Physicians.[1] It was followed by many others during the sixteenth and early seventeenth centuries. The first official pharmacopoeia in Britain, the *London Pharmacopeia* (LP), was published in 1618. Yet it was not the first list of medicinal materials published in England, nor was its content limited to items available locally.

THE INTERNATIONAL DRUG TRADE
AND THE COLUMBIAN EXCHANGE

The importation of medicines into Britain from across the world predates both the preparation of pharmacopoeias and the emergence of European colonial empires. Many were introduced to Britain by the Romans between 43 and 410 CE. They originated from a vast geographical area. In *Drug Recipes* Scribonius Largus – who accompanied Claudius on the British invasion – listed 271 recipes and 249 vegetable, 45 mineral, and 36 animal substances. These were 'drawn from the Mediterranean region or imported from further east or from Africa via Alexandria'.[2] Largus's aim was 'to discover what works', and his recipes came from lay practitioners as well as physicians.[3] Many items reached Europe from China having travelled along the Silk Road; some are still listed in herbals today.

Anglo-Saxon physicians had access to medical works of the classical and late antique periods.[4] *Bald's Leechbook* – a collection of recipes – contained a wide range of remedies that were widely shared and copied. Similarities in forms and substances suggested that 'at least as early as the late ninth century there had grown up a sort of corpus of remedies in Old English'.[5] By the tenth century some 'exotic' medicines – non-native items imported from abroad – were in regular use in England, and medicinal items became valued objects of commerce. Trease notes that the trade in exotics was well established by the eleventh century, with pepperers importing them from Mediterranean cities including Montpellier, Marseilles, and Venice, and spicers subsequently distributing them to towns and cities across Britain.[6] By the fourteenth century concern about adulteration had led to consignments of drugs being inspected at ports.[7] But towards the end of the fifteenth century the international trade in medicines expanded rapidly and exotic drugs become more widespread.

The discovery of the New World of the Americas and the West Indies was possible because of advances in ship construction; larger ships with improved sail formations could sustain crews for longer periods. Columbus's voyage marked the beginning of the transoceanic exploration that led to the discovery of previously unknown territories by Western adventurers and a process of biological globalization in the fifteenth and sixteenth centuries. It was followed by many other voyages: John Cabot arrived in Newfoundland from Bristol in 1497;

8   Pharmacopoeias, Drug Regulation, and Empires

Magellan completed his circumnavigation of the earth in 1522. Following the discovery of the New World a transatlantic drug trade quickly developed between the West Indies, Central America, and Spain.[8] The first New World drugs 'discovered' were tobacco and coca. Columbus's crew witnessed locals smoking tobacco on Hispaniola in 1492, and in 1503 Panamanians were seen chewing coca.[9] Medicinal plants harvested in Bermuda, Virginia, and the Carolinas included sarsaparilla, sassafras, ipecacuanha, and Jamestown weed.[10] Jalap was encountered by Spanish conquistadores whilst enslaving and robbing Indigenous Mexican people and was introduced to Europe in 1565 as a medicinal herb used to treat an array of illnesses.[11]

The search for items of potential trade value soon became more systematized and formalized. Londa Schiebinger has shown how epic scientific voyages sponsored by European imperial powers explored the natural riches of the New World with the aim of uncovering the botanical secrets of Indigenous peoples.[12] The import of increasing numbers of plant medicines followed European expeditions throughout the Caribbean, North, Central and South America over many decades, as illustrated by Francisco Guerra (figure 0.1). He noted that there was often a time lag between discovery and introduction into Europe and that new sources of recently recognized plants were frequently discovered elsewhere soon after.[13]

The Columbian Exchange had a profound impact on world history in the centuries that followed, especially in the Americas, Europe, and Africa.[14] It involved the widespread transfer of plants, animals, precious metals, commodities, culture, human populations, technology, diseases, and ideas between the New World and the Old in the late fifteenth and subsequent centuries.[15] In 1574 the Spanish physician and botanist Nicolas Monardes (1493–1588) described forty-seven new drugs, with another twenty or so added over the next fifty years. The most profitable were guaiac, sarsaparilla, sassafras, and tobacco. Balsam of Peru, dragon's blood, and pepper fell out of favour in the early nineteenth century, and guaiac had all but disappeared from medical practice by 1830. Sarsaparilla became a popular ingredient of home remedies, and sassafras became a popular folk remedy.[16] Trading in these items began before the first English North American colonies were established. Planters and explorers actively sought out potential new drugs that might have a large European market.[17] In 1602 Walter Raleigh returned to England with a cargo that included sassafras, China root, Benjamin (benzoin), sarsaparilla, and cassia lignea.[18] The transatlantic drug trade

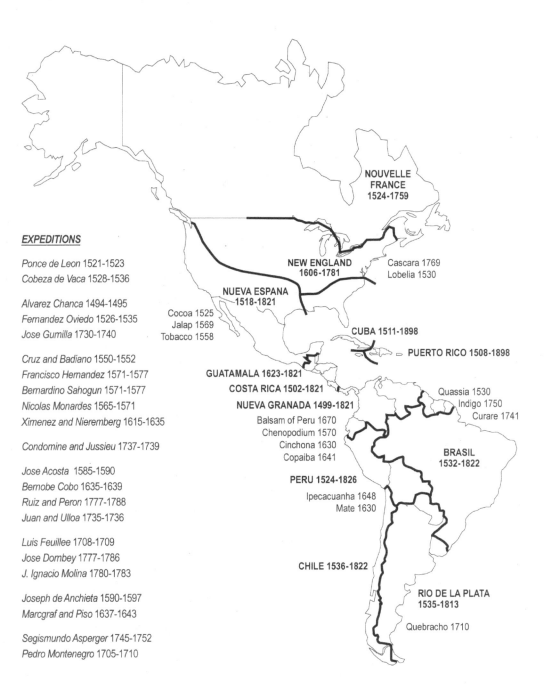

Figure 0.1 Expeditions to the New World, 1494–1788.

between the West Indies, Central America, and Spain was well established by the seventeenth century.[19]

By the mid-seventeenth century large numbers of medicinal plants were being imported. Settlements in Jamestown, Plymouth, Cupids, and Ferryland in Newfoundland relied heavily on imported medicines from England.[20] Between the 1570s and the 1770s the value of medicinal drug imports – mostly of plant origin – increased over fifty times.[21] Cinchona from Peru reached British shores in 1640, and Culpeper included it in his *The English Physitian* in 1652. Ipecacuanha arrived from North America in 1670, and both this and cinchona were included in the next edition of the *LP* in 1677. Early exchanges laid the foundation for European colonization, for global trade, and for the rise of slavery. Whilst many exchanges were deliberate, others were accidental or unexpected. The arrival of communicable diseases of European origin resulted in an 80 to 95 per cent reduction in the number of Indigenous peoples in the Americas from the fifteenth century onward, most notably in the Caribbean. European colonists and enslaved Africans replaced Indigenous populations across the Americas, with the migration of free and enslaved people having a significant impact on cultures in both hemispheres.[22]

Supplying the slave trade and plantations became an important part of the business of many apothecaries. Quaker networks and London merchants such as Thomas Corbyn and Joseph Gurney Bevan played an important part in this trade.[23] Others involved in supplying the American colonies included Samuel Storke, Thomas Mayleigh, and William Jones.[24] Mark Jenner and Patrick Wallis have demonstrated that the changing content and scale of commercially available drugs – particularly those imported from abroad – were crucial factors in the emerging medical marketplace of the early seventeenth century. Drug imports have been posited as a major factor driving changes in the form and level of demand for medicine; but they played a very minor role in the early medical marketplace historiography, where 'interest in commercialization overshadowed the material culture of medicine.'[25] This literature makes little mention of the impact of imperial and exotic goods on medicine, although Hal Cook and Roy Porter – among others – have identified a number of drugs as being important factors in its growth; they found that opium, quinine, and guaiacum transformed therapeutics.[26]

MEDICINAL PLANTS
AND INDIGENOUS KNOWLEDGE

Early European settlers acquired knowledge of the use of local plant medicines from Indigenous people, although the extent of this may have been overstated.[27] Indigenous knowledge of plant medicines included where and how to grow them, when best to harvest them, as well as which medical conditions to use them for. This knowledge was intimately linked to Indigenous medical cultures and beliefs, often tied up with religious practices. The purloining of Indigenous medical knowledge raises many questions, including ownership of rights to such knowledge and how they should be recognized and compensated. Yet these are not just historical questions; much Indigenous knowledge remains untapped. Letitia McCune and Alain Cuerrier, for example, note that 'apart from work done on common juniper, blueberry, and birch, few phytochemical or pharmacological analyses of medicinal plant populations have been undertaken based on traditional knowledge of North American Indigenous peoples.'[28] These authors discovered that a number of traditional medicinal plants found in the boreal forests of Canada contained antioxidants and were used to treat diabetes.[29] They noted that their presence could 'link anti-diabetic medicinal plants both to the traditional healer's knowledge and to specific locales on the land.'[30] They concluded that Western scientific documentation could have a key role in land-use conflicts by emphasizing the importance of particular harvesting sites for medicinal plants.[31] Similar observations have been made regarding Indigenous populations elsewhere.

Indigenous peoples were often keen to try out remedies used by the Europeans they came into contact with. Audrey Martin found that – at larger settlements around Hudson Bay trading posts in Western Canada in the 1730s – stores were provided where Indigenous people could exchange furs for Western items.[32] These included clothing, utensils, tools, and medicines. 'The most successful trader was naturally the one who knew best how to appeal to the popular taste. The chief articles of barter were ammunition, blankets, knives, print, shawls, nails, handkerchiefs, tobacco, bacon, flour, tea, jam, sugar, and white man's medicines.'[33] Locally available items of pharmaceutical value soon came to the attention of settlers, including isinglass – a gelatin product obtained from freshwater fish first mentioned in 1679. It was mainly used for clarifying wine and beer, but it also found pharmaceutical and culinary uses.[34]

The appropriation of Indigenous medical knowledge has received considerable attention from scholars. The organization of knowledge about medicinal substances was a vital part of the scientific and colonial enterprises of European powers in the early modern period.[35] From the early sixteenth century substantial quantities of flora and fauna were taken home by European explorers from their newly discovered lands. But during the early modern period much healing knowledge from both Native American and African cultures was not only appropriated by Europeans but also presented as their own in medical and natural history texts published in European centres.[36] From the start of the seventeenth century, drugs travelled freely around the world and were easily assimilated within different cultural traditions.[37] Drug use in countries of the Middle East, Asia, and the Far East had a great deal in common with that in Europe. Indeed, as Bhattacharya states in relation to India, 'prevailing distinctions drawn between Indigenous and Western drugs in colonial India are misleading.' Such distinctions are premised on an understanding of cultural nationalism, and 'do not take into account the heterogeneous nature of the trade, manufacture, and consumption patterns in the market.'[38]

The British planters, explorers, and naturalists who actively sought out new species or economically valuable drugs that had a large European market also sought out Indigenous medical knowledge.[39] Medical knowledge was shared across societies tied to the Atlantic world. In her study of processes of plant trade, therapeutic exchange, and 'epistemic brokerage' from Lima to Canton and Paris to Constantinople – focusing on Peruvian bark –Stefanie Gänger found that not only the bark but also recipes, stories, and understandings about its use moved between and across societies, into Peruvian academies, Scottish households, Moroccan court pharmacies, and Louisiana plantations.[40] The networks that facilitated these movements were extensive and diverse. Newly established scientific networks played important roles in facilitating the transition of Indigenous remedies to European medical practice.[41] Londa Schiebinger noted that the practice of learned men sending questions to travellers was well established in naturalist traditions, that colonial physicians replied by letter, that observations were discussed in learned societies, and that European publications found their way back to the colonies. Medical knowledge was concentrated in repositories such as the Colleges of Physicians in London and Edinburgh, universities, and royal societies.[42]

Botanical gardens played a crucial part in the journey of Indigenous drug to European practice and eventually to official pharmacopoeia. Lucille Brockway identified politically significant effects resulting from scientific research in the field of economic botany during the nineteenth century.[43] The British botanical garden network developed and transferred economically important plants – particularly cinchona, rubber, and sisal – to different parts of the world to promote imperial prosperity. Botany and the entwined relation between science and politics played an important social role in the age of empire. Chandra Mukerji – writing about French plant collections – noted that because of the spiritual and political significance of health and illness, writers prescribed the development of herb gardens devoted to pharmacopoeia, thereby placing botanical gardening squarely in the tradition of territorial politics.[44] Mukerji notes that the proliferation of botanical gardens in France resulted in a dearth of these sites in the colonies.[45] In India prospecting for drugs became highly organized and systematic, but only some of the many Indigenous drugs found their way into European pharmacopoeias. Pratik Chakrabarti has shown that by the eighteenth century collecting and observing plants had become the hallmark of European natural history.[46]

It was important not only for trade but also to help colonists become self-sufficient. Sir Hans Sloane emphasized that the purpose of his activities was to make British colonists self-sufficient, by instructing them in the uses of plants 'growing spontaneously or in gardens' for medicines and foods. 'It is very hard to carry thither', he noted, 'such European simples as are proper for the cure of all sorts of diseases' – especially since most drugs lost their effects in transport. But an equally important purpose was to enrich the range of medicines available at home. Sloane noted that whilst useful West Indian herbs did not grow naturally in England, many were brought over and employed in medicines every day.[47] He hoped to find remedies as widely applicable as Peruvian bark, which had been included in the *LP* in 1677.[48] As president of the Royal College of Physicians between 1719 and 1735 he understood better than anyone how colonial drugs such as ipecacuanha and cinchona passed into the official pharmacopoeias of London, Paris, and Amsterdam.[49]

PHARMACOPOEIAS AND KNOWLEDGE TRANSFER

The processes by which local curiosities became disseminated across Europe, how exotic drugs came to be known, used, recognized as useful, and included in official pharmacopoeias, have received some attention from historians.[50] Pratik Chakrabarti cites a letter sent by Patrick Russell (1727–1805), a physician and naturalist based in southern India, to Joseph Banks (1743–1820) at the Royal Botanic Gardens, Kew, about Tabasheer, an exotic substance obtained from a bamboo extract much used in Arab medicine. The letter was published in *Philosophical Transactions*. Russell obtained samples from the bazaars of Hyderabad and Masulipatnam and submitted them to the Royal Society of London for examination. Chemical tests were carried out and reported in *Philosophical Transactions*. New drugs and botanical discoveries were reported in new medical compilations. Andrew Duncan Sr (1744–1828) published the journal *Medical and Philosophical Commentaries* from 1773 as a means of keeping practitioners abreast of new developments. His son Andrew Duncan Jr (1773–1832) reformulated it as the *Annals of Medicine*, which 'catered more widely to the Empire, explicitly seeking medical news from the East and the West Indies.'[51] He was closely associated with medical discoveries in other parts of the world and became the author of the *Edinburgh New Dispensatory*.

In the preface to the 1803 edition of the *Edinburgh New Dispensatory* Duncan noted that the period 1789 to 1803 had witnessed great developments in chemistry, pharmacy, and natural history 'so as to render a complete reform absolutely necessary'. This was essentially 'the Edinburgh tradition', although on the Continent attempts had been made to bring 'a new language of chemistry into pharmacy'.[52] Duncan claimed that the credit for composing a pharmacopoeia in the 'pure and unmixed language of science belongs indisputably to the Royal College of Physicians of Edinburgh'.[53] The *New Dispensatory* and its supplement drew on the research of colonial botanists and surgeons scattered across the empire; its sources ranged from bazaars to the 'Mussulman Fakir of Calcutta'.[54] In his 1829 supplement he noted that 'the richness and complexity of the Empire was apparent in discussion of the "confusing commercial varieties" of cinchona bark, the different cloves of Barbados and Cayenne, the several forms of Ipecacuanha collected from the various parts of the Empire, and the spurious Columba roots from the state of Barbary'.[55] Problems in obtaining samples from distant parts related to dubious quality, source, and identity. Duncan was instrumental in bringing the empire into the pharmacopoeia and making the pharmacopoeia more empire-facing in the late eighteenth and early nineteenth centuries.

The impact of New World medicines was still felt in British medical practice three hundred years after their discovery. Of 218 plant medicines used in England in 1874, twenty-seven (one in eight) came from the New World, although some were introduced much later: cinchona and ipecacuanha in the seventeenth century, cocaine in 1884, and curare only in 1942.[56] But whilst many New World drugs were later included in pharmacopoeias, many were not. How and why these decisions were reached are important historical questions. As Nandini Bhattacharya points out in relation to India 'the exclusions and marginalization from the official formularies are of as much historical consequence as the inclusion of Indian drugs within the British Pharmacopoeia and the publication, finally, of an Indian Pharmacopoeia.'[57]

Many accounts of the interconnectedness of trade, empire, and science – often under the umbrella of 'colonial science' – made reference to pharmacopoeias as instruments for the collation and transfer of scientific knowledge.[58] But, as Mark Harrison noted, by the 1980s historians were finding that a single model of colonial science 'could not encompass its varied trajectories in different parts of the empire.'[59] The term 'colonial science' seemed 'little more than a label of convenience, lacking precise definition and of questionable utility.' Harrison emphasized the value of Roy MacLeod's concept of a 'moving metropolis' in portraying the colonial relations of science by recognizing the diversity and dynamism of the periphery in the late nineteenth century.[60] MacLeod argued that local centres such as Sydney and Calcutta could take on a measure of autonomy and authority whilst remaining within a framework of imperial dominance.[61] It is a concept that has utility in examining the use of metropolitan pharmacopoeias in empires and their relationship with drug regulation. So, too, has Michael Worboy's concept of 'constructive imperialism', where he argues that the chief function of colonial science in the late nineteenth and early twentieth centuries was 'the location and evaluation of new resources for the purposes of imperial development.'[62] This has resonance in the gathering of suggestions of local medicinal materials for inclusion in an imperial pharmacopeia.

In *Matters of Exchange* Hal Cook argued that the medical marketplace was the site where objective knowledge and commercial interests coalesced.[63] This is mirrored in the importance of the bazaar as a place where information and material were exchanged in nineteenth-century India.[64] Cook uncovered direct links between the rise of trade and commerce in the Dutch Empire and the flourishing of scientific investigation. Dutch commerce – not religion – inspired the rise of science in the sixteenth and seventeenth centuries. The preference for accurate information that accompanied the rise of commerce also laid the groundwork for the rise of science globally, wherever the Dutch engaged in trade. Medicine and natural history were fundamental aspects of this new science, as reflected in the development of gardens for botanical study, anatomical theatres, curiosity cabinets, and books about nature. Global science began with the rise of a global economy.[65]

Anna Winterbottom used the term 'hybrid' to describe commonalities in the different ways of knowing that she found in her study of the development between 1660 and 1720 of the English East India Company, which played a central role in the movement of medicinal items from India and the Far East. They involved a mixture of information drawn from diverse sources brought together to make something new. Such hybridity applied to animals, plants, and people, and 'also has an element of the wild.'[66] Connections between scholarship, patronage, diplomacy, trade, and colonial settlement abounded in the early modern world. Patronage links between cosmopolitan writers and collectors and scholars associated with universities and the Royal Society of London were essential components in the transmission of Indigenous medicines to metropolitan pharmacopoeias. Innovative works of scholarship – covering natural history, ethnography, theology, linguistics, agriculture, and medicine – were created amid multi-directional struggles for supremacy in Asia, the Indian Ocean, and the Atlantic. Non-elite actors, including enslaved people, played important parts in transferring knowledge and skills between settlements. As Steven Shapin has argued, both scientific and social knowledge are in some sense inevitably hybrid, since what we know about natural phenomena is always mediated through our knowledge of the people who describe them, whilst our understanding of people is conditioned by the explanations they provide for natural things.[67]

EXOTIC MEDICINES
AND EUROPEAN MEDICAL PRACTICE

The medicinal value of exotic remedies was based on the prevailing medical philosophy, that based on Galenic principles – of ill health resulting from a lack of balance between the four humours stemming from the mix of primary qualities (hot, cold, dry, and moist) and elements (air, fire, water, and earth).[68] Early modern medicines were dominated by emetics, purgatives, diuretics, and cathartics. The discourse of such philosophies changed over time. Bhattacharya noted that the conventional divide had been between Western and Indigenous medicine,

Introduction

a convention that is equally applicable to medicinal substances.[69] That discourse related to 'inclusions and exclusions of drugs from the formal and informal formularies', and 'the principal themes of circulation, marginalization, and formalization of drugs in both text and praxis in colonial India'.[70] Laurence Monnais concluded that contemporary sources described the medical system they viewed as originating in Europe, and 'anchored in scientific validation and discovery', as either European, modern, or scientific. She uses the more neutral term 'biomedicine', which 'refers to the increasingly close relationships between medicine and biological sciences without making claims as to geographical origins, epistemological universality, or temporal status'.[71]

By the mid-eighteenth century the process of international integration of medical understanding, practices, and materials was already underway. This followed the almost continuous search for new drugs of natural origin in overseas territories, a process described as 'colonial bioprospecting'.[72] Iatromechanics was the rival concept to iatrochemistry towards the end of the seventeenth century. Boyle's corpuscular chemistry provided the theoretical framework for explaining the actions of drugs and poisons by their content of specially shaped particles.[73] By the eighteenth century, pharmacology – the scientific study of the actions and uses of drugs – was becoming established. Sir Hans Sloane provided a direct link between Indigenous medicines and European pharmacopoeias, at a time of increased scientification and shifting medical philosophies. By the early nineteenth century treatises on pharmacology were being published as supplements to official pharmacopoeias.[74]

By the mid-seventeenth century the use of exotic medicines was an essential part of the status, esteem, and authority assumed by physicians. In 1649 Culpeper noted, 'Would it not make both a man's ears glow to hear a man affirm that God hath created no remedy for such a disease nearer than the East Indies?'[75] The use of such items set physicians apart from those supplying Indigenous medicines or domestic remedies, many of which had been in use for centuries.[76] Gabrielle Hatfield listed nearly three hundred plants employed domestically. Most were in use in the late sixteenth century, and a substantial number appeared in the LP 1618. Many plants were listed more than once, with different parts of the plant being used for different purposes.[77] Many others appear in the large number of domestic recipes that survive.[78]

But it was not only natural products from the colonies that entered European medical practice; chemical medicines and metals emerged from alchemists' laboratories, and their use was heavily promoted by

Pharmacopoeias, Drug Regulation, and Empires

Paracelsus and other physicians. By the early nineteenth century chemists and pharmacists succeeded in extracting active ingredients from plant medicines –such as morphine from opium and quinine from cinchona – and these chemical medicines began replacing medicinal plants in pharmacopoeias.

MEDICINE, PHARMACY, AND PROFESSIONALIZATION

In England in the early years of the Columbian Exchange – the first decades of the sixteenth century – the role of making medicines was in the hands of apothecaries, then a distinct group within the Grocers' Company.[79] Their incorporation as a separate Society of Apothecaries in 1617 gave them a degree of professional autonomy.[80] As new colonies were settled, apothecaries were among the early colonists. Pharmacy professionalization in the British Empire was modelled on that of the metropole, where the discipline had evolved very differently to that in other European countries, particularly with regard to its separation from medicine – which only occurred in the mid-nineteenth century.[81] As Jenner and Wallis note 'the early modern medical marketplace has generally been represented as being supplanted by the advent of professionalized medicine in the nineteenth century, notably the advent of medical registration in 1858.'[82] Its ending was accompanied by the 1841 foundation of the Pharmaceutical Society of Great Britain, the demise of the *London*, *Edinburgh*, and *Dublin Pharmacopoeias*, and their replacement by a single *British Pharmacopoeia* in 1864.

Patrick Wallis has shown that a major factor in the emergence of the official pharmacopoeia was the shifting relationship between practitioners of medicine and pharmacy, between those who prescribed and those who made medicines, and the boundary between those roles. In the early seventeenth century there were often informal relationships between different medical practitioners. Wallis found that 'brief combinations between practising apothecaries and surgeons seem to have been a particularly common way of treating patients.'[83] In 1600, when an apothecary treated a patient in their home, he did so in association with a surgeon. Such associations served an important purpose where medical practitioners supplied both medicines and advice, or when they wished to prescribe medicines that they had invented.[84] There was then a need to find a trustworthy supplier. 'The College and medical guilds provided only limited assurance about the quality of medicines. The fragmentation and diffusion of production, limitation of assaying techniques, and the legitimacy of substitution and variation in some recipes

Introduction

meant that fraud was widely suspected, Wallis writes.[85] Whilst the physicians were anxious to control the activities of the apothecaries in the early seventeenth century, the poor quality of many medicines and the need for standards provided a strong incentive for a pharmacopoeia. Physicians and apothecaries were motivated to comply with its requirements to encourage patients to return, since repeat business would be undermined if poor-quality medicines were repeatedly supplied.

Although boundaries between medical and other practitioners were frequently porous, some delineation was necessary. Wallis notes that 'although the medical treatments employed by practitioners were not complex or resource-intensive ... most still relied on some division of labour in order to supply different elements such as drugs, knowledge, bleeding, and nursing'.[86] Without this, practitioners would have found it much harder to practise. The pharmacopoeia was aimed as much at physicians making their own medicines as at apothecaries. The battle between the two groups in the seventeenth and eighteenth centuries was as much about doctors practising pharmacy as apothecaries practising medicine. In a pamphlet attacking apothecaries, physicians were encouraged to make their own medicines, on the grounds that 'it was necessary if the physician was to emulate the observational practices of the natural philosopher'.[87]

Medical practice in the New World maintained close parallels with those in the Old. It changed remarkably little in transit from the established societies of Spain, France, and England to these countries' new settlements in the Americas. This applied as much to the medicines used as anything else.[88] As Numbers notes in his conclusion, 'although the discovery of indigenous medical plants led to some additions to the pharmacopoeia, medical theory and practice scarcely changed. Instead of relying on expensive and sometimes scarce European drugs to induce vomiting, sweating, and evacuation of the bowels, the medical men of New Spain simply substituted comparable herbal remedies borrowed from the Aztecs'.[89] The same was true in Britain's imperial world. He concludes that 'medical substitution and practice in New England tended to become increasingly English as the years passed'.[90]

THE BRITISH EMPIRE
AND OFFICIAL PHARMACOPOEIAS

The origins of the British Empire are usually traced to Cabot's arrival in Newfoundland in 1497, although at first there were only short-lived settler communities. The empire grew in a largely unplanned

Table 0.1
British dependencies and colonies, 1914

Division	Colonies
Indian Division	Ajmer-Merwara, the Andamans, Assam, Bengal, Bihar and Orissa, Bombay, Baluchistan, Burma, the Central Provinces and Berar, Coorg, Delhi, Madras, the North-West Frontier Province, the Punjab, United Provinces of Agra and Oudh
African Division	Basutoland, Bechuanaland Protectorate, Gambia, Gold Coast, Nigeria, Northern Rhodesia, Southern Rhodesia, Saint Helena, Sierra Leone, Swaziland, The Union of South Africa (provinces of Cape of Good Hope, Natal, Orange Free State, Transvaal)
Australasian Division	New South Wales, Queensland, South Australia, Tasmania, Victoria, Western Australia, Northern Territory of Australia, Federal Capital Territory; forming the Commonwealth of Australia. New Zealand, Fiji Islands, Papua, Western Pacific
Eastern Division	Ceylon, Hong Kong, Labuan, Mauritius, Seychelles, Straits Settlements, Weihaiwei
Mediterranean Division	Cyprus, Gibraltar, Malta
North American Division	Alberta, British Columbia, Manitoba, New Brunswick, North-West Territories, Nova Scotia, Ontario, Prince Edward Island, Quebec, Saskatchewan, Yukon; forming the Dominion of Canada. Newfoundland
West Indian Division	Bahama Islands, Barbados, Bermuda Islands, British Guiana, British Honduras, Jamaica and Turks and Caicos Islands, Leeward Islands (Antigua, Dominica, Montserrat, Saint Christopher and Nevis, Virgin Islands), Trinidad and Tobago, Windward Islands (Grenada, Saint Lucia, Saint Vincent)
South Atlantic	The Falkland Islands

Source: British Pharmacopoeia 1914 (London: General Medical Council, 1914), xxii.

manner over several centuries. Territories were acquired through occupation, settlement, and treaties following wars with other European powers. England began acquiring overseas possessions from about 1583, resulting in territories in America, the Caribbean, and Africa. Then followed an institutionalized and highly organized slave trade, and conflict with other European colonial powers – a period lasting throughout the seventeenth century. The empire expanded substantially following the end of the Spanish War of Succession and the signing of the Treaty of Utrecht in 1714. For most of the eighteenth century the American states constituted a key part of the empire, but this 'First British Empire' came to an end in 1775 with the start of the American Revolutionary War.

The short period between 1775 and 1815 saw the rise of the 'Second British Empire' following James Cook's exploration of lands in the Pacific and his claiming of territories for Great Britain. But the period was dominated by war with France, and at the end of the Napoleonic Wars in 1815 Britain expanded its empire through a series of peace treaties with other European powers. The hundred years between 1815 and 1914 are often described as 'Britain's imperial century'. It encompassed the expansion of control in India, following the 'Indian War of Independence' of 1857 and the start of the British Raj the following year; the growth of British settlements in Canada, South Africa, Australia, and New Zealand; and the acquisition of vast expanses of Africa following 'the scramble for Africa' in the nineteenth century.[91] When consultations began about 'imperializing the pharmacopoeia' in the late 1890s, the British Empire consisted of seventy colonies administered in seven divisions (table 0.1).

The period between 1914 and 1945 was largely defined by the two world wars, but it also witnessed the rise of nationalism in many colonies, as well as difficulties in maintaining order and addressing the needs of diverse subject populations whilst expanding trade. In population and territorial terms, the British Empire reached its peak in 1921 following further acquisitions at the end of the First World War. The period from 1945 to 1997 witnessed the process of decolonization and the decline of empire; India was divided and granted independence in 1947, and independence was awarded to former colonies in the Caribbean, in Africa, and elsewhere mainly in the 1950s and '60s.

It was against this multifaceted background – of a growing empire, the appropriation of Indigenous remedies, bioprospecting, and increasing international trade in drugs, coupled with shifting boundaries between medical and pharmaceutical practitioners, professionalization, medical belief systems, and the rise of science – that official pharmacopoeias appeared in Britain in the shape of the first *LP* in 1618. It was to be followed by one for Edinburgh in 1699 and for Dublin in 1807. The first proposal for an 'imperial British Pharmacopoeia' was made in 1813. A *British Pharmacopoeia* (*BP*) replaced those of London, Edinburgh, and Dublin in 1864, and by 1914 the *BP* was described as 'suitable for the whole Empire'. An exploration of the processes involved in that transition offers a better understanding of the relationship between pharmacopoeias, trade, and drug regulation – and the distinction between official and statutory pharmacopoeias – and is described in this book.

Matthew Crawford has suggested that one way to assess pharmacopoeias and their impact on healing knowledge is to view them as a genre of medical writing.[92] They were 'a genre of texts that listed medicinal substances and provided the recipes to prepare them for therapeutic use'.[93] In *Drugs on the Page*, Crawford and Gabriel focused on 'reframing pharmacopoeias and their histories'. They took a broad view of what counted as a pharmacopoeia, suggesting that 'such an approach embraces the ambiguity of the term itself'.[94] They elucidated two meanings of the word: firstly, in referring to 'a genre of medical writing that lists simple and compound medicaments as well as the techniques for preparing and administering'; and secondly, in referring to 'the collective knowledge of medical virtues and therapeutic preparations of different substances as held by any society, culture, or group of specialists within a society or culture'. Yet neither definition makes reference to whether such volumes had official status. Pharmacopoeias are best understood, they suggest, 'not as finished and stable products but as stages in the larger processes of collecting, co-opting, organizing, revising and controlling knowledge about healing goods'.[95] They 'were often the subject of editing and revision just as the knowledge they represented changed over time and across space'. *Drugs on the Page* also demonstrated 'the ways in which pharmacopoeias were produced and were the products of colonialism, globalization, and the rise of the nation-state'.[96]

Large numbers of examples of the genre exist, but many writings about them make little or no distinction between traditional and official pharmacopoeias, for which many definitions also exist. Thompson, for example, defined an official pharmacopoeia as 'a collection of formulas for medicinal preparations issued under the authority

Introduction

of some publicly recognized body'?[97] Discussion by historians has usually focused on particular countries or specific time periods, such as Bhattacharya's work on Indian pharmacopoeias,[98] and Crawford and Gabriel's volume on the early modern period. Yet pharmacopoeias – whether official or not – have received scholarly attention from many disciplines, not only history and anthropology. There are often significant differences in the meaning attached to the word.

Scholars have drawn attention to difficulties in the use of other terms frequently used in the history of medicine. Jenner and Wallis, for example, noted that by the early 2000s use of the term 'medical marketplace' – which came to prominence in the early 1980s – was then so broad as to be more of a hindrance than a help. It was, they found, being used in at least three different ways, and was employed as a shorthand for claims about the fundamental transformation of the medical economy during the early modern period.[99] They suggested that, 'given these divergent means and approaches, it might be argued that it would be best to abandon the terminology of the medical marketplace altogether'.[100] However, they suggested that a more helpful approach might be a more rigorous engagement with what is meant by the medical marketplace.

In this book I suggest that a similarly rigorous engagement with what is meant by pharmacopoeia is now required. The book problematizes issues concerning the official and statutory nature of pharmacopoeias through the prism of the origins, purposes, and processes of imperialization of the pharmacopoeia in the British Empire over the course of 350 years, from publication of the first edition of the *London Pharmacopoeia* in 1618 to the replacement of a Pharmacopoeia Commission with a Medicines Commission in 1968. In doing so it draws on a wide range of secondary and primary sources, including General Medical Council and Royal Pharmaceutical Society archives and others available mainly at the British Library, the National Archives, and the Wellcome Collection in London.

The book is aimed at all those who study and write about pharmacopoeias from any perspective, from any time period, and from any geographical region. Its purpose is to raise awareness of the problems that can arise from lack of clarity, and to draw attention to the opportunities that exist for interdisciplinary collaboration and new areas of research from more informed use of the term. In the next chapter I examine the many meanings currently attached to it.

I

The Many Meanings of 'Pharmacopoeia'

Today the term 'pharmacopoeia' – derived from the Greek *pharmakon* (medicine) and *poiein* (to make) – has come to have a wide range of meanings, although its origins are ancient. George Urdang showed that it was first used by the Greek writer Diogenes Laertius in the second or third century CE.[1] But this was a book about the preparation of medicines, not a list of simple and compound remedies. Antoine Lentacker points out that, as a newly coined Latin term derived from Greek roots, it was really a creation of the Renaissance.[2] The first volume to appear under this title in Europe was the book *Pharmacopoeae, libri tres*, published in 1548 by the French physician and Galenist Jacques Du Bois (1478–1555). But this was not the first 'official' pharmacopoeia, and not all subsequent official pharmacopoeias were described as such. Paula de Vos has demonstrated that early pharmacopoeias included different elements and genres, but that over time, they developed into 'official, legally enforced regional, national, and imperial standards'.[3] Although the instructions given in the 1498 *Ricettario Fiorentino* were directed at apothecaries, this work is of significance because it was a joint collaboration between apothecaries and physicians.[4] It was greatly expanded between the first and the third editions in 1567.[5]

The *Dispensatory* of Valerius Cordus was published in Nuremberg in 1546 on the instructions of the civil authority and directed at dispensers. It was a collection of formulas taken from the works of previous writers, and contained a wide range of remedies of plant, animal, and vegetable origin. It was the first pharmacopoeia to have 'received the stamp of any public authority'.[6] It went through many editions; the first drugs from the New World – including sassafras, sarsaparilla, and tobacco – appeared in 1592.[7] Nuremberg's example

The Many Meanings of 'Pharmacopoeias'

was soon followed by other European cities. In 1564 the medical officer of health of Augsburg issued a dispensatory under the name *Enchiridionia*. A second edition followed, and in 1613 it became the *Pharmacopoeia Augustana*. This quickly became the template for many of those compiled elsewhere, including the *London* (1618), *Paris* (1637), and *Edinburgh* (1699) *Pharmacopoeias*. Richard Powell (1767–1834) later noted that 'on account of the facilities and advantages they afford in the practice of medicine' similar works were introduced in all the countries of Europe.[8]

Other genre of pharmaceutical texts continued to be published after the appearance of official pharmacopoeias.[9] Many books describing medicinal plants had appeared earlier, including Garcia da Orta's *Treatise on Simples and Drugs of India* in 1563.[10] 'Books of secrets', such as that published by Juan de Cardenas in Mexico in 1591, were both popular and influential.[11] Printed herbals and formularies were published in England prior to the first pharmacopoeias. Many locally available simples later included in the *London Pharmacopoeia* (LP) had been used as domestic remedies for centuries and were mentioned in John Gerarde's (ca 1545–1612) *Great Herball*, first published in 1597 when work on the LP was already underway. This largely reproduced English translations of Rembert Dodoens's (1517–1585) herbal of 1554, although Gerarde added some plants from his own garden and others from North America, which had reached London by the late sixteenth century. Many were already included in other European pharmacopoeias.

An examination of the geographical origins of items included in early pharmacopoeias indicates that many had undergone the transition from Indigenous remedy to item of international trade many years earlier. Records of such transitions are to be found in ancient texts. Sumerian, Chinese, and Egyptian physicians left lists of items they used as medicines, to be followed by Greek and Roman scholars. In Europe texts were usually written in Latin as the lingua franca and easily crossed national boundaries, although translations into the vernacular were common. The situation was transformed with the invention of printing after Johannes Gutenberg (ca 1400–1468) published his Bible in 1455. Herbals and formularies were among items published before 1501 (the incunabula). The first herbal printed in German – written by a Frankfurt physician at the request of a Mainz official – was the *Gart der Desundheit*, published in 1485 by one of Gutenberg's apprentices.[12]

George Urdang noted that it was not until 1573 that the term 'pharmacopoeia' was used as the designation of an official pharmaceutical standard, appearing in the title of the second edition of the book issued as the legally enforceable pharmaceutical guide for the pharmacists and physicians of the City of Augsburg – the *Augsburg Pharmacopoeia*.[13] Although other terms including *antidotarium* (from the Greek for 'given against') and *dispensatorium* survived, the designation 'pharmacopoeia' became predominant from the end of the sixteenth century. Urdang reported that it was originally used 'for all kinds of formularies, issued with and without official recognition. It gradually gained the distinctive quality of an official term for a legally enforced book.'[14] But whilst pharmacopoeias may or may not have been official, 'official' ones may or may not have been statutory.

In *Drugs on the Page* Matthew Crawford and Joseph Gabriel note that the term 'pharmacopoeia' is now most commonly found in anthropological and ethnobotanical scholarship.[15] However, a cross-disciplinary search of the literature reveals that it is also found in the writings of a wide range of researchers including geographers and economists, as well as medical and pharmaceutical historians. Scholars are interested in them for many reasons, whether with regard to the discovery of remedies, their role in addressing political, economic, and cultural questions, or their place in the history of science, medicine, and technology. Some of this literature is multidisciplinary with multiple authors, but much of it is not.

Whilst Crawford and Gabriel suggest that 'pharmacopoeia' normally refers to lists of 'simple and compound medicaments as well as the techniques for preparing and administering these',[16] a brief examination of the literature indicates that many of the pharmacopoeias referred to are limited to simples rather than compounded medicines, and rarely provide instructions for preparation. There is great diversity in the nature of pharmacopoeias, whether official or not. This chapter considers the origins, meanings, and uses of 'pharmacopoeia' by researchers across a broad range of scholarship. It addresses the following key questions, among others: What meanings are attached to 'pharmacopoeia' by the scholars of disparate disciplines? Are there differences between them? How has its meaning changed over time and space? What are the consequences of differences in the use of the term? And what can one discipline learn from others?

PHARMACOPOEIAS, ANTHROPOLOGY, AND MEDICAL SOCIOLOGY

Anthropologists have long been interested in materials from the natural environment used by Indigenous communities in the treatment of sickness and disease. Yet they have often been of peripheral interest, and use of the term 'pharmacopoeia' by them is of relatively recent origin. Early histories of anthropology rarely make reference to materia medica or pharmacopoeias. Franz Boas in 1904 made a clear distinction between 'the speculative anthropology of the eighteenth and early nineteenth centuries' and what he called the science of anthropology, on the grounds of both scope and method.[17] 'Up to ten years ago', he claimed, 'we had no trained anthropologists'. Students drifted into anthropological research from a wide range of other disciplines. 'The multifarious origin of anthropology is reflected in the multiplicity of its methods', he noted.[18] Anthropology appropriated from other disciplines a range of methods and terms it found useful, including a word that encapsulated the materia medica of Indigenous communities – their 'pharmacopoeia'. Yet 'materia medica' is also problematic, as it infers use in medicine and therefore by medical practitioners – including traditional practitioners – but excluding lay use. Yet pharmacopoeias barely received a mention in later histories of anthropology. Alfred C. Haddon's (1855–1940) 1934 history makes no mention of them.[19] Neither do Eriksen and Nielsen's 2013 *History of Anthropology*[20] or Efra Sera-Shriar's *Making of British Anthropology, 1813–1871*.[21]

It was only after 1963 that 'pharmacopoeia' began to appear regularly in anthropological writing. In the 1976 edited volume *Medical Anthropology* several contributors used the term. Francis Clune explored the relationship between witchcraft, the shaman, and what he described as 'active' pharmacopoeias, in which locally available materials were combined with other approaches in the treatment of diseases. In the same volume Janet Belcove discussed the primary curative agents in the 'pharmacopoeia of Spanish-American traditional medicine' in Taos, New Mexico, which included herbs that were used by the *curanderos* (traditional Native healers or shamans).[22] Herbs were used for disorders including cancer and influenza as well as more minor ailments. With this volume pharmacopoeias entered mainstream anthropological discourse. Anthropologists' interest was principally in the range of materia medica used by Indigenous communities. For them pharmacopoeia often included charms, chantings, and rituals in addition to materials from the plant, animal, and mineral kingdoms. Pablo Gomez has described these pharmacopoeias as 'social pharmacopoeias'.[23]

References to pharmacopoeias in medical sociology date from around the same time. The field of medical sociology studies some of the same phenomena as medical anthropology, although medical anthropology has different origins, originally studying medicine within non-Western cultures and using different methodologies.[24] The term 'medical anthropology' has been used since 1963 as a label for 'empirical research and theoretical production by anthropologists into the social processes and cultural representations of health, illness and the nursing/care practices associated with these'.[25] Peter Conrad argued that there was some convergence between the disciplines, as medical sociology adopted anthropological methodologies such as qualitative research and began to focus more on the patient, and medical anthropology started to focus on Western medicine.[26] Yet the etiological, philosophical, and textual roots of pharmacopoeias were all firmly rooted in Western cultures. He argued that more interdisciplinary communication could improve both disciplines.

Pharmaceutical anthropology emerged as a sub-discipline within medical anthropology with the 1988 publication of Sjaak Geest and Susan Reynolds White's edited volume.[27] In her account of herbal and biomedical pharmaceuticals in Mauritius Linda K. Sussman reviewed the anthropological literature on pharmacopoeias, noting that 'there is a growing body of literature that makes note of the enormous pharmacopoeias of some cultures and the propensity of peoples to use relatively straightforward, non-ritualised physical treatment for some types of illness'.[28] Nina L. Etkins explored the cultural context of pharmacopoeias in relation to Indigenous populations. She asked, 'what does the content, size, internal consistency, variability, and potential for change of a given pharmacopoeia *mean*? Does a large and varied herbal pharmacopoeia reflect the skilled elaboration of a broad-based and effective therapeutic regimen, a botanically rich environment, or a host of other factors?[29] These questions have resonance with historical studies on these issues.

PHARMACOPOEIAS, ETHNOBOTANY, AND ETHNOPHARMACOLOGY

But it was not just anthropologists and sociologists who were interested in traditional remedies used by Indigenous communities. The 1980s saw renewed interest in medicinal plants in the West fuelled both by the rising cost of prescribed drugs and by bioprospecting of new plant-derived drugs. As Siva Krishnan has pointed out, an impressive number of modern drugs have been isolated from natural sources, many of which were based on materials used in traditional medicine.[30] Plant-based, traditional medicine systems continue to play essential roles in health care, with about 80 per cent of the world's inhabitants relying mainly on traditional medicines for their primary health care. Modern pharmacopoeias still contain at least 25 per cent drugs derived from plants, and many synthetic analogues are built on prototype compounds isolated from plants.[31] Traditional pharmacopoeias have received close scrutiny from scholars, including ethnobotanists screening the plant kingdom for potentially useful compounds. The term 'ethnobotany' was coined in 1896 by the American botanist John Harshberger to describe 'studies of plants used by ... aboriginal people', although by then they had already been studied for some time.[32] The term 'ethnopharmacology' was coined much later, and concerns the intersection of medical ethnography and biological studies of therapeutic action.[33] Its main goal has been the discovery of novel compounds, derived from plants and animals used in Indigenous medical systems, which can be employed in the development of new pharmaceuticals. Much of this literature describes medicinal plants used by people who have lived in the same ecological niche for generations. Ethnopharmacologists also aim to improve the ethno-medical systems of the people who they study by testing Indigenous medicines for efficacy and toxicity.

References to 'traditional', 'Indigenous', and 'herbal' pharmacopoeias abound in the *Journal of Ethnopharmacology*, which has been reporting studies on Indigenous plant medicines for over forty years. In 1981 Nina L. Etkin undertook a biomedical evaluation of the Hausa (northern Nigeria) herbal pharmacopoeia with reference to its prevention of malaria infection.[34] Peter Delaveau published an evaluation of traditional pharmacopeia in the same year.[35] In 1983 Joseph W. Bastien in his 'pharmacopoeia of the Kallawaya Andeans' presented a list of eighty-nine medicinal plants employed by this Indigenous group in Bolivia, who were well known as herbalists in South America.[36] Exotic botanicals played a vital role in their culture, providing some of their most important remedies, treating a wide variety of body systems, and having a number of pharmacological properties. They existed alongside species that had persisted in the pharmacopoeia since pre-Columbian times. Since the 1990s some authors have described such pharmacopoeias as 'ethno-pharmacopoeias'.[37]

Janni and Bastien have noted that 'pharmacopoeia' is now used extensively in the anthropological and ethnobotanical literatures to describe 'the collective knowledge of medical virtues and therapeutic preparations of different substances as held by any society, culture, or group of specialists within a society or culture'.[38] However, the interest of ethnobotanists is limited to materials of vegetable origin; items of animal or mineral origin are outside their remit. They usually use the term 'pharmacopoeia' to describe such knowledge rather than the narrower term 'herbal'. Yet to do so would also be misleading, as herbals embrace botanical materials with both culinary and medicinal uses. These pharmacopoeias also tend to only include 'simples', items used as found in nature unprocessed. They may include 'galenicals' (botanical medicinal items processed by physical means) but not 'pharmaceuticals' (medicinal items processed by chemical means), rarely including 'compounded' medicines or instructions for making formulations.

Similarities and differences between the pharmacopoeias of ethnic groups in close proximity have been studied by many scholars. In a study of wild medicinal plants included in the pharmacopeia of the Wichí people in a region of Argentina where native forest persists, similarities between their pharmacopoeia and that of neighbouring ethnic groups related more to geographical proximity than to cultural affinity.[39] Much of their 'wild plant pharmacopoeia' was novel, resulting from the continuing search for solutions to old and new health problems in native forests. Many medicinal plants came from neighbouring criollos, whilst traditional remedies were simultaneously preserved. The author tested the 'diversification hypothesis', which suggests that exotic plant species are selected to fill therapeutic vacancies in an ethno-pharmacopoeia due to novel bioactivity, thereby diversifying available treatment options.[40] The hypothesis was found to apply – at least in a modified form – as new wild medicines were added to old ones to fill therapeutic vacancies that appeared for various sociocultural and historical reasons. Others who

The Many Meanings of 'Pharmacopoeias'   31

have tested the diversification hypothesis found that exotic and native plants contained significantly different proportions of certain compounds, supporting it.[41] The diversification hypothesis may have utility for historians interested in how exotic plants came to be included in traditional pharmacopoeias.

Whether 'insular pharmacopoeias' – those existing in island communities – differed significantly from those in mainland communities has also been studied.[42] The extent to which local pharmacopoeias were impoverished by their insular nature has been investigated using a model that takes account of all the phenomena associated with being on an island. The historical and social trajectories of each island were the most important factors. The similarity of neighbouring islands with each other suggested that there had long been an exchange of medicinal knowledge between them. One of the most important forces influencing local pharmacopoeias on some islands was the presence of local herbal specialists. Such individuals helped to maintain the general knowledge of medicinal herbs. Korčula stood out as an island with an active local community interested in preserving its traditions and using local resources. This island had the longest list of medicinal herbs in active use, as well as the most widespread use of wild vegetables.[43]

Pharmacopoeias as 'expressions of society' have been explored in a variety of contexts. Using an ethnopharmacological approach emphasizing biological, social, and cultural aspects of the pharmacopoeia, Laurent Pordié showed how, in the Himalayan context, materia medica (and medicinal plants in particular) can be used to illustrate social change and contemporary perceptions, as well as to convey cultural expression and as symbols of the challenges between tradition and modernity. 'Pharmacopoeia' was 'a dynamic object refusing the dualistic approach between bio-therapeutic entity and socio-cultural form.'[44] Pordié highlighted diverse aspects of Ladakhi society by reversing the perspective, 'by seeing the society from a fundamentally biological object but located at the interface of the swings between the social and the biological.' Studying the world through plants 'widens our understanding and reveals pharmacopoeia as a social expression.'[45]

Pharmacopoeias have also been used to illustrate geopolitical differences. The history of medicinal plants in the Russian pharmacopoeia has been investigated, involving a critical appraisal of data concerning plants used in Russian medicine.[46] The authors described the pharmacological effects of specific plants in the Russian pharmacopoeia not included in its European counterparts. Phytotherapy was an official and separate branch of medicine in Russia; herbal medicinal preparations were considered official medicaments. Due to its location between West and East, Russian phytotherapy accumulated and adopted approaches that originated in European and Asian traditional medicine.

PHARMACOPOEIAS AND ECONOMIC BOTANY

Economic botanists have highlighted the impact of introduced plants on Indigenous pharmacopoeias as a result of the drug trade. The movement of plant medicines between Indigenous communities and Western colonizers was a two-way process. Many Indigenous communities tried out and absorbed into their own practices materials that originated elsewhere and which were often introduced to them by Europeans. Researchers have investigated the extent to which Indigenous communities depended on plant materials readily available to them in their immediate surroundings using the apparency hypothesis. This predicts that the apparent plants (those most easily found in the local vegetation) will be the most commonly collected and used by Indigenous people, and hence the most likely to be used as medicines.[47] However, following its application to a local pharmacopoeia in north-eastern Brazil researchers concluded that it did not have predictive potential to explain the use and commercial value of medicinal plants. Exotic (non-native) plants were found to be disproportionately represented in the Indigenous pharmacopoeia.[48]

In 2000 economic botanists examined the abundance and importance of introduced plants in the pharmacopoeias of northern South America. Introduced species were commonly employed as medicines throughout the region, and included at least 216 Eurasian, North American, African, and Pacific species that had been introduced over several centuries.[49] Among the Shuar of lowland Ecuador, four introduced plants were included in their most commonly prescribed remedies. The widespread use of introduced plants was found to be partly due to the medicinal value of plants whose primary use was as food. Similarly, they found that many introduced ornamental plants also had therapeutic value. Some species had been introduced specifically as medicines during the early years of colonial occupation.[50]

PHARMACOPOEIAS AND KNOWLEDGE TRANSFER BETWEEN COMMUNITIES

The flow of knowledge between communities is reflected in many scholarly contributions. Migrant pharmacopoeias have received considerable attention, including an ethnobotanical survey of four Caribbean communities in Amazonia (French Guiana).[51] French Guiana had long been at the crossroads between Amazonia and the Caribbean, and knowledge moved freely across the Caribbean to South America. Where medicines had become established through the settlement of migrants from the Antillean islands, the different migrant communities 'maintained a common background in terms of perception of the body and disease (in particular humoral systems and magical beliefs) and modes of administration of the medicinal species used.'[52] Nevertheless, differences in plant-based practices and knowledge were seen in the communities, largely resulting from factors such as the urban or rural origin of the populations, their length of time in the country, and the level of intercultural interactions that they experienced.

A study of the Mexican migrant pharmacopoeia has described the ethnopharmacological knowledge of women in an urban community in the us state of Georgia.[53] Mexican migrant women used medicinal plants in combination with commercially produced medicines, but most had a strong preference for the herbal remedies that they made themselves over drugs prescribed by physicians. Some of their descriptions of the actions of medicines were supported by the pharmacological literature, but many of the attributes ascribed to them have not been investigated. In a study of the Colombian folk pharmacopoeia, adaptation related to health-care practices was found to be a multifaceted process. Persistence, loss, and incorporation of remedies into the folk pharmacopoeia after migration were influenced by practical adaptation strategies as well as by motives of ethnic identity.[54]

'Traditional pharmacopoeias' in Western developed countries have now received considerable attention. In 2005 a cross-cultural comparison between traditional pharmacopoeias and medicine use among Albanians and Italians in southern Italy was undertaken. Traditional household remedies and ritual healing practices were compared in two economically and socio-demographically similar communities, one inhabited by ethnic Albanians – who migrated to the area during the fifteenth century – the other inhabited by autochthonous inhabitants of southern Italy. In the first they found that the number of traditional natural remedies (mainly derived from local medicinal plants) was only half that of the local folk pharmacopoeia of the other. Ritual magic-healing practices still played a central role among the Albanians but not the Italians. Differences were explained by factors affecting cultural adaptation and transition, including age and previous residence.[55] Dermatological remedies were found to make up at least one-third of the traditional pharmacopoeia. Identification of folk remedies was considered important both for the preservation of traditional medical knowledge and for the search for novel antimicrobial agents in the treatment of skin infections.[56]

PHARMACOPOEIAS, ETHNOBOTANISTS, AND HISTORY

Ethnobotanists taking a historical perspective have discussed the entry of plant medicines into both Indigenous and Western official pharmacopoeia. The field of historical ethnobotany is now well established. In 2014 Christina da Silva and others presented an overview of past studies. They defined 'historical ethnobotany' as an area of research responsible for understanding past interrelationships between people and plants using written records and iconography.[57] Over half of the 103 studies they identified began in the modern age, with 17 relating to antiquity. They covered a broad geographical range, although almost half of the studies focused on the Western Hemisphere, particularly South America. Many referenced pharmacopoeias, both Indigenous and official.[58]

A study of ethnobotanical traditions in Albacete, Spain, found that in 1526 all the compound medicines in use appeared in official pharmacopoeias, notably the 1498 *Ricettario Fiorentino*. A total of 101 medicines (29 simple drugs and 72 compound medicines) comprised 187 ingredients (85 per cent botanical, 7.5 per cent mineral, and 7.5 per cent zoological substances). Most were no longer in use in pharmacy practice by 1750, and they were completely absent in popular herbal medicine in 1995.[59] 'Old medicine' in Mediterranean Europe, as reflected in the Albacete 'tariff of medicines', involved strict formulations and preferences for certain ingredients, despite other ingredients being available locally but undervalued. The authors concluded that medical systems did not use all the resources available to them.

Records of materia medica in rural areas of Albacete described medical systems with a high degree of stability and resilience, where the use of locally available wild and cultivated resources predominated, in contrast to the emphasis on imported exotic products in pharmacy.[60]

The historical origins of incorporative pharmacopoeial processes have received some attention from scholars. Researchers found that Xhosa healers in southern Africa utilized Western medicines for their symbolic value, allowing them to negotiate some of the historical precedents that had the effect of marginalizing their profession.[61] Others have examined the pharmacopoeia of the Benedictine monks in a study of the use of medicinal plants in north-eastern Brazil during the early nineteenth century.[62] Data obtained from a prescription book in the archives of an Olinda monastery provided evidence that has found relevance in modern pharmaceutical research.

THE UNIVERSALIZATION OF PHARMACOPOEIA

In ethnobotanical writing use of pharmacopoeia has expanded from a community focus to a regional, national, and international perspective. This 'universalization' of the pharmacopoeia is illustrated in Veronica Davidov's 2013 description of 'Amazonia as pharmacopoeia', where she analysed the commonly deployed imaginary of the Amazon as a cornucopia of ethno-medicinal cures unheard of in the Old World.[63] More recently Kerri Brown has explored the conflict between enhancing Indigenous pharmacopoeias and environmental issues.[64] During the nineteenth century, Brazilian materia medica included products of both animal and mineral origin, but a much greater contribution was made to medicine by plant products.[65] Although there is written evidence showing that plants were widely used in Brazilian medical practice, few studies have identified which plant species were used in nineteenth-century medical practice.[66]

Some authors have suggested that there may have been a 'universal' pharmacopoeia evident across cultures and especially in the therapeutic resources adopted by conventional medicine. An examination of surviving prescription books suggested that there is a list of plants that, since ancient times, have been commonly accepted in both academic and traditional medicine. The most significant medicinal plants included rhubarb, ipecacuanha, opium, quinine, and guaiacum. Rather than Indigenous pharmacopoeia being distinct, separate, and unique, pre-European international

36 Pharmacopoeias, Drug Regulation, and Empires

trade may have resulted in at least some elements of an 'international ethno-pharmacopoeia'.[67]

The historical development of a 'global pharmacopoeia' has been explored by several other scholars. A Brazilian team examined the development of herbal medicine and pharmacopoeias in relation to the inclusion of 'exotic' herbal drugs in the New and Old Worlds based on the different epidemiology and cultural evolution of Europe and Brazil. They found that 'in spite of the rich bio-cultural diversity found in the neotropics, relatively few herbal drugs native to South America are included in the global pharmacopoeia'.[68] Yet this article is open to misinterpretation. They compared the share of exotic and native herbal drug species included in the 'Brazilian Pharmacopoeia' with the share included in the 'European Pharmacopoeia'. Both terms are capitalized, suggesting reference to specific pharmacopoeial texts. Are the authors referring to official volumes, or to the totality of Brazilian and European materia medica, respectively? Such lack of definition is a source of potential confusion and a possible hindrance to further scholarly study.

PHARMACOPOEIAS
AND SOCIAL HISTORIANS OF MEDICINE

Pharmacopoeias have received considerable attention from social historians of medicine. Their research has embraced both Indigenous and official pharmacopoeias, although too often little distinction is made between them. Thus, in describing them as 'a genre of texts that listed medicinal substances and provided the recipes to prepare them', Crawford and Gabriel make no reference to whether or not they were issued under the authority of a recognized body before going on to describe pharmacopoeias that were official. 'Several pharmacopoeias of the time used virtually the same categories in organizing ... materia medica used in their prepared medicaments ... the *London Pharmacopoeia* (1618) grouped its materia medica' under certain headings.[69] Other scholars refer to pharmacopoeias without indicating whether they mean 'traditional' or 'official'. Thus, in describing early modern French plant collections, Chandra Mukerji notes that 'the territorial ambitions of this regime had complex connections to pharmacopoeia and botanical collection'.[70] We have to assume that she is referring to the range of materials used by Indigenous communities for medicinal purposes rather than to the official publications.

The Many Meanings of 'Pharmacopoeias'   37

Londa Schiebinger has made important contributions to the literature on pharmacopoeias, but the meaning she attaches to the word is not always clear. She notes, for example, that 'Europeans moving into the tropics encountered illnesses completely unknown to them; their standard pharmacopoeia proved largely ineffective against new diseases.'[71] Does this refer to the official pharmacopoeias that physicians brought with them from their homelands, or to the wider materia medica available to them? Later, in discussing the movement of traditional Indigenous knowledge to European mainstream practice, she notes that 'most women ... whose cures were eventually adopted and published in the various European *Pharmacopoeia* remained nameless.'[72] How are we to interpret the italicization and capitalization of 'pharmacopoeia' here? Is she referring to official European pharmacopoeias, to the large number of unofficial dispensatories, or to other publications such as lists of materia medica? It is an important point, as the former represents a much smaller range of drugs than the latter.

In discussing the role of Jean-Baptiste René Pouppé-Desportes (1704–1748) in St Domingue, Schiebinger records that he presented what he called 'an American pharmacopoeia' offering an extended list of Carib remedies.[73] Was this an official pharmacopoeia, and if so, which one? She explains that 'Europeans had begun producing pharmacopoeia – official compendiums of drugs for major cities – in the sixteenth century in an effort to secure uniformity in remedies. Pouppé-Desportes's is one of the first to record Amerindian remedies.' This indicates a direct link between Indigenous medicines and official pharmacopoeias. As a royal physician Pouppe-Desportes's own publication, *Histoire des maladies de Saint Domingue*, was 'official', having been published 'with the approval and privilege of the king', but the status of the American pharmacopoeia referred to is not clear.

Social historians have used 'pharmacopoeia' in a variety of ways. It has been used to describe the drug options available for a specific condition. In his discussion of the treatment of venereal disease in eighteenth-century England, Bill Bynum notes that 'antimony was occasionally flirted with, but the botanical world produced most of the alternative pharmacopoeia syphilitica.'[74] Others have suggested that pharmacopoeias have an important part to play in analysing imperial expansion, global trade, and contact with Indigenous populations. Crawford and Gabriel note that 'collections of curiosities and pharmacopoeias served, in part, as tools for making sense of the encounters with a diversity of peoples, places, and things provoked by the commercial and colonial expansion of early modern Europe.[75] Paula de Vos notes that pharmacopoeias slowly evolved from unofficial to official publications. As a genre, they were in effect the culmination of earlier ones since they 'brought together elements from these genres into one comprehensive work.'[76]

Historians have extended the spatial boundaries of pharmacopoeias beyond the city, region, or nation. Mark Jenner and Patrick Wallis, for example, found that employees of the English East India Company 'expended immense intellectual, economic and social energy on appropriating substances from their indigenous contexts into the Western pharmacopoeia.'[77] By 'Western pharmacopoeia' they presumably mean the transfer of Indigenous medicinal substances into general Western medical practice, but this statement could equally be interpreted as meaning inclusion in the official pharmacopoeias of European colonial powers. They add that 'English medicine and health care practices were transformed by the process of transplantation into new environments', and that 'particularly in the seventeenth and eighteenth centuries British, imperial, and other transnational dimensions affected medicine more than many other areas of life.'[78]

They were, however, by no means the first to refer to a 'Western pharmacopoeia.' In 2001, Mark Harrison noted that 'from the late 1850s Western pharmacopoeia were standardized.'[79] He quotes Poonam Bala in suggesting that this process led Western practitioners to take an increasingly critical view of Indian remedies.[80] Harrison notes that the fact that many well-known Indian medicines were not included in Western materia medica meant that they were considered by many as beyond the pale. But what exactly does he mean by 'Western pharmacopoeia were standardized'? Is he referring to the fact that in Western countries such as Britain regional and city official pharmacopoeia were 'standardized' into a single national one? Or is he referring to Western pharmacopoeias transforming from lists of simple and compound medicines to compendia of specifications for quality 'standards'? And in referring to Western materia medica does he mean official Western pharmacopoeia, any Western written text concerning medicines, or the items actually used in day-to-day medical practice?

Nandini Bhattacharya has written extensively about the history of pharmacopoeias in India. In discussing 'the inclusions and exclusions of drugs from the formal and informal formularies' she states that 'an official Indian Pharmacopoeia was first published in 1955.'[81] Here 'official' implies that the pharmacopoeia was not only issued by an authorized body (the Indian government) but was also underpinned by legislation with enforcement and sanctions (the 1940 Drugs Act). It was statutory as well as official. Yet the 1868 *Pharmacopoeia of India* was no less official in being published under the authority of the Government of India; that it was not underpinned by legislation meant that it was not also statutory. The publication of the official *British Pharmacopoeia* (BP) in 1864 was mandated in the 1858 Medical Act, but it predated the 1868 Pharmacy and Poisons Act and was given no statutory authority under that act. Bhattacharya is also in good company in using the term 'materia medica' to describe both the materials used in medicine and publications listing them. In her recent book she refers to 'the journey from numerous materia medica to the Indian Pharmacopoeia',[82] but on the next page defines materia medica as 'the content of the drugs themselves'.[83] Such terms provide considerable opportunities for confusion and misunderstanding.

Differences in meaning of 'formal' or 'informal', 'official' or 'non-official', 'statutory' or 'non-statutory' are important and are a potential barrier to further insightful scholarship in this field. When she describes the 'eventual substitution [of China root] in the Western pharmacopoeia with sarsaparilla in the nineteenth century' she presumably means its substitution in the long list of items in regular use in medical practice across Europe, rather than in the shorter list of items selected for inclusion in official European pharmacopoeias.[84] But in the same paragraph she indicates that 'pharmaceutical science and political and economic opportunism both facilitated the expunge of the China root from the British pharmacopoeia by 1914'. It is not clear whether she means its total removal from British medical practice, or simply its exclusion from the BP.

This confusion is apparent in the work of many other scholars, particularly with regard to terms such as 'European pharmacopoeia'. Thus, Sara Press reports that psychedelic plants 'were never integrated into European pharmacopoeia'.[85] She notes that the cures of healing women 'were frequently adopted and published in European *Pharmacopoeia* [her italics]'.[86] Is she referring to unofficial texts listing materia medica, to official pharmacopoeia published by European governments, or to a specific text, a *European Pharmacopoeia*? The same usage is made by Ashley Buchanan. She reports that 'the association of contrayerva root with the treatment of fevers was likely first introduced into the European pharmacopoeia in 1582'.[87] She appears to be referring to use in regular practice rather than indicating any official publication, as she also refers to an 'important plant from the Nahua pharmacopoeia' used in this way.[88]

Yet other articles imply official status where it may not be intended. In her article Ellen Amster writes that 'Pharmacopoeia in Morocco reveals a new dimension – colonial pharmacy as gender history and colonial history.'[89] Again, is she referring to official pharmacopoeia or not? She notes that 'traditional pharmacopoeia remains a popular therapy in post-colonial Morocco.'[90] Such confusion is a hindrance to further elucidation of these themes. In her contribution Rachael Hill reports uncertainly over the variety of wormwood observed by Francisco Alvarez, noting that 'all are staples of Ethiopia's herbal pharmacopoeia.' Again it is not clear whether she is referring to a written text or to Indigenous materia medica, especially when she adds that 'the surrounding forests were also valuable sources of incense, honey, and herbs – all important components of highland Ethiopia's traditional pharmacopoeia.'[91] These examples serve to illustrate how loose use of the term 'pharmacopoeia' can lead to confusion, uncertainty, and error – particularly in the interpretation of the role of official pharmacopoeias in the standardization of medical practice and the regulation of drug use.

PHARMACOPOEIAS AND PHARMACEUTICAL HISTORIANS

Pharmacopoeias have been a central topic in the history of pharmacy since such histories were first written. Successive histories have devoted extensive chapters to the subject. They are invariably narrative accounts of official pharmacopoeias; they usually described the preparation and publication of successive editions of official pharmacopoeias, often reflecting changes in their intended purpose, their underlying medical philosophy, and their content, but rarely explored the social, political, economic, or imperial contexts in which they were developed. John Mason Good in his 1795 publication noted that 'the Royal Edict prefixed to the *London Pharmacopoeia* ... as well as the commentaries of Dr Pemberton and Dr Healde ... are all addressed to apothecaries.'[92] The solution to widespread medicinal incompetence and fraud, he claimed, was association and medical reform, not the tighter imposition of pharmacopoeial requirements.[93] Jacob Bell in his 1880 *Historical Sketch* provided a chronological account of the evolution of pharmacopoeias in Britain. Yet he, too, had much to say about the regulation of poisons and medicines, the professionalization of pharmacy, and their interconnectedness.[94] Bell saw no need to

The Many Meanings of 'Pharmacopoeias'

define what he meant by a pharmacopoeia, to identify the source of its authority, or to explain its purpose.

Wootton's 1910 *Chronicles of Pharmacy* included an extensive chapter on pharmacopoeias, as did C.J.S. Thompson's 1929 *Mystery and Art of the Apothecary*.[95] In defining a pharmacopoeia as 'a collection of formulae for medicinal preparations issued under the authority of some publicly recognized body' he noted that its main purpose was 'to ensure uniformity in the composition of the preparations and the purity of the substances used'.[96] It was the first of many such definitions. James Grier's 1937 *History of Pharmacy* followed the established pattern in having a separate chapter on pharmacopoeias.[97] He drew attention to the distinctiveness of the British experience; the 1498 *Receptario Florentino* had been compiled jointly by pharmacists and doctors, as had the 1535 *Concordia Pharmacopolarum* in Spain, which had been the first pharmacopoeia to receive royal assent.[98]

In 1944 George Urdang undertook an analysis of the two issues of the 1618 first edition of the *London Pharmacopoeia*.[99] He located pharmacopoeias within their wider social and political context and linked them directly to drug regulation. He noted that responsibility for ensuring compliance with their instructions fell to the College of Physicians. Munk had earlier described its implementation: 'Four persons (Censors) were to be chosen yearly to whom was consigned the correction and government of physic and its professors, together with the examination of all medicines and the power of punishing offenders by fine and imprisonment, or by other reasonable ways'.[100] In a 1946 article Urdang concluded that the trend towards greater unification in the fields of politics and culture would 'undoubtedly be mirrored by pharmacopoeias in the future'.[101]

In 1951 Urdang offered a revised definition for a pharmacopoeia. It was, he suggested, 'a pharmaceutical standard intended to secure uniformity in the kind, quality, composition, and strength of remedies approved, or at least tolerated, by the representatives of medicine within a particular political unit and made obligatory for this unit, especially for its pharmacists, by the authorities concerned'.[102] Their functions included the 'economic needs of the area concerned by including products of its own soil and industry, and excluding, as far as possible, products of foreign origin'.[103] The conditions required for a pharmacopoeia to function successfully included its obligatory use by a group of pharmaceutical specialists, although this 'could not be expected until such a group existed and had grown into general recognition.'

There were two prerequisites: the separation of medicine from pharmacy, 'at least as a matter of principle'; and the existence of a public welfare system of which pharmacy was an inherent part. This emphasized pharmacy professionalization and organized health care; effective pharmacopoeias operated within drug regulation frameworks.

The American pharmaceutical historian David Cowen carried out extensive studies of both the Edinburgh dispensatories and the *Edinburgh Pharmacopoeia*.[104] He subsequently described what he considered to be the key characteristics of an official pharmacopoeia. It was, he suggested, 'a compendium of drugs and formulas which is intended to secure uniformity and standardization of remedies and which is made legally obligatory for a particular political jurisdiction, especially upon the pharmacists and pharmaceutical manufacturers of that jurisdiction'.[105] He noted that an additional criterion was often added, that it 'must be prepared by an official pharmaceutical commission'.[106] But these criteria described the official pharmacopoeia of the twentieth century and represented the later stages of pharmacopoeial development. They are less helpful in exploring the transition of the nature and function of pharmacopoeias over time. Cowen noted that the influence of the *Edinburgh Pharmacopoeia* and the dispensatories extended far beyond the borders of the United Kingdom, across Europe and the British Empire.[107] He differentiated between official pharmacopoeias, foreign imprints, private dispensatories, hospital and pauper's compendia, military and surgical compendia, and conspectuses; pharmacopoeias were one genre of many forms of pharmaceutical texts.[108]

Three histories of pharmacy in Britain published in the 1960s had much to say about official pharmacopoeias. Leslie Matthews defined a 'national pharmacopoeia' as 'a compilation reflecting the accepted practice of the medical and pharmaceutical professions in the use of, and standards for, medicinal substances in a country at the time of its compilation'.[109] He cited Robert Multhauf's use of the term with reference to medical philosophies: 'from the middle of the sixteenth century the pharmacopoeia of medical chemistry attained a popularity which approached, if it did not equal, that of the Galenic Pharmacopoeia'.[110] In his book George Trease took a chronological approach describing the various iterations of the *London, Edinburgh, Dublin*, and *British Pharmacopoeias*, describing the reasons why drugs disappear from the materia medica of a particular country.[111] Finally, Poynter's 1965 edited volume included a chapter by Betty Jackson in which she emphasized the role of pharmacopoeias in establishing standards for drugs. The pharmacopoeia became 'an official book of standards which could be used

The Many Meanings of 'Pharmacopoeias'   43

to assess the quality of the drugs appearing on the market.[112] For pharmaceutical historians 'pharmacopoeias' were invariably 'official.'

CONCLUSION

This brief review of the literature on pharmacopoeias highlights a range of issues that merit further attention. Anthropologists and ethnobotanists mainly use the word very loosely to describe the range of traditional or Indigenous items used for medicinal purposes, although their discussions sometimes extend into official pharmacopoeias without this being clear. Recent ethnobotanical research has shown how so-called Indigenous pharmacopoeia are constantly changing and respond to new knowledge obtained both from neighbouring Indigenous communities and from further afield. There is much in this literature that offers fruitful avenues for collaborative research with historians and others, including the use of contemporary hypotheses to explore historical questions. I return to these issues in the book's conclusion.

But if the boundaries between traditional and official pharmacopoeias are not always well delineated in scholarly writing, the distinction between those official pharmacopoeias that were also statutory and those that were not is barely recognized at all. Examination of many apparently 'official' pharmacopoeias indicates that Cowen's criteria are rarely met in their entirety, and indeed that many comply only with one – that they were published by a relevant authority. Recent research has highlighted that important differences exist between pharmacopoeias that are official on these grounds alone and others that are not only official but statutory, having the full backing of legislation. But here again important differences exist; a great diversity of legislation can be applied to pharmacopoeias. A pharmacopoeia might be statutory only in that a law required it to be produced; others may be subject to comprehensive legislation providing for enforcement, inspection, prosecution, and sanction.

The role and use of official pharmacopoeias can only be fully understood in the context of drug regulation; they are inextricably linked, although drug regulatory processes may be weak, incomplete, or absent. Those processes are the result of interaction between a wide range of factors ranging from medical and pharmaceutical professionalization and relations between the two professions to the role of the state in defining them. I consider the relationship between official pharmacopoeias and drug regulation in the next chapter.

2

Pharmacopoeias and Drug Regulation

Thompson's definition of an official pharmacopoeia, 'a collection of formulae for medicinal preparations issued under the authority of some publicly recognized body' with the aim of ensuring 'uniformity in the composition of the preparations and the purity of the substances used,'[1] said nothing about how such an aim might be enforced. Whether or not such a pharmacopoeia was complied with in practice depended on many factors, especially the powers available to that authority and its willingness and capacity to apply them. Historically, both in European metropoles and their corresponding empires, compliance with official pharmacopoeias has ranged from very little to full compliance, with a wide range of compliance or noncompliance in between. Full compliance was almost invariably associated with detailed legislation, where pharmacopoeias were not only official but statutory. Yet relevant legislation could also extend across a broad spectrum, from laws requiring that a pharmacopoeia be published, to ones specifying inspection regimes, offences, and penalties.

Cowen's expanded definition of an official pharmacopoeia as 'a compendium of drugs and formulas which is intended to secure uniformity and standardization of remedies, and which is made legally obligatory for a particular political jurisdiction – especially upon the pharmacists and pharmaceutical manufacturers of that jurisdiction,'[2] along with the additional criterion that 'a pharmacopoeia must be prepared by an official pharmacopoeial commission', effectively established two categories of official pharmacopoeia: those that were 'legally obligatory' and those that were not. For many pharmacopoeias recognized as official did not meet all or even most of Cowen's criteria. Whilst all official pharmacopoeias were published by a recognized body – whether king, government, Parliament, or college of physicians – their legal authority varied greatly. That authority might be conveyed through an edict or an Order in Council, or it might be elaborated in statutory law – written law passed by a legislative body. Thus, pharmacopoeias might be official but not statutory – that is, 'decided or controlled by law, enacted, regulated, or authorized by statute.'[3] But even where pharmacopoeias were included in laws, such legal obligation might extend only to its publication or to apothecaries and others being required to comply with it.

This chapter explores the relationship between pharmacopoeias and drug regulation. It considers its historical development, describes key models of drug regulation, and asks what role pharmacopoeias historically played in controlling the quality, purity, potency, efficacy, and safety of medicines. How effective were they in doing so? Who was involved in their compilation, use, and compliance monitoring? And how important was being statutory as well as official to compliance with pharmacopoeial standards?

PHARMACOPOEIAS AND THE LAW

In Britain official pharmacopoeias were often not 'legally obligatory' either in the metropole or the colonies. Of the official pharmacopoeias in use before 1864, only the Dublin one had a legal basis. As the 1928 Macmillan Report later noted, 'prior to the Medical Act of 1858 [the] Irish Statute of 1760 was the only enactment in the three Kingdoms giving statutory effect to a pharmacopoeia,' and that 'it was not until 1807 that the first *Dublin Pharmacopoeia* appeared.'[4] Macmillan noted that the 'observance of the *London Pharmacopoeia* by all apothecaries in the making and compounding of medicines was enjoined by an Order-in-Council … the *Edinburgh Pharmacopoeia* possessed no legal sanction, although "custom" no doubt gave it a certain authority; and the *Dublin Pharmacopoeia*, on the other hand, enjoyed the sanction both of the Irish Act of Parliament of 1760 and of an Irish Order-in-Council of the 22nd August 1850.'[5] Thus no official British pharmacopoeia was statutory before the first *Dublin Pharmacopoeia* appeared in 1807.

With the decision to replace the three pharmacopoeias with a single volume, the Medical Act of 1858 required that a British Pharmacopoeia be published but gave it no legal authority. In Britain there was no link between pharmacopoeias and drug regulation before 1868; there was no effective legal basis for drugs and poisons control

46 Pharmacopoeias, Drug Regulation, and Empires

before the 1868 Pharmacy and Poisons Act, which linked pharmacy regulation with poisons control.[6] That act required that where a drug listed in the *British Pharmacopoeia* (BP) was supplied, it must be presented in a form also described in the BP. Whilst many colonies subsequently passed ordinances based on this act, its successful implementation depended on having adequate inspection regimes, followed by prosecutions and harsh penalties. Implementing these was often a tough challenge. In colonies (such as India) where no such acts were passed the pharmacopoeia was little more than another guide to drugs and their preparations. Legislation – whether through laws or ordinances – was the essential prerequisite to drug regulation.

The term 'drug regulation' is a product of the late twentieth century, although the issues with which it is concerned have been around for many years. In exploring drug regulation historically, it is instructive to start with a twenty-first-century definition, since this embraces the wide range of drug-related issues that state and other officials have grappled with for centuries. Drug regulation is underpinned by legislation. In a 2003 World Health Organization publication Lembit Rägo and Budiono Santoso indicated that 'medicines regulation demands the application of sound medical, scientific, and technical knowledge and skills, and operates within a legal framework.'[7] Today the principal medicines regulatory functions include licensing the manufacture, import, export, distribution, promotion, and advertising of medicines; assessing their safety, efficacy, and quality, and issuing marketing authorizations for individual products; inspection and surveillance of manufacturers, importers, wholesalers, and dispensers of medicines; controlling and monitoring the quality of medicines on the market and their promotion and advertising; monitoring their safety, including collecting and analysing adverse reaction reports; and providing independent information on medicines to professionals and the public.[8]

Many of these functions – monitoring the quality of medicines on the market, controlling their import and export, and inspecting dispensers of medicines – were as much concerns of early seventeenth-century authorities as they are today. Indeed, the need to address these concerns date from antiquity. Items used for medicinal purposes were usually of high value and low bulk and were invariably a non-discretionary purchase. They were subject to every kind of fraud from adulteration, substitution, and counterfeiting, to poor preparation such as contamination with other items, inaccurate measuring, and inadequate storage. Drugs have been subject to adulteration for millennia. Pliny (23–79 CE) complained that 'nature has revealed … most remarkable properties to mortals, were it not that the fraudulent propensities of man are apt to corrupt and falsify everything.'[9]

ADULTERATION AND SUBSTITUTION

Ernst Stieb has pointed out that the concept of adulteration had different meanings in different times and contexts, but may be considered to have included – 'always in association with intent or neglect – the secret addition of extraneous substances, whether deleterious or merely to increase bulk and weight, the subtraction of constituents usually considered part of the substance; or deterioration from an accepted standard of strength or quality.'[10] Adulteration could also include preparing a substance in such a way as to conceal its defects and to make it appear better than it was. Bhattacharya has shown that, in India, the term 'adulteration' came to be used by the consuming public as a catch-all for any kind of problem resulting in commodities that 'were not of the quality that they expected.'[11] It had several meanings, was frequently used indiscriminately, and could include cases of poisoning that were not deliberate. The adulteration of food and drink was widespread, and an outbreak of epidemic dropsy in Calcutta in 1878 was blamed on adulterants in mustard oil. The production and sale of both therapeutic drugs and cosmetics were subject to counterfeiting, 'where the packaging of a reputed brand was replicated to resemble the original.'[12]

But the problem of adulteration was universal and taxed the authorities in settler communities as much as in colonies with diverse Indigenous populations. In Australia at the first meeting of the Victoria Pharmaceutical Society in 1857 the vice-president, Joseph Bosisto, devoted much of his speech on the 'unholy' practice of adulteration. He placed the blame firmly not on the English wholesale druggists who had sent them, but on unscrupulous foreign dealers – 'the proud Arabian, the intelligent Persian, and the cunning Chinaman' preying on and profiting from 'these English pharmaceutists.' He concluded that the remedy was education, particularly 'a more correct knowledge of botany.'[13] But education was no substitute for legislation. By 1865 a correspondent for the *Melbourne Medical and Surgical Review* was suggesting that an act of Parliament was necessary to bring about immediate reforms in pharmacy 'to protect the public from the effect of cheap and therefore adulterated drugs, and from garrulous and therefore untrustworthy chemists.[14]

The issue of drug substitution has received considerable attention from historians. It is most frequently discussed as a source of conflicting policy, as in India, where debates raged for much of the eighteenth and nineteenth centuries about the substitution of European medicines – particularly those included in pharmacopoeias – with locally available equivalents, many of which were considered to be equally effective as their European counterparts. They were also invariably cheaper and fresher than those imported from England or elsewhere. Whilst British doctors in India were often keen to use such items, others felt that they should not be used until they had been subjected to the same level of scrutiny as the European items. At the same time a powerful trade lobby fought to retain the lucrative trade in medicines between Britain and India.[15] Whilst support for legitimate and policy-driven substitution with local remedies was shared by practitioners in other colonies with large Indigenous populations, the greater concern in settler communities such as Canada and Australia was with fraudulent substitution, with one item being passed off as another.[16]

Whilst historians of medicine typically discuss official pharmacopoeias in relation to the quality or otherwise of medicines (whether adulterated, substituted, counterfeit, or substandard), historians of drug regulation emphasize their role with regard to the safety and efficacy of medicines as well as quality. Concern with drug safety had been an issue from the earliest civilizations, where the emphasis was on deliberate poisoning, resulting in an early genre of pharmaceutical texts, the *antidotaria*, although this title was also used to describe antidotes to diseases.[17] But state authorities also took an interest in other issues of drug safety, such as accidental overdosage due to imprecision in the quantity of active substance included and of unwanted serious side effects when known.[18]

Before humans began trading with each other all medicines were Indigenous. People used whatever was to hand, whether plant, animal, or mineral, to soothe pains, treat illnesses, and reduce fears. The 1618 *London Pharmacopoeia* (LP) contained a large number of simples that would have been familiar to country people. In the home people prepared simple remedies from readily available items (figure 2.1). The difference between domestic remedy and pharmacopoeial medicine was often little more than the complexity of the preparation

Pharmacopoeias and Drug Regulation 49

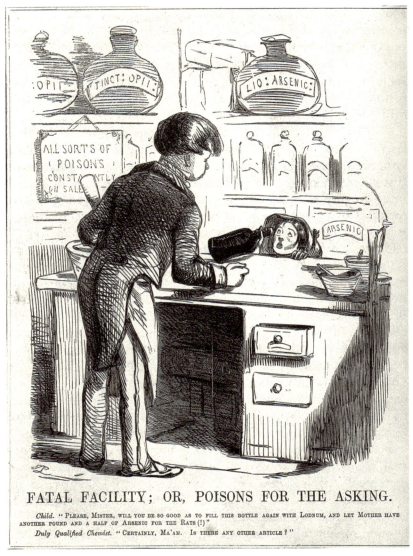

Figure 2.1 An unscrupulous chemist selling a child arsenic and laudanum. Wood engraving after J. Leech.

made and the dose used. Physicians' prescriptions usually contained many and bitter ingredients along with colourants and flavourings. Barbara Griggs noted that 'almost all the standard professional treatments for illness were at best unpleasant; at worst they meant agony.

Most medicines tasted vile.[19] Doses could only be reliable and safe if identity and quality was assured; the margin between safe dose and poisoning was often perilously thin.[20] Physicians had a range of treatments available to them according to severity; the *LP* included formulas for ten 'gentle' purgative pills with long lists of ingredients, and a further fourteen for 'purgative pills fortified with scammony or colocynthide and other items'.[21]

The impact of overdosage of potent drugs only received serious attention after 1785, when William Withering described in detail the symptoms of digitalis intoxication, an account now recognized as the first systematic paper on a medicinal drug.[22] Some historians of pharmacovigilance locate its origins in the mid-nineteenth century and to the death of a young girl following the administration of chloroform. It led to a commission of inquiry instigated by *The Lancet* and the initiating of a reporting system for adverse effects to drugs.[23] The harmful effects of many common medicinal agents – including arsenic, mercury, and nicotine – were revealed only in the twentieth century. According to Mann 'modern concepts of the control of drug safety in Britain derive from the Therapeutic Substances Act of 1925', which regulated the manufacture and sale of substances requiring biological testing.[24] He notes that toxic impurities in drugs such as arsphenamine (Salvarsan) could only be detected by biological testing.

Concepts of efficacy and purity in relation to drugs have been recognized if not fully understood for centuries. Instructions in ancient texts gave details of what time of day or what season of the year to collect certain plant items for maximum benefit. Eighteenth-century merchants were well aware that impure medicines – whether adulterated, counterfeit, or rotten – would be unlikely to have the desired therapeutic effect. Their supply by others would undermine the apothecaries' profits, and if supplied by themselves was unlikely to generate repeat business. But the principle of *caveat emptor* (buyer beware) applied in English law, and neither criminal nor civil law was effective in addressing the circulation of fraudulent or adulterated medicines. As Dorner has pointed out the requirement to inspect drugs at the ports was abolished in 1708 at the same time as corporate oversight over the medical marketplace was being seriously weakened.[25] He notes that some legal protections for patients did apply through common contract law, but that these dealt more with attendance and advice than the sale of medicines. For unscrupulous merchants adulteration was an easy way of undercutting their more

Pharmacopoeias and Drug Regulation

Table 2.1
Models of drug regulation

Model of drug regulation	Territorial scope	Location of responsibility	Mechanism of redress
consumer sovereignty	local	customer/patient	complaint to supplier
consumer sovereignty	national	customer/patient	complaint to manufacturer
occupational control	local	health professional	complaint to health professional
occupational control	national	health professional	complaint to health professional organization
bureaucratic regulation	local	local council	prosecution under by-law
bureaucratic regulation	national	state	prosecution under legislation

Source: Adapted from S.W.F. Holloway, "The Regulation of the Supply of Drugs in Britain before 1868," in *Drugs and Narcotics in History*, ed. Roy Porter and Mikulás Teich (Cambridge: Cambridge University Press, 1997), 77.

honest competitors; Thomas Corbyn argued that adulteration was the only way that some wholesale apothecaries and chemists could undercut his prices.[26]

MODELS OF DRUG REGULATION

Historically, authorities have thus had a wide range of medicine-related issues to contend with, and over the centuries they have deployed a variety of strategies and instruments to deal with them, including the publication of pharmacopoeias. In Britain the history of the regulation of medicines has received considerable attention from scholars, and a number of models of drug regulation have been proposed and studied. Sydney Holloway constructed three distinct models, which he described as 'consumer sovereignty', 'occupational control', and 'bureaucratic regulation'.[27] In consumer sovereignty responsibility for checking that the quality of medicines was 'of the standard expected' was left in the hands of patients: anyone supplying poor quality or fraudulent medicines would, it was assumed, soon find themselves out of business and subject to prosecution. In occupational control responsibility was lodged in the hands of health professionals, initially physicians and doctors but later chemists and druggists and pharmacists. In bureaucratic regulation responsibility for the control of medicine quality was assumed by the state – usually by the passage of appropriate legislation. Holloway added a local/national dimension to these three models, developing a six-fold overall classification (table 2.1).[28]

Whilst these models often existed in parallel with each other with different degrees of emphasis, the historical evolution of drug regulation typically entailed the movement of responsibility from the patient to the health practitioner, and then from professional bodies to the state. Gradmann and Simon, for example, note that 'for centuries, each individual apothecary was responsible for guaranteeing the quality of the medicines he sold in his pharmacy in a context where he prepared the majority of these himself.'[29] Personal responsibility and professional regulation continued as other modes of regulation emerged. Gradmann and Simon note that the 'principle of the personal responsibility of the apothecary for the quality of his wares changed at the end of the nineteenth century' in response to new ways of organizing and legislating for public health, innovations in therapeutics, and the influence of industrial methods of production on the pharmaceutical market.[30] In Britain, poisons legislation became the main mechanism for drug regulation with passage of the Arsenic Act in 1851.[31] However, Corley suggests that 'the first government initiative of any note to regulate drugs [in Britain] was the Pharmacy Act of 1868.'[32]

Whilst it is often suggested that there were no such national controls in Britain before this, a number of mechanisms and sanctions were in place locally. Indeed, ordinances addressing some of the issues had been passed before the end of the fourteenth century. In 1393 the Mistery [sic] of Grossers, Pepperers, and Apothecaries secured an ordinance requiring that – before weighing or sale – drugs had to be inspected by a 'garbler', who was chosen by the grocers but financially disinterested.[33] His task was to detect and remove any impurities found.[34] After garbling, each bale was marked, and the common weigher could only weigh bales so marked. Measuring and weighing gave an indication of specific gravity or density and hence offered some protection against adulteration.[35] Sanctions were available and were applied. In 1394 a London merchant found guilty of supplying 'divers false powders for good ginger and tansy seed for good wormseed' was condemned to the pillory and the false powders were burnt under it.[36]

In 1429 the Grocers' Company became incorporated, and the task of garbling was vested in its wardens. A royal order of Henry VI in 1447 gave the Grocers' Company powers to examine 'anis, wormseed,

Pharmacopoeias and Drug Regulation 53

rhubarb, scammony, spikenard, senna, and all sorts of drugs belonging to medicine, so as not in the buying of these to be hurt in their bodily health.'[37] The grocers were authorized to confiscate adulterated samples.[38] But the physicians continued to claim that the apothecaries were selling and using adulterated drugs, and persuaded Henry VIII to enact an Apothecary, Wares, Drugs, and Stuffs Act in 1540.[39] Section 2 provided for the appointment of physicians to visit apothecaries' shops in London and to destroy any found to be adulterated.[40] A further act in 1553 confirmed the transfer of responsibility for the regulation of medicines from the apothecaries to the doctors.[41] It was nearly two hundred years before the act was amended – in 1727 – to allow officers of the Society of Apothecaries to accompany the physicians on their visits.[42]

When the Society of Apothecaries was founded in 1617 some of the grocers' powers were transferred to them.[43] Its master and wardens were empowered to inspect any pharmacy and 'to burn before the offender's door all drugs and preparations deemed corrupt or unwholesome'.[44] At first the physicians and apothecaries worked amicably together, but by the 1630s issues of professional boundaries and drug regulation had become intermingled. The physicians seized the stock of an unknown powder invented by an apothecary and judged it to be 'defective'. In 1632 a man died of mercury poisoning having been prescribed it by an apothecary without consulting a physician. Two years later an apothecary was found guilty of supplying faulty milk of sulphur, a medicine not included in the LP and therefore not 'official', despite the fact that it was widely used and prescribed by the royal physician, Sir Theodore Turquet de Mayerne. In the same month milk of sulphur sold by another apothecary was judged to be faulty by the physicians, and the apothecary was sent to Newgate Prison. Drug regulation in the early seventeenth century was driven more by inter-professional rivalry than by concern for the public's health and safety.

In the early eighteenth century the powers of the College of Physicians were strengthened by making them statutory. In 1724 'an Act for the better viewing, searching and examining all drugs, medicines, waters, oils, compositions, used or to be used for medicines, in all places where the same shall be exposed to sale, or kept for that purpose, within the City of London and suburbs thereof, or within seven miles circuit of the said city'[45] empowered the College of Physicians to visit and examine the shops of apothecaries. Cases

54 Pharmacopoeias, Drug Regulation, and Empires

involving doubtful drugs were judged by a court composed of both physicians and apothecaries.[46] The first to be visited by the college's censors was an unincorporated apothecary, James Goodwin. They 'commenced the destruction of his goods, turning out one drug after another, and burning them in the street.'[47] Scotland also placed the inspection of apothecaries' stock in the hands of physicians in the seventeenth century.[48]

STANDARDIZING MEDICINES

Lists of formulas or recipes (formularies) for making compound medicines date from antiquity, but – as Colin Dollery pointed out in 1994 – there is little evidence of systematic attempts to standardize their composition before the mid-sixteenth century.[49] The London College of Physicians was conscious of the need to bring some order to the chaotic prescribing situation in the city, leading to publication of the first edition of the LP in 1618. For Dollery this 'was the beginning of an attempt to standardize drug therapy' by an authorized medical body. The 1542 Nuremberg pharmacopoeia had been published under the authority of the city's Senate – not the College of Physicians – whilst the dispensatories published by other cities were texts on pharmacy and therapeutics rather than pharmacopoeias aimed at standardizing the composition of the medicines in use.[50]

This role in standardizing the composition of compound medicines was distinct from their role in specifying standards for the quality of medicines. Standards specified for medicines gradually became more detailed and explicit, and pharmacopoeias only came to be regarded mainly as books of standards in the late eighteenth century, when methods of testing became more robust, supplementing the organoleptic tests of appearance, colour, smell, and taste previously available. Tests for detecting impurities and adulterants were introduced into the LP 1836, although they applied mainly to chemical preparations. It was 'less necessary' and 'more difficult' to apply such tests to vegetable and animal substances. But thereafter the BP became more scientific during the nineteenth and twentieth centuries, although organoleptic tests remained a feature of pharmacopoeial monographs. Analytical tests were a feature of the BP from the 1864 first edition. Subsequent editions followed a similar format, although the 1898 edition added an appendix on 'tests for substances mentioned in the text of the pharmacopoeia, which included qualitative tests for metallic ions and chemical radicals.

Ernst Stieb attributed the change in complexity apparent with the 1898 edition of the BP to the increased participation of pharmacists in preparing the pharmacopoeia, and to its editor, John Attfield. Thus by 1898, at the time the pharmacopoeia was being actively 'imperialized', its nature had already undergone a major transformation, from collection of remedies to compendium of standardized medicines. Whilst the metropole was focused on quality and testing, practitioners in the colonies were concerned about having local remedies – mainly of plant origin – included in the pharmacopoeia. The BP of 1914 added quantitative limit tests for lead and iron;[51] until that edition macroscopic descriptions without the use of a microscope dominated the criteria used to examine vegetable drugs. Quantitative measures including refractive index, optical rotation, acid value, saponification value, and iodine value were first mentioned in the 1914 edition of the BP, in which the first mention of microscopes also appeared.[52]

Pharmacopoeias could provide descriptions and standards for identity and purity, but in the absence of legislation they often had little or no impact. To be effective they needed to be supported by an inspection regime, prosecutions, severe penalties, and strict enforcement, underpinned with the legal authority of statutes passed by legislative bodies. These were largely lacking in the eighteenth century and were really only addressed with passage of the 1868 Pharmacy and Poisons Act. The link between the regulation of the pharmacy profession and poisons controls was no accident; it was a necessary compromise to obtain passage of a Pharmacy Act.[53] The 1868 act placed conditions on the access by the public to certain substances designated as poisons. It provided no control over the quality of the substances thus sold.

Its passage was followed shortly after by enactment of the Adulteration of Food and Drugs Act in 1872, which required local authorities to appoint persons 'possessing competent medical, chemical, and microscopical knowledge' as analysts 'of all articles of food and drugs purchased within the local authority's boundaries'. But the act did not specify standards for drugs, nor the methods for their analysis. Authorities simply had to report the number of items tested and the nature of the adulteration detected in the drugs. It did, however, specify penalties for those found guilty of adulterating food or drugs or who sold them.[54]

During the nineteenth century the dominant model of drug regulation in Britain and the empire shifted from 'occupational control' to 'bureaucratic regulation', although differences in the rate at which this transformation took place were often as stark between London and the provinces as they were between the metropole and the periphery. Holloway notes that the time lag between the rise of the chemist and druggist in London and in the provinces was nearly half a century, roughly over the period 1780 to 1830, and was reflected in pharmacy practice.[55] Apothecaries increasingly obtained medicines in ready-to-sell forms, shifting responsibility for quality and safety to manufacturers. Gradmann and Simon note that as the number of these increased 'a nascent pharmaceutical industry flourished in a legal grey area, in which informal rules more than any formal legislation dictated acceptable conduct.'[56]

Pharmaceutical company representative bodies played increasing roles in drug regulation in association with the state as – with the development of biological medicines such as vaccines and sera in the late nineteenth century – government institutions became increasingly involved in their development and regulation. As animal tests were developed 'it was no longer enough to know what the ingredients were and how much of each was in the medicament in question.'[57] Potency, purity, efficacy, and safety all became essential features of drug quality in the nineteenth century, and central to debates around both the regulation of medicines and the role of pharmacopoeias.

DRUG REGULATION AND PROFESSIONALIZATION

Legislation for drug regulation and the implementation of pharmacopoeias were intimately bound up with the professionalization of medicine and pharmacy. It would not be possible to curtail the adulteration or counterfeiting of medicines if anyone could set themselves up as a chemist and druggist without any recognized training, education, or registration. Across the empire pharmaceutical societies were established following the lead of the 'mother country'. In Sydney, Australia, plans to form such a society were circulated in 1844. The aim of the society was 'to raise the standard of pharmacy chiefly by establishing controls over entry'. Candidates were to be examined at the

Pharmacopoeias and Drug Regulation 57

standards set by the Pharmaceutical Society of Great Britain (PSGB), and the examiners were to be chemists rather than doctors.[58] But there would be no quick fix; a Select Committee of the Legislative Council was established in 1849 to inquire into the Medical Practices Bill. It found that adulteration and short weighing of expensive drugs, and the judicious substitution of cheaper drugs in place of more expensive ones, was common practice in the Australian colonies at the time.[59]

The rise of the chemist and druggist in the late eighteenth century further complicated the relationship between the physicians and the apothecaries. Their vastly increasing numbers presented a serious threat to the livelihoods of the apothecaries. The 1704 Rose case had given the apothecaries the right to diagnose and treat patients provided that they charged only for any medicines supplied and not for services rendered.[60] The situation was further clarified in the 1815 Apothecaries Act, which enabled apothecaries to act as general medical practitioners whilst allowing chemists and druggists to supply and dispense medicines, a move that led ultimately to the foundation of the PSGB in 1841.[61] In his history of the society, Holloway notes that it 'took the lead in establishing the BP as a reliable standard for drugs and drug preparations'. Its increasingly scientific orientation in the late nineteenth century was 'primarily the result of the increased involvement of leading members of the Pharmaceutical Society in its production'.[62]

With the passage of the 1851 Arsenic Act 'the close association between poisons and pharmaceutical regulation was established'.[63] Peter Bartrip argued that that act was 'a first legislative step towards pharmaceutical reform'. But as Holloway points out, 'there was, and is, a world of difference between the mode of regulating the sale of drugs advocated by the Pharmaceutical Society and that enshrined in the Arsenic Act. It is the difference between professional and bureaucratic forms of control'.[64] Indeed, it presaged the Pharmacy Act of 1852 and the much more significant Pharmacy and Poisons Act 1868. The sole concern of the British government in promoting poisons legislation, he argued, was the prevention of crime – mainly murder by poisoning – rather than any broader aim. If the link between the regulation of the pharmacy profession and the control of medicines was established in 1851, it became cemented with passage of the 1868 act, and remained a feature of legislation until the 1968 Medicines Act.[65]

From the 1830s reformers began to articulate a vision of the medical profession as a unitary and democratized body of practitioners connected by common ideals, knowledge, and practices.[66] The pre-1855 British Medical Association aimed to 'unite the scattered members of our profession into one body.'[67] This body would consist of four sections: those devoted to physicians, surgeons, apothecaries, and chemists and druggists. For a growing band of medical radicals the elimination of quackery and unlicensed practice, including the counter-practice of druggists, became part of a grand vision of the medical profession as a united and democratized body with a state-sanctioned hegemony over health care.[68] Thomas Wakley, editor of *The Lancet*, and other radical medical reformers argued that the popularity of patent medicines and unlicensed practitioners proved that consumers were in no position to judge the latter's merits or skills. As Michael Brown points out, to ensure the health of the community it was consequently necessary for the state to protect the public from itself, by preventing anyone without appropriate qualifications from practising medicine.[69]

Regulating medicines was not a gradual transition into increased control and standardization, but a circuitous journey often prompted by disasters, public outcries, or medical demands about the quality of medicines. But to protect the public from exposure to dangerous drugs and poisons it was necessary to regulate not only who could practise medicine but also how medicines and poisons might be accessed. The focus was on regulating practitioners rather than medicines. Between 1857 and 1859 the PSGB successfully fought off attempts by the government to impose detailed poisons regulations. Its Committee on the Sale of Poisons Bill concluded that 'the chief security of the public consists in the discretion and intelligence of the qualified vender of poisons, who, in self-defence as well as from higher motives, is constrained to adopt precautions which no Act of Parliament could define so completely as to constitute a safeguard equal to the moral responsibility now existing.'[70]

The sale of medicines and poisons required the exercise of judgement and discretion. Detailed regulations would take away from the person selling the poison 'that responsibility which at present is a great safeguard to the public.'[71] As Sydney Holloway has shown, when the PSGB was founded in 1841 'any person in this country could sell and advertise practically any medicine he liked, could put into it whatever he pleased, could call it by any name he fancied, and claim for it anything and everything he wished the public to believe'.[72] Likewise, the public were free to buy any drug or pharmaceutical preparation they wished, in any quantity, without restriction from the chemist or needing a doctor's prescription. In Britain before the 1841 foundation of the Pharmaceutical Society, the 1864 publication of the BP, and the 1868 Pharmacy and Poisons Act, professional judgement and the power of medical authorities formed the basis of public protection with regard to medicines rather than legislation.

PHARMACOPOEIAS AND DRUG REGULATION

The use of pharmacopoeias as a tool for tackling adulteration has a long pedigree. In his history of drug regulation Penn noted that, in an attempt to rectify the problem of adulteration in medieval Muslim countries, 'standards were officially laid down by means of a pharmacopoeia and tests described to detect adulteration' in a range of drugs. Official pharmacopoeias were one element in the toolbox available for standardization and control, but their effectiveness depended on whether or not they were underpinned by legislation. England, Scotland, and Ireland had introduced pharmacopoeias in 1618, 1699, and 1807, respectively, with little statutory backing, and there were no revisions to any of them between 1851 and 1864, when the BP was published.

Penn noted that 'save for a brief period between 1872 and 1875 the BP never achieved status as describing legally enforceable standards. The 1875 Sale of Food and Drugs Act failed to provide legal recognition to the BP in cases of adulteration, but it nevertheless offered a presumptive standard for the Courts'.[73] Clinical pharmacologists writing about the history of drug regulation almost invariably link it to pharmacopoeias. Sir Derek Dunlop noted that 'until 1864 when the first BP was published there was little real control over medicines in the UK'.[74] But historians of drug regulation have themselves occasionally been less than clear when using the term 'pharmacopoeia'. Thus, in his monumental *Modern Drug Use: An Enquiry on Historical Principles*, George Mann appears to use it in its more general sense, writing that 'the bulk of the present-day pharmacopoeia is, in historical terms, very recent indeed', although he is in fact describing the BP.[75] The arrangements he subsequently described relied heavily on a licensing system and an inspectorate, providing for in-process control and batch-by-batch record keeping. It laid the foundations for much post-1968 legislation.[76]

Pharmacopoeias played a key role in the standardization not only of drug use but also of nomenclature. It was necessary to ensure that a particular term meant the same thing to different practitioners, as well as ensuring that they used a common list of drugs and preparations, and that standards – however minimal – were established for the quality of those medicines. But the concerns of both practitioners and state changed over time; Dorner notes that the purity of drugs had been a matter of concern to medicine merchants around the turn of the eighteenth century, but by mid-century their main issue was with the adulteration of compounded medicines.[77] Bhattacharya shows that in India one category of adulteration was 'the sale of therapies in all forms that did not comply with the BP'. She notes that this was an ambivalent category, and one that was difficult to identify or to prosecute legally. She argues that the BP was not the 'official' pharmacopoeia, but that it did serve as 'an unofficial mark of quality. The potency or the lack of adequate potency in any drug, therefore, was seen as adulteration in official, medical, and often in public discourse.'[78] Stieb suggests that the emergence of pharmacopoeias needs to be considered within the context of attempts to control adulteration, and to provide a way of establishing means of assessing drug identity and quality. From the sixteenth century onward, he notes, official pharmacopoeias increasingly set standards for the preparation and evaluation of drugs; previously, standards were largely implicit and varied from place to place.[79] But advances in the control of adulteration and in methods for its detection were extremely slow; few occurred before the nineteenth century.[80]

In tracing the early history of drug regulation Gradmann and Simon noted that the aim of a model of drug regulation that placed responsibility in the hands of the individual apothecary was 'to protect the apothecary's customers against poisonous substances, although … the amounts of the ingredients that went into any prescription were precisely dictated by the pharmacopoeia.'[81] They added that 'as a general rule, the contents of the pharmacopoeia, which often determined what could be legally dispensed by an apothecary, were fixed by groups of elite doctors and pharmacists who transcribed the combinations of ingredients, with quantities specified to the nearest grain, that formed the contemporary standards.'[82] This description of pharmacopoeias in relation to both regulation and standardization has echoes in John Pickstone's 'technoscience' way of knowing. He notes that 'States became involved as consumers of these scientific commodities and in some cases as producers, but also as regulators, especially for standardization.'[83]

DRUG REGULATION
IN THE COLONIAL CONTEXT

Drug regulation became a matter of considerable concern in the colonial context, where alarm emerged particularly around the use of addictive narcotics. Indeed, James Mills and Patricia Barton went so far as to suggest that 'drugs were at the heart of the empires of the modern period.'[84] They were referring to psychoactive drugs – those affecting the mind and resulting in intoxication. Contributors to their edited volume agreed 'that colonialism increased drug use by expanding the supply on which revenue depended. As supply increased and prices fell, millions of new consumers entered the market'.[85] But there were limits to the freedom of European colonial powers to control drugs, as William Walker has demonstrated. He illustrated how drug regulation in colonies involved engaging with international politics. Following the Opium Wars with China the trading networks that supplied the market became caught up in the politics of imperial rivalry. Britain, the United States, Japan, and China all fought to secure their own interests.[86] William McAllister showed how dealing with the opium trade caused divisions within individual governments as well as between them. This was the case for most of the major participants in the diplomatic process from the beginning of the twentieth century to the end of the Second World War and was a particular problem for Britain.[87]

Such accounts rarely make reference to pharmacopoeias, yet opium preparations were to be found in the pharmacopoeias of all the European colonial powers.[88] Issues including international disputes, political disagreements at home, and trade pressures all complicated attempts at drug regulation in the colonies. If it was difficult to reach agreement on the regulation of narcotic substances it was much more so for other medicines. The British approach was to pass local ordinances based on the 1868 Pharmacy and Poisons Act in the colonies, including its requirement that drugs included in the BP must only be supplied in the form of preparations described in its pages. It placed the majority of opium in use firmly outside the remit of pharmacopoeia-backed drug regulation. Shifts in 'ways of regulating' medicines occurred at the same time as the pharmacopoeia was being imperialized.

In the countries of the British Empire drug-related prosecutions under medicines legislation varied greatly, although there were large differences in the number of prosecutions made between settler and non-settler colonies. Two issues that resulted most frequently in prosecution were practising as chemists and druggists without qualification and offences under narcotics legislation, which were often rigorously enforced. In the South African state of Transvaal in 1906 a chemist and druggist, L. Gerschung, was convicted in a Civil Court of contravening the Opium Ordinance; one of his assistants had sold surplus opium stock to a Chinese client. Both Gerschung and his assistant were censured and heavily fined, and their prosecution was referred to the statutory body for disciplinary action.[89] The Transvaal Pharmacy Board concluded that their actions had brought discredit to the profession, and both were severely reprimanded and cautioned, although no further action was taken as it was a first offence. It illustrated once again that to be effective, drug regulation and professionalization needed to be embedded in legislation, and any infringements prosecuted vigorously. Successful action on drug-related issues in both the metropolitan and colonial contexts necessitated a solid framework built on the three pillars of drug regulation, pharmacy professionalization, and pharmacopoeial standards.

CONCLUSION

As the British Empire expanded during the course of the nineteenth century, and Britain moved to unify separate pharmacopoeias for England, Scotland, and Ireland into a single British one, thoughts turned to compiling a single 'British imperial pharmacopoeia' that would apply throughout the empire. How this was achieved proved to be a uniquely British experience. Most European colonial powers simply elected to impose the metropolitan pharmacopoeia throughout their colonies. Britain followed the pharmacopoeial developments of its rivals closely; as early colonizers the Spanish, Portuguese, and French had previous experience of new drug discoveries and the need to codify and regulate their use both at home and in the colonies. Key features of the British approach that made it stand out from its rivals can be identified by considering the approaches taken by other European colonial powers to the place of pharmacopoeias in their empires. These I explore in the next chapter.

3

Pharmacopoeias
in European Colonial Empires

The role and use of pharmacopoeias in the colonial context has now been studied by a number of scholars. Nandini Bhattacharya and others have written about pharmacopoeias in British India, whilst others have explored their role in the empires of other European colonial powers. In *Drugs on the Page* Matthew Crawford explored ways in which the *Pharmacopoeia Matritensis*, published in 1739, might be considered 'an Imperial Pharmacopoeia'.[1] It had been prepared by metropolitan physicians appointed by the body that regulated the medical professions (the Royal Protomedicato) in Spain, and published under the authority of the Spanish Crown. A royal decree that accompanied it exhorted officials in 'all the Provinces and subject Kingdoms' to ensure that all pharmacists had a copy and followed all the rules and production methods for medicaments described in it.[2] They were to enforce its stipulations throughout Spain's territories, including the Americas. Pharmacists who failed to do so would be fined and would lose their licence to practise pharmacy.[3]

This statement raises many questions about the use in colonies of pharmacopoeias developed in metropoles. To what extent were they the work of doctors working alone? Did they seek the advice of pharmacists? Did the two groups, doctors and pharmacists, work together? Was the metropolitan pharmacopoeia simply imposed in all colonies without regard to local circumstances, and to what extent was it imperialized? And were colonial practitioners consulted regarding its content? Questions also arise concerning its content. Were items native to particular colonies incorporated into the metropolitan pharmacopoeia? Was any account taken of tropical conditions? To what extent were colonies allowed to compile their own pharmacopoeias? Did the pharmacopoeia include all medicines routinely prescribed by doctors and dispensed by pharmacists, or was it a selection of the most common? And was the pharmacopoeia embodied in legislation (was it statutory as well as official)?

Asking these questions of a number of European colonial powers helps to identify whether there were differences in the approaches taken, and, if so, what these were. Answers to them provide a vital context for an examination of Britain's approach to both the compilation and use of pharmacopoeias in its empire. Identification of features that are peculiar to the British approach illuminate the historical origins of these and enables the distinction between official and statutory pharmacopoeias to be explored.

This chapter considers the development and use of pharmacopoeias in the empires of Britain's European imperial rivals. The British Empire was built in a context of extreme competition among the European colonial powers. Yet the political and pharmacopoeial histories of those countries were very different, as were the nature, size, and longevity of their empires. Portugal, Spain, Holland, and France all had colonies from the early modern period, but others came late to empire. Germany and Italy, for example, only become sovereign states themselves in the late nineteenth century.[4] Colonies changed hands as European powers engaged in wars with each other; the overseas territories of some expanded as others shrank. Denmark had a small number of colonies based around trading posts. Yet despite their many differences occupying powers faced similar problems in maintaining the health of their armies and navies, assuring supplies of essential medicines, and safeguarding their quality. Some had colonies before the first pharmacopoeias were published; others had national ones before expanding overseas.

PHARMACOPOEIAS
IN THE SPANISH EMPIRE

The *Pharmacopoeia Matritensis* was not the first official Spanish pharmacopoeia; that distinction belongs to the *Concordia Pharmacopolarum Barchinonensium*, published in 1511. It had been written by the Society of Apothecaries with the consent of doctors in Barcelona. Further editions followed in 1535 and 1587.[5] In 1546 apothecaries in the city of Saragossa published a pharmacopoeia, of which an expanded edition appeared in 1553 under the title *Concordia Aromatariorum Caesar-augustanemsium*. The title *concordia* (harmony) reflected the consent or binding agreement reached with the physicians. In 1593 a royal decree ordered the Protomedicato to prepare a national pharmacopoeia, after which local pharmacopoeias would cease to apply. But work on it was delayed, and the Protomedicato asked the Valencia College of Apothecaries to produce a pharmacopoeia. The *Officina Medicamentorum* was published in 1603 by the College of Physicians. The college published further editions until 1698.[6] Before 1739 official pharmacopoeias were in the hands of the apothecaries.

Paula de Vos noted that the early modern pharmacopoeia, written by physicians, reached its culmination with Felix Palacios's 1706 *Palestra pharmaceutica*, which served as the basis for the standard formulary for the Spanish Empire.[7] It was the basis for the 1739 *Pharmacopoeia Matritensis*, which represented the Crown's official policy regarding the preparation of medicines.[8] New editions followed in 1762 and 1775, but in 1780 responsibility for its preparation was transferred to pharmacists. The Protopharmaceutical (the government institution representing pharmacists) published a *Pharmacopoeia Hispana* in 1794, with new editions appearing until 1817. But after 1850 responsibility for compiling it was removed from the pharmacists and entrusted to the Royal Academy of Medicine, consisting only of doctors and surgeons. It was published by authority of the government. Further editions followed in 1865 and 1889. The 1905 edition included several tables intended for use by pharmacists. The 1955 ninth edition remained effective in all Spanish territories until enactment of the Medicines Act in 1997.

The *Pharmacopoeia Matritensis* was an imperial pharmacopoeia, imposed by state authorities and made mandatory in all territories under the Spanish Crown. Early modern pharmacopoeias included items imported from far and wide, reflecting centuries of medicine trading. The *Pharmacopoeia Matritensis* divided 'simples' into 'official simples' and 'exotic simples'. In 1739 the highest proportion of substances included originated in Asia.[9] Its content also reflected advances in scientific knowledge, but no consultation with doctors and pharmacists in the colonies appears to have taken place. It incorporated some items of American materia medica. Limited accommodation of local needs was probably allowed, such as the substitution of some items with local materials, but pharmacists were otherwise required to follow the pharmacopoeia. It is clear, however, that often they did not always do so, possibly as a result of lack of proper materials or an interest in using local methods.[10] Pharmacists in Spain's

South American colonies such as Peru were adaptable and made use of what resources were available locally.[11] Substitution of Spanish medicines with Indigenous ones was a necessity. Mexico printed compilations of medicinal substances that had been available prior to the arrival of Europeans. Mexicans had a deep understanding of the medicinal value of local flora and wrote treatises about them.[12] These included the 'little book of Indian medicinal herbs' and the *Codice de la Cruz Badiano* completed in 1552.[13]

Learning acquired from Indigenous practitioners soon entered European discourse. In 1791 Cervantes published an essay on Mexico's vegetable materia medica in which he described 293 plants of therapeutic value. He also proposed 108 species that could be used as substitutes for Spanish plants. In 1832, Antonio de la Cal y Bracho published a list of additional items from the animal and mineral worlds. Spanish pharmacopoeias remained in force until the first edition of the *Farmacopoeia Mexicana* was published in 1846.[14] This reinstated large numbers of Indigenous remedies; of the 180 plants listed in de la Cal y Bracho's text, only 32 were not included in the 1846 pharmacopoeia.[15] In Spain imposition of an 'imperial pharmacopoeia' was tempered by necessity.

PHARMACOPOEIAS IN THE PORTUGUESE EMPIRE

Portugal was the first of the European powers to establish an overseas empire and the last to withdraw from all its occupied territories.[16] The first Portuguese pharmacopoeia was the *Farmacopoeia Lusitana*, written by an apothecary and published in 1704.[17] It was followed by a number of translations during the eighteenth century.[18] These were variously authorized by church authorities, the Inquisition, or by other agencies and bodies. The first official pharmacopoeia approved by royal decree was the *Pharmacopoeia Geral para o Reino e Dominios de Portugal*, published in 1794. It was 'an aid to education, and to guide apothecaries in the preparation of medicines.'[19] An updated version, the *Codigo Pharmaceutico Lusitano*, was published in 1824.[20] Further editions followed between 1836 and 1858, mostly written by individual physicians, but occasionally with help from apothecaries. In September 1876 the first official pharmacopoeia prepared jointly by physicians and pharmacists, the *Pharmacopoeia Portugueza*, was approved by royal decree. Its purpose was 'to perfect and standardize the exercise of pharmacy.'[21]

The pharmacopoeia quickly became outdated thanks to rapid developments in science and technology. Several efforts were made to replace it, but none succeeded, due to wide-ranging social, political, and professional factors that coincided with technical and scientific problems.[22] In 1903 an official commission was appointed to prepare a new edition. It laboured for seven years, but as it was nearing completion revolution occurred. In 1910 the new government replaced the commission with individuals who shared its political aims. The work was not completed, and the new volume never appeared. In 1913, a new commission was formed consisting of doctors from the various faculties of medicine and science. No attempt was made to engage with pharmacists, and in the absence of pharmaceutical expertise, the commission was dissolved.[23] Twenty years later a committee of pharmacists was asked to produce a pharmacopoeia.[24] The *Farmacopeia Portuguesa* was published in 1935 but it went unchanged for thirty years, and remained in force for over fifty years until a new edition based on the *European Pharmacopoeia* was published in 1986.

Portugal's colonies became constitutional parts of Portuguese territory and subject to its laws and rules. This applied as much to medicines and pharmacopoeias as to any other field. The metropolitan pharmacopoeia was thus applied throughout its empire. Until the late seventeenth century Portuguese apothecaries – whether at home or abroad – relied on foreign pharmacopoeias, but with its publication in 1794 the *Farmacopoeia de D. Maria I* was implemented in the colonies. In Brazil, it was the official pharmacopoeia until 1835, when it was replaced with the *Codigo Pharmaceutico Lusitano*, which remained official until 1851. In Goa the sale and supply of medicines was regulated through metropolitan laws, with legislation passed at regular intervals between 1893 and 1946. Medicines were supplied only against *possao* (prescriptions) written by doctors, with pharmacists receiving a fee for dispensing prescriptions.[25] The metropolitan pharmacopoeia applied.

In the early twentieth century it became extremely difficult to impose metropolitan pharmacopoeias in colonies that relied on the services of physicians and others who were not of the nationality of the colonial power. In the 1920s the concessionary company that operated in north-eastern Angola employed doctors from France, Belgium, and Serbia.[26] Portuguese pharmacopoeias played no part in their prescribing. When the company attempted to eradicate sleeping sickness it did so in collaboration with a Belgian mining company.[27] Those infected were treated with newly developed chemical medicines, none of which were listed in either the Portuguese or the Belgian pharmacopoeias.[28] By the 1930s the contents of European pharmacopoeias bore little relationship to needs or practices in the colonial context; pharmacopoeial requirements were effectively ignored.

PHARMACOPOEIAS
IN THE DUTCH EMPIRE

The Dutch were among the earliest European colonizers, following Spain and Portugal. By the 1590s they were trading with Brazil, had settlements on the Gold Coast, possessed bases around the Indian Ocean, and had established a lucrative spice trade in the East Indies.[29] The Dutch colonial empire initially comprised overseas territories and trading posts controlled by the Dutch East India Company (Verenigde Oostindische Compagnie, or VOC) founded in 1602, and the Dutch West India Company founded in 1621. By the 1650s the Dutch had overtaken Portugal as the dominant player in the spice and silk trades and founded a colony at the Cape of Good Hope in 1652. Some Dutch outposts remained undeveloped, isolated trading centres dependent on local host nations.[30] Between 1602 and 1796 the VOC sent almost a million Europeans to work in the Asia trade. The Dutch lost possessions in Bengal to Britain in 1757 and others following the Fourth Anglo-Dutch War (1780–84). Parts of the empire including the Dutch East Indies and Dutch Guiana survived until after the Second World War.

Dutch pharmacopoeias initially had only local legal authority.[31] The first one, the *Pharmacopoeia Amstelredamensis* (*PA*) was published in Amsterdam in 1636.[32] Its sources included the Augsburg, Cologne, and London pharmacopoeias, and it was official throughout the Dutch Empire. In Ceylon a colonial compendium of materia medica was published in 1679, but this did not have official sanction. By 1686 a third edition of the *PA* had been published and was in use across the empire. This was 'considered binding on the basis of the rules that the fatherland employed.'[33] Physicians in the colonies often knew little Latin, and Dutch translations were used. The pharmacopoeia had the effect of increasing the drug trade as pharmacists were obliged to stock the simples listed in their pharmacies.[34] The *Pharmacopoeia*

Amstelredamensis renovate, published in 1726, added seventy-two new simples including ipecacuanha, ginseng, and cinchona from the East and West Indies. Pharmacopoeias also enabled self-taught individuals in the Dutch colonies to function as apothecaries, and determined which drugs they could prescribe.[35] The *PA* had been imperialized to a limited extent by the incorporation of useful items from the colonies. For medicines not described in the *PA* apothecaries in the colonies used other Dutch publications, such as the 1702 *Pharmacopoeia Harlemensis*.

The publication of Dutch national pharmacopoeias was part of a broader European trend.[36] The *Pharmacopoea Batava* – published in Amsterdam in 1805 and prepared by pharmacists and doctors working together – was followed by the *Pharmacopoea Neerlandica* in 1851, revised in 1871 and again in 1889.[37] In the Dutch East Indies the authorities intended to fully imperialize it.[38] Plans were made to transform the pharmacopoeia through a process of consultation, but nothing came of them.[39] Despite the lack of local consultation 'this pharmacopoeia was put into effect by special decree of the Governor General.'[40] Further attempts were made at local consultation; in the 1920s a supplement to the metropolitan pharmacopoeia was prepared taking account of the wishes of practitioners in the East Indies. P.H. Brans reported that – at the same time as the fifth edition became official in August 1929 – 'a supplement was published which gave different regulations for the Dutch East Indies, including different standards for the scales, etc. Many proposals and advice had been received from East India for a pharmacopoeia of their own.'[41]

But despite these measures very little changed. Dutch metropolitan authorities were reluctant to accept large numbers of local substitutes for plant medicines. Brans noted that few of the suggestions from the colonies were taken up: 'a number of Indian "simplicia" were considered ... Mylabrides were approved instead of Cantharides ... Gall apples do not need to come from Cynips tinctoria ... Mel [honey] need not be derived from *Apis mellifica* but must otherwise comply with the provisions of the pharmacopoeia.'[42] Most of the approved changes related to climatic conditions and included giving specific gravities at higher temperatures and allowing modifications to ointment bases.

In the end nothing came of the intended colonial addendum to the *Dutch Pharmacopoeia*, despite engagement with practitioners across the empire. Brans recorded that 'In preparing the fifth edition, physicians and pharmacists in the Dutch East and West Indies were asked for their requirements. The intention was to publish a supplementary volume for overseas. However, when the colony separated from the mother country as the Republic of Indonesia in 1949, this volume had not yet appeared.[43] At the end of the nineteenth century the Dutch national pharmacopoeia was to be used both at home and in the East and West Indies. By the early twentieth century it had become more a book of standards for industry than a recipe book for retail pharmacists,[44] although the Netherlands shared international concerns about both the efficacy and safety of drugs.[45]

PHARMACOPOEIAS
IN THE FRENCH EMPIRE

The French colonial empire began in 1605 when Port Royal was founded in what is now Nova Scotia, with further colonies established in North America, the Caribbean, and India in the seventeenth century. A second phase of French colonialism began with the conquest of Algiers in 1830, but after 1850 France focused on Africa, Indochina, and the South Pacific.[46] The French were desperate to find their own source for cinchona to avoid the Spanish monopoly.[47] Many new medicines from the colonies entered the French metropolitan pharmacopoeia. The French colonial machine has been described as a 'research engine' that deployed experts to solve colonial problems.[48]

The earliest French pharmacopoeias date from the mid-sixteenth century and were published by particular cities – Paris in 1639, Lille in 1640, Bordeaux in 1643, and Lyons in 1674.[49] Others followed in the eighteenth century, including Strasbourg in 1725 and Douia in 1732. Although regarded as pharmacopoeias these were in fact described as codices because they were considered to be 'codes of laws' applying in their specific areas.[50] The large number of official pharmacopoeias created challenges for the authorities in the colonies. Before the 1789 French Revolution, the *Parisian Pharmacopoeia* of 1758 was dominant throughout the empire (figure 3.1); following it, steps were taken to regularize arrangements in all French territories. In 1803 the National Assembly approved uniform standards and regulations for the pharmacy profession, together with the founding of three state-regulated schools of pharmacy to monopolize pharmacy education and training. The pharmacists established professional

CODEX
MEDICAMENTARIUS,
SEU
PHARMACOPŒA
PARISIENSIS,

EX MANDATO FACULTATIS MEDICINÆ
Parifienfis in lucem edita,

DECANO, M. JOANNE-BAPTISTA BOYER,
Equite Ordinis Regii S. Michaelis, Regis Confiliario Medico in fupremo Senatu, ac in generali Præfecturâ Parifienfi, Militarium Regni Nofocomiorum Infpectore, Regio librorum Cenfore, & Societatis Regiæ Londinenfis Socio.

EDITIO QUINTA.

PARISIIS,
Apud PETRUM-GUILLELMUM CAVELIER,
viâ San-Jacobæâ, fub infigne Lilii Aurei.

M. DCC. LVIII.
CUM PRIVILEGIO REGIS.

Figure 3.1 Codex Medicamentarius seu Pharmacopoeia Parisiensis, 1732 Cum Privilegio Regis.

associations and a peer-reviewed journal, giving them a firm basis on which to build an academic discipline.[51]

In Britain the position of the pharmacist was much less formalized than in France; neither was there any serious attempt to reform pharmacy there in the late eighteenth century as there had been across the

Pharmacopoeias in European Colonial Empires 73

English Channel. As Jonathan Simon noted 'the schism in nineteenth century British pharmacy was between those who remained apothecaries and those who became physicians.'[52] The French pharmacist evolved directly from the apothecary of the seventeenth century into the pharmaceutical chemist of the late eighteenth century; pharmacists were predominantly chemists. Indeed, Simon wondered whether pharmacists practising at that time were chemists who practised pharmacy or pharmacists with an interest in chemistry.[53] It would be at least fifty years before the same could be asked of a British pharmacist. Yet the transformation of pharmacopoeias in both Britain and France was driven by developments in chemistry. There were frequent calls to redefine the relationship between pharmacy and chemistry. In post-revolutionary France, where key chemical discoveries had been made by Lavoisier, Berthollet, and others, chemists such as Antoine-Francois de Fourcroy declared that pharmacists 'needed to recognize the position of the pharmacist as subordinate to chemistry.'[54] Chemistry would in fact dictate the nature of pharmacy. But with few apothecaries in England taking much interest in chemistry it fell to physicians and chemists to take the leading role in driving the scientification of the pharmacopoeia.[55]

At the start of the nineteenth century plans were made in France for an 'imperial pharmacopoeia'. It was to be a collaboration between doctors and pharmacists. The Germinal Law of year XI (1803) declared that 'the Government will ask professors of medicine, jointly with members of the schools of pharmacy, to write a Codex or Formulary that will contain medical and pharmaceutical preparations that should be in the hands of all pharmacists. This Formulary will have to include sufficient different preparations to be adapted to climate and production differences according to the different parts of the French territory; it will be published only with the authorisation of the French Government and according to its orders.'[56] It would take account of colonial conditions but made no allowance for local consultation.

Pressure to create a standardized national pharmacopoeia updated with the latest knowledge came from metropolitan doctors rather than those in the colonies. Article 38 of the 1803 act set out the method for its production. The commission charged with preparing the text was responsible to a minister, not a medical body. The consul for civil (public) hospices declared that 'We are impatient to see a volume which encompasses this knowledge, presenting it together with the developments which it may undergo; a pharmacopoeia where finally all the medicines will be adequately given their full place, and which will deserve the title of National Pharmacopoeia.'[57]

Despite the vision for an 'imperial' pharmacopoeia little action was taken. New ones were published in Angers in 1812, and in 1816 a commission was appointed to 'publish a new Formulary' for the Bas-Rhin region. In view of the 1803 law pharmacists in Paris decided 'to stop the publication of specific pharmacopoeias'. Science and politics had combined to produce a change in thinking. Jonathan Simon notes that French pharmacists created a new professional identity and institutions around ideas generated from the two revolutions in political and scientific thought.[58] But in 1816 a royal ordinance 'obliged the Home Office to publish and to print this Codex', with pharmacists obliged to own a copy within six months of publication. The *French Pharmacopoeia* was published in 1818, with each copy stamped by the Faculty of Medicine of Paris.[59]

As Antoine Lentacker points out, the *Codex Medicamentarius, sive Pharmacopoeia Gallica* of 1818 was the first to be given the full force of laws in France that were applied uniformly across the nation's territories.[60] It was both official and statutory. Its main object was to standardize preparations, along with weights and measures. But it was an entirely metropolitan work. Any plan 'to include sufficient different preparations to be adapted to climate and production differences according to the different parts of the French territory' had long been abandoned. France imposed its metropolitan pharmacopoeia throughout its territories, with little account taken of local conditions and no consultation with local practitioners. However, exceptions were made for the army and navy; the chief medical officer was authorized to prepare a formulary adapted to the location of the mission concerned.[61]

French pharmacopoeias had nevertheless been used in French overseas settlements from the start of the empire. Christopher Parsons has shown how in relation to Canada and the French Atlantic world the pharmacopoeia became an important genre in which claims about colonial space were produced and consumed. He notes that 'the abstract colonial spaces of metropolitan maps were mobilized and contested in the pages of medical and pharmaceutical texts'.[62] But his description of a list of remedies written by the Mother Superior of the nuns providing medical care in New France as a 'sort of pharmacopoeia' seems unlikely to have been an 'official' one. It seems more likely that it was simply a list of medicines that may or may not have been available. 'Lists of medicines' requested by the Hotel-Dieu appear to have been no more than orders for replenishment.[63]

Legislation was passed in French colonies to regulate the use of medicines. Between 1913 and 1926 a series of acts were passed in Indochina aimed at imposing 'on non-biomedical therapists and druggists some of the same rules that governed the practice of metropolitan pharmacy'.[64] Whilst mandating use of the *French Pharmacopoeia*, these 'prohibited the sale of chemicals and medicines used by the European, American, and Japanese pharmacopoeias'; only twenty-two substances widely used in Vietnamese therapeutics were exempt. In 1920 Vietnamese 'auxiliary doctors' were authorized to prescribe medicines in 'doses [no] higher than the maximal doses set by the pharmacopoeia for 24 hours'.[65] Their petition to be allowed to prescribe any medicine included in the pharmacopoeia was finally granted in April 1924.[66] The imposition of metropolitan medicines legislation across the empire meant that French pharmacists could move freely between colonies and the metropolis. Many did so. Marcel Kerboriou, for example, established a pharmacy in Nha Trang in 1952 and later moved to Senegal, where he opened a pharmacy in Kaolack. Maurice Buisson founded a company in Vietnam, bought Kerboriou's pharmacy in 1956, and left Vietnam in 1960 to run a pharmacy in Paris.[67]

PHARMACOPOEIAS
IN THE GERMAN EMPIRE

The first German pharmacopoeias were produced by city states, with a variety of health practitioners involved.[68] The first – the *Nuremberg Dispensatory* of 1546[69] – was followed by those of Augsburg in 1564 (compiled by four doctors and a pharmacist) and Cologne in 1565. From the late seventeenth century local medical administrations were required to produce their own pharmacopoeias; smaller ones adopted those of neighbours. The 1698 *Brandenburg Dispensatory* was the first to apply to a state rather than a city state. Its 1713 second edition followed establishment of the Kingdom of Prussia in 1701, with further editions following until 1781. A first edition of the *Wurttenberg Pharmacopoeia* was published in 1741 after local physicians, pharmacists, surgeons, barbers, and midwives were invited to submit written proposals.[70] A *Dispensato-*

rium Lippiacum was produced by the medical officer for Lippe. Regulations in 1789 prescribed the use of a local pharmacopoeia rather than the *Dispensatorium Brandenburgicum*, and in the absence of a local volume the physician Johann Scharf was instructed to write one. It was published in two parts and appeared in 1792 and 1799, respectively. Scharf attempted to introduce his pharmacopoeia into other German states but was unsuccessful.

Countries being created through the unification of many smaller states often had great difficulty in agreeing on a single pharmacopoeia. In 1797 a commission consisting of four doctors and three pharmacists was convened to produce a Prussian pharmacopoeia - the *Pharmacopoeia Borussica* – published in 1799. Pharmacists were involved in the development of all subsequent German pharmacopoeias, with further editions being published between 1804 and 1854. The 1862 edition was officially accepted by all the countries of the North German Federation in 1868, but several other states opted to produce their own pharmacopoeias rather than adopt the Prussian one. These included Oldenburg (1801), Kurhessen (1806), Hamburg (1818), and Saxonia (1820). Plans for the *Bavarian Pharmacopoeia* were announced in 1808, with publication occurring in 1822. A second edition in 1856 differed significantly from that of Prussia's in extent, format, and structure. It was updated in 1859 and remained in effect alongside the *Pharmacopoeia Borussica*. In 1840 the Baden pharmacists produced a *Baden Pharmacopoeia* replacing the Prussian one, despite being ordered to use the latter text.

Renewed efforts were made to agree on a single pharmacopoeia, and in 1865 a *Pharmacopoeia Germaniae* was published. By 1868 the second edition was declared to be the official pharmacopoeia of the Kingdom of Saxony. But a Berlin committee in 1869 accepted neither the *Pharmacopoeia Borussica* nor the *Pharmacopoeia Germaniae* as the national pharmacopoeia. It was agreed that a new one should be prepared, with its scope extended so as to reflect the unified country from 1871. A pharmacopoeia commission was appointed, chaired by a Prussian physician and consisting of five pharmacists, three physicians, and two professors of pharmacy and chemistry. The *Pharmacopoea Germanica* was published in 1872, with a second edition following in 1882. The following year German pharmacists established a commission to revise it, but in 1885 the authorities asked for an entirely new work to be written, and in 1887 a permanent commission was established to that end.

Pharmacopoeias in European Colonial Empires 77

The 1890 third edition of the *Pharmacopoea Germanica* was published in German. A supplement containing additional monographs was published four years later, to be followed by several more. Pharmacologists and representatives of the German pharmaceutical industry joined the commission to prepare the next edition published in 1900. The 1910 fifth edition, compiled by a commission that included leading pharmaceutical scientists, was the last produced during the German colonial period.[71] The changed composition of the commission transformed the resulting text's content. During the nineteenth and early twentieth centuries pharmacognosy (the study of medicinal substances of natural origin) flourished in Germany, resulting in an extensive literature, mostly in German. This contextualized the history of ethnomedicine with the latest discoveries in chemistry and pharmacology.[72] Whilst the 1872 first German pharmacopoeia contained 255 herbal drugs, the 1910 edition included only 167. At the same time the presence of chemical preparations increased from 53 in 1872 to 98 in 1910.[73]

The use of pharmacopoeias in German colonies has been explored by several scholars. Josef Ketteler showed that throughout the period of the German Empire no attempt was made to produce an imperial pharmacopoeia.[74] Günter Klatt reviewed the legal framework for medicines and pharmacopoeias applying at the time and found no evidence of colonial accommodation.[75] André Schön's study of regulations for pharmacies and medicines distribution in the former German colonies in western and south-western Africa highlighted the role of the military.[76] In the early years of German colonialism few metropolitan regulations were implemented in the colonies, and drugs were delivered by military depots, mission pharmacies, and other enterprises, usually supervised by physicians. But when concessions for civilian pharmacies were issued in German East Africa in 1893 and 1897, they were obliged to follow Prussian law, which required that the preparation and storage of medicines complied with the *Pharmacopoea Germanica*.[77] The same was true of German pharmacies in south-east Asian missions.[78] After the German Colonial Office was established in 1907 a pharmacist – Alfred Adlung (1875–1937) – was made responsible for supplying the colonies with medicines, and for implementing regulations concerning concessions for pharmacies.

The *Pharmacopoea Germanica* was imposed on the colonies from 1911 under a new decree. It applied to German-protected areas throughout

Africa and the South Seas, with the exception of German South West Africa, which was controlled by the military. German colonies were permitted to issue additional rules according to local circumstances. In Togo government pharmacies supplied medicines to the people, and no private pharmacies were established until 1914. The *Pharmacopoea Germanica* and German medicine taxes took effect within the colonies three months after their implementation in the German Reich itself.[79] Studies of pharmacopoeias in the German colonial context have illustrated many of the issues that other European authorities had to resolve, and particularly the relationship between pharmacy professionalization, pharmacopoeias, and drug regulation.

PHARMACOPOEIAS
IN THE DANISH EMPIRE

The Danish Empire illustrates the approach of state authorities to the role of pharmacopoeias and drug regulation in small, localized colonies. Between 1620 and 1953 Denmark had colonies in Asia, Africa, the Caribbean, and the North Atlantic.[80] A colony at Tranquebar became a centre for trade in sugar, indigo, pepper, cinnamon, cardamom, cotton, and silk; others were established at Serampore and the Nicobar Islands but were later sold to Britain.[81] Denmark acquired three islands in the West Indies to establish sugar plantations between 1672 and 1733: St Thomas, St John, and St Croix. These were sold to the United States in 1917. In 1728 Denmark had also founded a colony in Greenland, which became part of the Kingdom of Denmark in 1953.[82]

The first official pharmacopoeia, the *Dispensatorium Hafniense* (Dispensatory of Copenhagen) was published in 1658 for use by pharmacists in the capital. The first national pharmacopoeia, the *Pharmacopoea Danica*, was prepared by doctors of the Collegium Medicum and published in 1772. It provided Danish pharmacists with a list of the simple and compound medicines that they were required to stock. Editions in 1805, 1840, and 1850 received strong criticism – mainly about omitted items – but in later ones the number of drugs was reduced, formulas were simplified, and increasing numbers of chemical medicines were included, although often without instructions for preparation. The 1868 edition was the first since 1772 to be well received. The 1893 edition was published in Danish, all preceding editions being in Latin. Further editions followed until 1948.

Danish colonies in Tranquebar, Serampore, and the Nicobar Islands were small communities, and none passed specific legislation regarding medicines; doctors and pharmacists used the *Pharmacopoea Danica*. Legislation in Denmark applied equally to pharmacies in the Danish West Indies. Two pharmacies were established in St Croix and one in St Thomas between 1826 and 1839. All three were functioning when the Danish West Indies were sold in 1917.[83] They operated under licences issued by the Danish king, under whose authority the *Pharmacopoea Danica* was made official.[84] Jensen has noted that the Danish West Indian authorities implemented health policies with considerably greater effectiveness than either the French or British administrations, including those covering the supply of medicines.[85] No pharmacies opened in Greenland during the colonial period; medicines were supplied by a private pharmacy in Denmark until 1931, when the Copenhagen Military Hospital took over. Only the *Pharmacopoea Danica* was in use in Greenland during this time.[86]

PHARMACOPOEIAS
IN THE ITALIAN EMPIRE

The Italian experience of pharmacopoeias illustrates the great diversity of both the official and statutory nature of pharmacopoeias that might exist. The consolidation of states on the Italian Peninsula into a single Kingdom of Italy was completed in 1871, although some states joined the kingdom only at the end of the First World War. Italy's first overseas territory was Assab Bay on the Red Sea, which was taken over by the Italian government in 1882. It acquired various colonies, protectorates, concessions, and dependencies in Africa in the late nineteenth century, including territories in Eritrea, Somalia, Libya, and Ethiopia. Italy held Albania as a protectorate from 1917 to 1920 and again from 1925 to 1939, and it also had concessions in China.

At the end of the eighteenth century, Italy had a bewildering array of pharmacopoeias in use.[87] Each state produced its own, usually written by apothecaries. This was the result not only of the political situation but also of the idiosyncratic nature of Italian apothecaries, who were imaginative and inventive.[88] Most pharmacopoeias were long lists of medicaments that often languished untouched on apothecaries' shelves. With the rise of chemical medicines they increasingly failed to meet the needs of medical practitioners. The pharmacopoeias in use in the four Italian states (Venice, Turin, Parma, and Naples), all published in the 1830s, differed widely in content and regulation. The Austrian pharmacopoeia, *Pharmacopoea Austriaca*, published in Vienna, was official in Lombardy-Venetia at the time.[89] All were published under different authorities: in Venice under that of the Ministry of the Interior; in Turin by the king; in Parma by Maria Luisa of Bourbon, daughter of the Duke of Parma; and in Naples, through the city's chief medical officer. They were all extensive volumes, containing between 1,200 and 1,570 items. Whilst all were official, only a small proportion were 'legally obligatory'. In Turin, 300 of the items listed could be supplied on prescription only; in Parma, 191 items had to be readily available in the pharmacy.[90]

Pharmacopoeias of the Kingdom of Italy were imposed in Italy's colonies. At the time of its creation in 1861, the official pharmacopoeia was the *Farmacopea per gli Stati Sardi*, printed in Turin in 1853.[91] This remained official until 1892, when the first edition of the *Farmacopea Ufficiale del Regno d'Italia* was published in Rome. It was reprinted with additions several times between 1902 and 1940. Separate arrangements were in place for the armed forces in the colonies. The War Ministry published a handbook on medicines in 1893 and again in 1903 for army use. Church authorities had a substantial presence in Italian colonies with priests, monks, nuns, and missionaries all producing their own handbooks. These included a guide to medicine, surgery, pharmacy, and botany produced for overseas missionaries by a Jesuit pharmacist, Pietro Antonacci. This was published in 1845 and reprinted many times. Antonacci also wrote other works about the use of medicines in Italian colonies, but none of these had the authority of an official pharmacopoeia.[92]

PHARMACOPOEIAS
IN THE BELGIAN EMPIRE

The modern state of Belgium was founded in 1830, and its history – and that of its pharmacopoeias – is interwoven with the history of the Netherlands, Germany, France, and Luxembourg. Its land was previously part of a larger territory or divided into smaller states. Between 1860 and 1960 Belgium controlled several overseas colonies, including Santo Tomas in Guatemala between 1843 and 1854; it also held concessions in China from 1900 until 1931. In the late nineteenth century King Leopold II assumed direct control over the Congo

Basin, and the Belgian Congo remained part of the Belgian Empire until 1960.[93] Belgium later acquired parts of the former German East Africa including Ruandi-Urundi, which became Rwanda and Burundi, respectively, on independence in 1962.

The pharmacopoeial histories of both Belgium and the Netherlands reflected the political and economic histories of those countries as they became important centres for the international drug trade. In Antwerp, a modified edition of the dispensatory of Valerius Cordus was published in 1568. It went through various editions and remained official for over a century.[94] The *Pharmacia Antwerpiensis* replaced it in 1661. Most cities in the region published pharmacopoeias in the seventeenth century. A Brussels pharmacopoeia – the *Pharmacopoeia Bruxellensis* – was published in 1641. Territory that came under Austrian rule in 1714 became subject to the Austrian pharmacopoeia. This was reprinted in Brussels in 1747, with a new Austrian publication appearing in 1774. A national pharmacopoeia was produced for the short-lived Batavian Republic (1795–1806), which included what became the Netherlands and Belgium. The *Pharmacopoeia Batava* was subsequently considered to be 'by far the best pharmacopoeia of its time.'[95]

In 1823 the *Pharmacopoeia Batava* was replaced by the first official publication to bear the title *Pharmacopoeia Belgica*. An official Dutch translation was published in 1826 under the title *Nederlandsche Apoteek*. In the 1850s both countries issued their own pharmacopoeias; these were the *Pharmacopoeia Neerlandica* in 1851 and the *Pharmacopoea Belgica Nova* in 1854.[96] Belgium thus had its own pharmacopoeia throughout its colonization period, and this applied throughout its empire.

CONCLUSION

This brief overview of the pharmacopoeias of European colonial powers has highlighted the diversity of situations and the variety of positions taken vis-à-vis pharmacopoeia use and drug regulation in overseas colonies. Most colonial powers made little attempt to imperialize their pharmacopoeias; the metropolitan one was usually imposed without reference to colonial circumstances. Neither was much attempt made to consult with practitioners and others in the colonies about what adaptations might be necessary. European countries that only recently completed the unification of their national pharma-

Pharmacopoeias, Drug Regulation, and Empires

Table 3.1
European colonial powers and pharmacopoeias, 1550–1920

Metropolitan pharma-copoeia	Applied to all colonies	Adapted to colonial needs	Colonial practitioners consulted	Published by medical authority	Pharmacists involved in preparation	Use required in dispensing prescriptions
Dutch	yes	no	attempts made	yes	yes	yes
Portuguese	yes	no	no	yes	varied over time	yes
Spanish	yes	no	no	yes	yes	yes
French	yes	no	no	yes	yes	yes
German	yes	no	no	yes	yes	yes
Danish	yes	no	no	yes	yes	yes
Italian	yes	no	no	no	varied over time	varied by region
British	yes	yes	yes	yes	subsidiary role	yes

Source: Compiled by the author.

copoeias were usually in no hurry to take on the process of imperialization. The status of doctors and pharmacists and relations between them varied greatly in different European countries and were reflected in the extent to which the compilation of pharmacopoeias was the result of collaborations between the two groups. For most the lead role was taken by pharmacists, although the level of collaboration between them and doctors varied considerably over time. Difficulties arose when one group prepared a pharmacopoeia without support from the other; in Italy, pharmacopoeias produced by pharmacists alone became unwieldy lists of drugs and preparations of little use to doctors; in Portugal a pharmacopoeia commission consisting entirely of doctors failed to deliver the required volume.

The precise status of official pharmacopoeias varied greatly (see table 3.1). Whilst some were statutory, many were not, and what was covered by statute also varied considerably. For some only the production of the pharmacopoeia was required by law; others mandated its use by some groups but not others. Very few were implemented alongside legislation regulating the access, use, and quality of medicines. Even the extent to which they were obligatory for dispensing prescriptions varied. For some their use was voluntary rather than mandatory. Their function was often more about persuasion than restriction, seeking to encourage practitioners to use items on a 'recommended list' as some assurance as to reliable quality. Metropolitan pharmacopoeias mainly served as sources of helpful information rather than as legally enforced statements about the range and quality of medicines to be available in colonies. In Dutch colonies the availability of pharmacopoeias enabled self-taught individuals to operate as apothecaries. Arrangements for their compilation changed over time and space. Pharmacopoeias soon became outdated, but the frequency of revision varied greatly. Between 1884 and 1954 Spain published six pharmacopoeias, one of which went through three editions; over the same period Portugal published only three, in 1876, 1935, and 1946.[97]

This review has identified themes that demand particular attention in examining the British colonial experience, and these run through the rest of this book. Among the questions raised are the following: What was the nature of the body giving the pharmacopoeia its authority? Was the metropolitan pharmacopoeia a work of doctors or pharmacists or of several groups working together? Did it include all medicines stocked by apothecaries, all those routinely prescribed by doctors, or only the most common ones? Was the published volume more a medical than a pharmaceutical work? Was it imposed unaltered across the empire? Was any effort made to 'imperialize' it? (by including items of colonial origin, allowing the substitution of European by Indigenous medicines, or adapting formulations to tropical conditions). Were colonial practitioners and others consulted about its content?

Answers to these questions are to be found in the early pharmacopoeial history of Britain – a history shaped by a wide range of issues, including the relationship between Indigenous medicines and European pharmacopoeias, and the substitution of European medicines with locally available ones. Drugs found their way into pharmacopoeias through many different routes; pharmacopoeias played important parts in the international drugs trade through which many new medicines of natural origin were imported, and official medicines were exported to the colonies. In the next chapter I consider the origin of official pharmacopoeias in England, Scotland, and Ireland from the late sixteenth century.

4

Pharmacopoeias for England, Scotland, and Ireland

Whilst England had settled overseas colonies by the seventeenth century, the long eighteenth century witnessed frequent battles between the European colonial powers over foreign territory, leading to changes of occupation, a growth in the slave trade, and massive movements of people, goods, and ideas between metropoles and peripheries.[1] Drugs were an important part of trade. With the Columbian Exchange new drugs reached European ports for redistribution to cities across Europe, including London, Liverpool, and Bristol. Exotic drugs claimed to have merit entered everyday practice, but their arrival presented questions of identity and purity, the answers to which often only came to light on use. Who was to blame for bad medicines, and what could be done to reduce their use? In the early seventeenth century these questions were among many others being asked about the roles of physicians and apothecaries, the relationship between them, and the impact of new medicines on medical practice, culminating in the founding of colleges of physicians and the publishing of pharmacopoeias.[2]

This chapter explores the nature and status of early British official pharmacopoeias. Over the seventeenth and eighteenth centuries separate ones were published in England, Scotland, and Ireland: the *London Pharmacopoeia* in 1618, the *Edinburgh Pharmacopoeia* in 1699, and the *Dublin Pharmacopoeia* in 1807. It examines the authority under which each was produced – whether king, medical college, or Parliament; considers whether each was also legally binding through an act of Parliament; and explores what incentives existed for compliance with its requirements. It seeks to understand the relationship between the pharmacopoeias and drug regulation. Were apothecaries prosecuted for offences and their drugs subject to regular inspection? And what sanctions existed for those found guilty?

The so-called British Empire was initially an English one. Before the early eighteenth century there was no 'Great Britain'; Scotland joined with England only in 1707; Ireland joined them in 1800. Prior to the establishment of the 'British' Parliament in 1707 England and Scotland had separate Parliaments whose role was to 'advise' the king, though the sovereign nevertheless required their consent to levy taxes. Whilst kings usually sought Parliament's advice before issuing royal decrees, the institution only ceased to be subservient to the English monarchy after the execution of Charles I in 1649.[3] Parliament's permission was not required for the king to impose a pharmacopoeia on apothecaries. Yet by the end of the sixteenth century a system of rudimentary drug regulation was already in place, allowing for the inspection of apothecaries' premises and the destruction of drugs judged to be of bad quality.

This chapter focuses on those issues where clear differences were found in the experiences of other European colonial powers, as described in the last chapter, to establish ways in which Britain's approach to pharmacopoeia use in its empire differed from that which obtained elsewhere: the extent to which they were the work of doctors or pharmacists, or of both groups working together; whether engagement with pharmacists and chemists was on an advisory or collaborative basis; whether early British pharmacopoeias were 'imperialized' by the inclusion of colonial items or the adaptation of formulas to tropical conditions; whether colonial practitioners were consulted about their content; and whether they included all medicines stocked by apothecaries, or only a selection of the most commonly used ones. The emergence of pharmacopoeias in Britain was intimately bound up with international trade, professionalization, and the regulation of poisons and medicines.

A PHARMACOPOEIA FOR ENGLAND

By the late sixteenth century the foundations of a pharmacopoeia for England had already been laid. The *London Pharmacopoeia* (LP) was published within a context marked by trade, international relations, medical philosophies, and professional rivalry between physicians and apothecaries. Physicians increasingly complained that apothecaries were practising physick without a licence.[4] Many Indigenous medicines had already reached European ports. The process by which the LP was first compiled set the pattern for subsequent editions, as well as how an 'imperial British pharmacopoeia' would be compiled two hundred and fifty years later. It would be produced by physicians and issued under their authority; advice would be sought but not necessarily accepted from apothecaries; and it would apply to the medicines prescribed by physicians and supplied by apothecaries. Initially the physicians saw no need to consult anyone else. Drugs from the colonies were gradually included, but practitioners in the colonies were expected to use the metropolitan pharmacopoeia.

The English physicians came to pharmacopoeias later than most of their European colleagues. In 1518 the king had signed a royal charter creating a Faculty of Physicians of London.[5] By 1523 it had become a college, incorporated by statute, and given additional powers that extended its remit to the whole of England. Its leading figure, Thomas Linacre, had been in Florence when the *Nuevo Receptario* was published and proposed the compilation of a London pharmacopoeia.[6] But it was only in 1585 that the college felt able to begin preparing 'one certain, uniform Pharmacopoeia for the use of all the apothecaries of London'.[7] Its aim was to counteract the fraud and deceit of those who sold 'filthy concoctions and even mud under the name and title of medicaments for the sake of profit'.[8] But a meeting intended to produce 'something complete and outstanding' had to be deferred when it was realized that 'the matter seemed weighty' and was 'a toilsome task'.

In the late sixteenth century the college experienced difficult relations with the apothecaries, who were exasperated by the lack of consistency in physicians' prescriptions. In July 1586 the Grocers' Company – which included the apothecaries – urged the physicians to set a fixed composition for Genoa treacle, although they considered publication of a pharmacopoeia unnecessary.[9] The apothecaries were more concerned about competition from unqualified charlatans, and pressed for 'the reformation of divers abuses' and the resolution of their 'griefes and complaints'.[10] In 1588 they petitioned the queen for a monopoly on the compounding and selling medicines. But it was opposed by the physicians and others; in the sixteenth century monopolies were considered unacceptable, and with the government preoccupied with the war with Spain the petition failed when Parliament was prorogued in 1589.[11]

The pharmacopoeia project was revived in October 1589. The college 'resolved that there shall be constituted one definite public and uniform dispensatory or formulary of medical prescriptions obligatory

Pharmacopoeias for England, Scotland, and Ireland   87

for apothecary shops.'[12] Ten committees of fellows were appointed to undertake the work, each dealing with different groups of medicaments.[13] But a committee appointed to edit the work was deferred as nothing had been submitted.[14] Conflicting medical philosophies added to political and religious turmoil in slowing progress. The teachings of Galen held sway over those of Paracelsus until the college's statutes were revised in 1601.[15] Candidates increasingly presented themselves well versed in chemical medicine but inadequate in Galenic medicine.[16] The tension between the two was reflected in existing fellows, but the impetus to complete the pharmacopoeia came not from the physicians but the apothecaries.[17] Increasing numbers became dissatisfied with the Grocers' Company and wanted to form their own. Gideon de Laune (1565–1659) presented a bill to Parliament in 1610 for the establishment of such a body with a monopoly of trade. The opposition from the Grocers' Company failed and in 1614 de Laune tried again with the support of the College of Physicians.[18] The resulting bill received the king's seal of approval on 6 December 1617, and the Worshipful Society of Apothecaries of London was founded.[19]

The prospect of a strong body of apothecaries prompted the physicians to revive the pharmacopoeia project. In 1614, eight fellows of the college were asked to examine the pharmacopoeias of Bologna, Bergamo, and Nuremberg and compare them with their own drafts.[20] In 1616 an editing committee was appointed and a final draft prepared. In inaugurating the Society of Apothecaries, the king had hoped to protect his subjects from unskilled empirics who compounded 'unwholesome, hurtful, deceitful, corrupt and dangerous medicines.'[21] He had anticipated that the Society of Apothecaries and the College of Physicians would work closely together, but the college expected the society to be subservient to it. Publishing a pharmacopoeia enabled them to control the apothecaries, and plans for the *LP* were therefore accelerated. The college's historian later noted that 'the invention of printing had made it possible to insist on a real uniformity of pharmaceutical standards.'[22] A pharmacopoeia would 'bring science to bear by standardizing and improving the dispensing of medicines.'[23] Differences remained between supporters of Galenic and chemical medicine, but Theodore de Mayerne (1573–1655) – an advocate of Paracelsian medicine – was instrumental in finalizing the *LP*.[24] He is thought to have been behind the inclusion of sulphur, iron, and antimony.[25] The manuscript was completed in April 1618 and

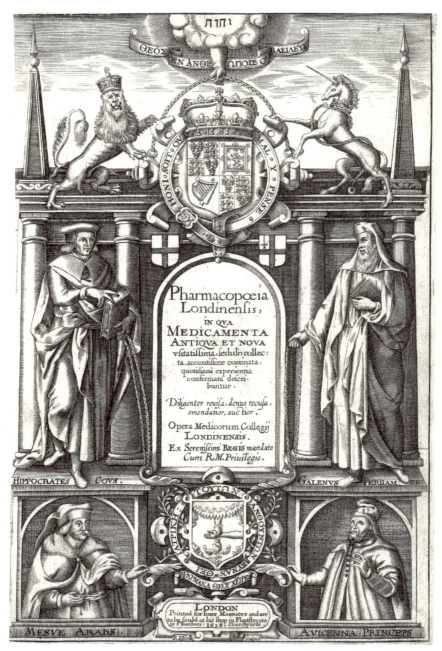

Figure 4.1 Frontispiece from the second issue of first edition of the *Pharmacopoeia Londinensis*, December 1618.

Pharmacopoeias for England, Scotland, and Ireland 89

two fellows were asked to correct the proofs. It was only at this stage that apothecaries were consulted.[26] Six prominent individuals were required to 'give daily attendance', which they assiduously did.[27] The *LP* was published in May, the king's proclamation requiring all apothecaries in the realm to compound their medicines in accordance with it.[28]

The publication, withdrawal, and subsequent reissue of the *LP* have been the subject of extensive debate.[29] The apothecaries claimed that the physicians did not take their advice, and as a result it contained a large number of errors.[30] Munk wrote that it was published 'surreptitiously and prematurely by the printer in the absence of the President',[31] who on his return 'found the book full of errors'.[32] In December 1618 a corrected issue was published, with an epilogue blaming the printer for the errors (figure 4.1).[33] This may have been to cover up serious differences of opinion within the college, some wanting to keep the pharmacopoeia simple, others wanting it to be more extensive.[34] The latter view prevailed, as the December edition combined a formulary with detailed text. Urdang noted that it represented the 'victory of baroque abundance over renaissance simplicity'.[35] He concluded that younger members of the college and dissatisfied practitioners had forced the shift. 'Change from the Renaissance to the Baroque spirit was taking place at the time. Effective display – not immediate practicality – dominated mind and action'.[36] Roberts concluded that the second issue represented 'an attempt by the College to widen the monopoly on medicines for the apothecaries' as a result of their dispute with the grocers.[37] Earles suggested that it was the version put together originally, and that last-minute efforts were made to produce a formulary that more closely reflected prescribing habits at the time.[38] The most plausible explanation has been provided by Clare Fowler. She suggested that de Mayerne gave his copy of the text to the printer before his departure to France, as his papers include a handwritten page listing the sections exactly as they appeared in the May version.[39]

The contents reflected accepted medical practice at the time. Fowler noted that in preparing it the London physicians aimed to emulate the 'formularies of Bergamo and Nuremberg', although it was the 1613 *Augsburg Pharmacopoeia* that had the most obvious influence, with the *LP* having a similar layout and using the same typeface.[40] Much of the content demonstrated a common lineage with the

Table 4.1

Drug imports into England by region of origin, 1567–1774

	Region					
Years	America	East Indies	North-western Europe	Southern Europe	Other (Africa, Northern Europe, and British Isles)	Total
1567–1609	–	–	75%	25%	–	100%
1617–38	1%	42%	22%	35%	–	100%
1662–86	6%	49%	7%	38%	–	100%
1699–1701	10%	42%	13%	33%	2%	100%
1722–24	35%	23%	12%	30%	–	100%
1752–54	35%	39%	5%	21%	–	100%
1772–74	28%	27%	10%	33%	2%	100%

Source: Adapted from Patrick Wallis, "Exotic Drugs and English Medicine: England's Drug Trade, c.1550–c.1800," *Social History of Medicine* 25, no. 1 (2011): 33.

Receptario Florentino of 1498 and 1567.[41] The college acknowledged its reliance on 'the old masters' for compounded medicines. Those of Mesue, Silvius, and Nicolaus were listed in the May issue, although Silvius and Nicolaus were excluded from that of December.[42] Ten formulas were taken directly from the *Augsburg Pharmacopoeia*, and a further five from the *Nuremberg Pharmacopoeia*. Three electuaries were credited to the 1565 *Dispensatorium Coloniensis* published in Cologne.[43] The inclusion of chemical medicines was significant for apothecaries as it aligned them with a relatively new and important aspect of medical treatment.[44]

The geographical sources of preparations reflected the textual sources. Patrick Wallis's analysis of the English drug trade, based on customs records, indicate the changing impact of England's overseas activities (table 4.1). In the early seventeenth century most imported medicines came from north-western Europe, although these included items re-exported from Amsterdam and elsewhere having originated from further afield. By 1618 the largest proportion of the medicines trade came from the East Indies. Physicians welcomed new exotic medicines not least because this gave them justification for higher prices. In 1649 Nicholas Culpeper observed, 'Would it not make both a man's ears glow to hear a man affirm that God hath created no remedy for such a disease nearer than the East-Indies?'[45]

Pharmacopoeias for England, Scotland, and Ireland   91

One of the features of the seventeenth-century drug trade was the growing range of commodities imported.[46] By the early eighteenth century over a third of imported medicines came from America – a substantial change over a fifty-year period. The medicine trade and inclusion in the pharmacopoeia were closely linked. Almost all the top twenty drugs traded between 1566 and 1774 were included in the *LP*; their geographical sources were diverse. There were just 11 in 1600 and 4 in 1604, but the numbers rose to 142 in 1686 and 174 by 1701. They included spices such as cardamum and coriander along with barks, roots, and gums. The value of most was low; in all but one time period the top ten drugs accounted for between two-thirds and three-quarters of all drug imports; the five most common drugs usually constituted about half of all drug imports by value.

Trade followed demand and demand followed use in practice, which was often followed by inclusion in the pharmacopoeia. Wallis listed the top ten drug imports by value over the two periods 1566–1610 and 1772–74.[47] The list included 30 drugs, most of which had been imported for many years, 24 appearing in the 1618 *LP* (table 4.2). Trade reflected changing use; only 3 of those in the top ten before 1610 were still in that list in 1774 – sarsaparilla, Benjamin (benzoin), and senna (the only drug to be included in the top ten throughout). Rhubarb was present in all lists except one and held first place in three periods. Most of the 30 drugs were of plant origin, although animal materials (ambergris and bezoar stone) and elements (sulphur) were also listed. All were 'simples' except theriac, which appeared in first place in the period 1566–1610. After 1618 English theriacs largely replaced imported ones.

The December 1618 *LP* sold in large numbers, and the College of Physicians saw no urgency in revising it.[48] Several reprints with minor corrections were published between 1621 and 1639, with a second edition eventually published in 1650, thirty-two years after the first. A third followed in 1677.[49] Both were little more than further reprints of the first, although some new medicines were added to the third edition.[50] Both showed little evidence of changing medical philosophies or the need to simplify many of the formulations. Over 200 compounded medicines contained more than 10 ingredients, with several containing over 50, including that of Matthiolus which contained 130 ingredients.[51] More than half continued to be ascribed to ancient authors. The *LP* continued to include a wide variety of remedies of animal origin – 35 in all – including 'the slough of a snake,

Table 4.2
Drug imports and inclusion in official pharmacopoeias, 1618–1775

English name	Other name	Source	First mention in import lists	First mention in LP
Theriac	*Theriacum*	compound	1610	1618
Sarsaparilla	*Smilax ornata*	root	1610	–
Wormseed	*Santanica artemisia*	flower	1610	1618
China roots	*Galanga*	root	1610	1618
Senna	*Cassia senna*	leaf	1610	1618
Spica celtica	*Valeriana celtica*	root	1610	1618
Sumatra benzoin	Benjamin	gum	1610	1618
Cassia pods	*Cassia fistula*	pods	1610	1618
Dragon's blood	*Sanguis draconis*	exudate	1610	1618
Agaric	*Amanita muscaria*	fungus	1610	–
Opium	*Papaver somniferum*	capsule	1638	1618
Rhubarb	*Rheum officinalis*	stalk	1638	1618
Scammony	*Radix scammonieae*	root	1638	1618
Spikenard	*Spica vulgaris*	root	1638	1618
Ireos	*Iris florentinae*	root	1638	1618
Gum tragacanth	*Tragacanthum*	exudate	1638	1618
Aloes cicotrina	Aloe	exudate	1668	1618
Ambergris	*Ambra grisea*	whale	1668	1618
Manna	*Fraximus ornus*	exudate	1685	–
Aloes hepatica	Aloe	exudate	1685	1618
Storax calida	*Liquidamber orientalis*	exudate	1685	–
bezoar stone	*Lapis bezoar orientalis*	animal part	1701	1618
Oil aniseed	*Oleum anisi*	seed	1701	1618
Lignum vitae	*Guiacum officinalis*	wood	1701	1618
Jesuit's bark	*Cinchona officinalis*	bark	1724	–
Sassafras root	*Sassafras albidum*	root	1724	1618
Jalap	*Ipomoea purga*	root	1754	1618
Camphor unrefined	*Cinnamonum camphor*	leaf	1754	1618
Sulphur	*Sulphur vivum*	mineral	1774	1618
Pyrmont water	–	Tonic water	1774	–

Source: adapted from Patrick Wallis, "Exotic Drugs and English Medicine: England's Drug Trade, c.1550–c.1800," *Social History of Medicine* 25, no. 1 (2011): 31.

Pharmacopoeias for England, Scotland, and Ireland   93

dung of various animals, and moss growing on a human skull.[52] It is unlikely that many were used in orthodox medicine by the seventeenth century despite still being used in folk medicine.[53] The 1650 LP included about twenty inorganic chemicals, although their nature and action were little understood.[54]

When the LP was published a royal edict declared that no other pharmacopoeia was permitted and that copying was banned, with those found to have done so facing a fine of five pounds per book.[55] Its use was to be exclusive, and it would be enforced by 'censors' appointed by the College of Physicians, who inspected apothecaries' premises and destroyed any drugs they considered 'bad'. The LP was official, having been authorized by royal edict, but was not statutory as no legislation had been approved by Parliament. Indeed, its implementation was not secure; when the English Civil War broke out in 1642 Parliament dissolved the prerogative courts, which removed the enforcement of censorship.[56] Those who failed to comply with the LP could not be prosecuted, and the LP could be copied and criticized without fear of recrimination. In 1647 Nicholas Culpeper was commissioned to translate it from Latin into English:[57] the result was published seven months after Charles I was beheaded in 1649.[58] The college was then close to completing the second edition of the LP, published in 1650 when Oliver Cromwell was lord protector of a 'Commonwealth of England, Scotland and Ireland'. Culpeper's *A Physicall Directory* was an immediate success. It was much more than a translation; it included information about materia medica and the indications for each remedy.[59] As well as commenting on errors, he was highly critical of the physicians, attacking both their greed and their attempt to monopolize medical knowledge. Further editions followed in 1650 and 1651. His translation of the new LP of 1650 was published in 1653 as the *London Dispensatory*, in which Culpeper ridiculed the catalogue of remedies derived from the animal kingdom.[60] It was his last work; he died in 1654 aged thirty-eight.[61] Culpeper was the pioneer of unauthorized translations of official pharmacopoeias; he demonstrated the merits of English as a means of communicating between prescriber and dispenser; he believed that medical information and knowledge were not the sole preserve of doctors – that patients had a right to access it; and he demonstrated that pharmacopoeias compiled without the collaboration of those with pharmaceutical expertise inevitably contained large numbers of errors.

The monarchy was restored in 1660, after which the college assumed the 'royal' epithet. The 1677 *LP* included details of weights and measures for the first time.[62] Besides the vegetable and animal drugs and compounded medicines in regular use by physicians, it reflected greater use of chemicals and minerals. Drugs were organized into three groups: metals, recrement, and *metallica nativa*. Irish whisky was added, reflecting growing trade with Ireland. Most animal remedies were deleted by the 1721 *LP*, although some continued into the late eighteenth century, and at least three survived into the twentieth (cantharides, leeches, and cochineal).

SCOTLAND'S BID FOR AN EMPIRE

A first edition of the *Edinburgh Pharmacopoeia* (*EP*) was published in 1699, eighty-one years after the *LP* first appeared. Its preparation was undertaken at a time of rising Scottish nationalism, strained relations with England, and growing conflict between physicians and apothecaries. Scotland was establishing its own empire and building a separate navy. These imperial ambitions predated foundation of the Edinburgh College of Physicians and publication of the *EP*. Yet when it was published it was more highly regarded in the British Empire than its English predecessor. In the sixteenth century religious conflict – with roots in the English Reformation – erupted in Scotland, and for long periods the two countries were at war.[63] Relations between Scotland and England had long been strained, particularly during the period between the 1603 Union of Crowns and the 1707 Act of Union.

Early in the seventeenth century, Scotland – then an independent country – took its first steps in building an empire of its own. A fishing enterprise in 1617 off Greenland was short-lived. Four years later a charter was granted to establish a Scottish colony in the territories between Newfoundland and New England, to be called Nova Scotia.[64] Settlement was finally achieved in 1629. T.M. Devine notes that this 'was the first serious attempt by Scotland to catch up with the established colonial powers.'[65] Others soon followed. One was briefly established on Cape Breton Island in 1625, but the French claimed sovereignty and the Scots stationed there either died or surrendered. Nova Scotia's charter made the colony legally a part of mainland Scotland. This allowed Scottish ships to avoid the English Navigation Acts, which required that trade with English colonies only be carried in English ships; Scotland could trade with North America by unloading at Nova Scotia ports.

Scottish involvement there ended in 1632, when it was surrendered to France. Efforts were then made to trade with Africa; a Guinea Company, founded in 1636, came to an abrupt end when its ship was seized by the Portuguese, its crew murdered, and its cargo stolen.[66]

Despite these setbacks Scotland continued its pursuit of an empire. The 1670s was a prosperous decade for the country, and 'for the first time in a wholly committed way, the Scottish state began to develop a strategy for independent colonization across the Atlantic.'[67] Plans were made to establish settlements in South Carolina and New Jersey.[68] Two counties in Carolina were purchased as a haven for Scottish Covenanters seeking freedom of conscience. About one hundred and fifty Scottish settlers arrived at Port Royal in 1682, but initial optimism soon faded as the town was burned by the Spanish and subsequently abandoned. There were some joint initiatives between the Scots and English; in 1683 a charter awarded the colony of New Jersey to twenty-four proprietors, half of whom were Scots. It was split between English West Jersey and Scottish East Jersey and was rather more successful than the Carolina adventure.[69]

The new strategy 'amounted to nothing less than the assertion of independent Scottish sovereignty in a world of intense global competition for territory and trade.'[70] In the 1690s Scotland initiated its most ambitious project, to establish a Scottish free port at the heart of the Spanish Empire. In 1693 the Scottish Parliament passed an 'Act for Encouraging of Forraign Trade,' and two years later a 'Company of Scotland Trading to Africa and the Indies' was founded. It would have exclusive rights to trade between Scotland and America for thirty-one years, and a monopoly of commerce with Africa and Asia in perpetuity. The company sent an expedition to Darien in Panama to establish a trading base, but by March 1700 it had ended in complete disaster, resulting from many factors including poor planning and the devastating effects of tropical diseases. But the Scots placed the blame squarely at the feet of the English; English investment had been withdrawn due to political pressure, largely caused by Scottish attempts to circumvent the Navigation Acts. An attempt to relieve the settlers in 1699 failed, largely as a result of the English Parliament's refusal to provide provisions and other support because of the need to maintain Spanish support against France.[71]

The unsuccessful attempt at creating a Scottish empire had enormous political and economic implications. A vast amount of the nation's wealth had been invested in these efforts, and their failure 'directly hit the pockets of many noblemen, lairds, and merchants represented in the Scottish parliament"[72] When the Royal Navy began searching Scottish waters for ships trading with English colonies the Scottish Parliament set up a Scottish navy; by 1703 it had three warships. The dire financial situation the Scots then found themselves in instigated a train of events that led inexorably to union with England.[73] On 16 January 1707 the Scottish Parliament in Edinburgh voted itself out of existence, and the Act of Union became law on 1 May 1707. Scotland was no longer independent, but Scottish doctors could at least demonstrate their independence from English medicine by producing their own pharmacopoeia. Most were in any case more concerned with competition from apothecaries than with building an empire.

A PHARMACOPOEIA FOR SCOTLAND

As Scotland fought to establish an empire its medical practitioners faced many challenges. In 1680 the country had neither a college of physicians nor a pharmacopoeia. Several attempts were made to establish a college in Edinburgh but these failed because of disagreements about its scope. The king had issued a warrant in 1621 entrusting the establishment of such an institution to the Scottish Parliament as part of his plan for a United Kingdom. It would include only physicians and supervise only those in Edinburgh, but an amendment was submitted proposing that it should have jurisdiction over surgeons and apothecaries as well as physicians across the whole of Scotland. This was opposed by surgeons in Edinburgh and physicians and surgeons in Glasgow, and no agreement had been reached before the king died in 1625.[74] A revised petition was put to his successor in 1630.[75] The Edinburgh physicians dropped their demand to have authority over the whole of Scotland, but again proposed that they should have jurisdiction over surgeons and apothecaries. The surgeons and others again objected, and this second attempt to form a college also failed. Resistance continued for another twenty-three years, and in 1642 civil war broke out in England.

Disputes with other practitioners resurfaced and medical politics again dominated the agenda. In 1645, the Incorporation of Surgeons and Barbers in Edinburgh began to admit apothecaries, and those who had served dual apprenticeships in surgery and pharmacy formed a new fraternity whose members were able to undertake all forms of medical activity. This represented a threat to the physicians, and in 1653 a third attempt was made to establish a college. Its advocates submitted a list of 'public abuses in matters of medicine', and a commission recommended that a college of physicians be founded. A draft charter would have given them jurisdiction over all physicians, surgeons, and apothecaries in Scotland except surgeons resident in Glasgow and Edinburgh. In 1657 the London College of Physicians shared their statutes with the Edinburgh physicians, but critics of the endeavour renewed their opposition and the plan died with Cromwell's demise in 1658.[76] The physicians faced competition from surgeon-apothecaries – who had become the largest medical group in Edinburgh – as well as the activities of those falsely presuming to 'profess and practise physic'.[77]

An attempt to join England with Scotland through an act of Parliament in 1667 failed. The 1670s witnessed growing prosperity and a strong sense of national identity, both of which were shared by Scottish physicians. They were led by Robert Sibbald, a staunch Scottish nationalist who as a young man had 'become determined to marshal the talents and resources of Scotland to carry his country forward into the modern world'.[78] In 1660 he studied medicine in Leiden and Paris before moving to London, where he met senior figures of the Royal Society. He returned to his birth country in 1662 with a 'grand design for the advancement of Scotland', which included the creation of learned institutions like those of London and Paris. In 1680 he began inviting Edinburgh physicians to meet at his lodgings to discuss matters of mutual interest. Many were from Scotland's landed gentry and had invested in the country's colonial projects.[79] Sibbald and several others, including Andrew Balfour, began drawing up a pharmacopoeia for use in Edinburgh. They agreed that there was an urgent need to protect their interests and those of a 'gullible public' against unqualified practitioners and unsafe medicines.[80]

An opportunity to revive the plans for a college of physicians arose in 1681. Sibbald and Balfour presented the warrant initially issued by James I in 1621 to the Duke of York (later King James II). In this renewed attempt they agreed that the proposed college would be 'metropolitan and not national'; that it would not rival the Edinburgh surgeons in 'trying to obtain the body of even one malefactor for dissection'; and that it would 'relinquish any idea of giving degrees' so as to placate the Scottish universities. The concessions were agreed, the charter was drawn up, royal approval was given, and the Royal College of Physicians (RCP) of Edinburgh was founded on 30 November 1681.[81]

Under its charter the college had a duty to 'examine and inspect the drugs and medicines sold within the jurisdiction, suburbs, and liberties of Edinburgh.[82] Limited drug regulation based on professional control operated before a pharmacopoeia was proposed. In order to clarify which drugs and medicines were acceptable a committee was appointed in March 1682 to prepare a new draft of the pharmacopoeia that Sibbald and others had previously drawn up.[83] It was the first item of business recorded in the college's minutes, and a manuscript was ready for the printer in 1683.[84] But it was sixteen years before it was published, a delay attributed by Sibbald to 'malice and obstruction by a faction'.[85] He was a committed Galenist sceptical of all post-Newtonian theories, regarded as a reactionary by his younger colleagues, and was later denied the right to teach at the university.[86]

Political and religious conflicts were also important factors in the delay. Cowen noted that 'religious controversy added fuel to professional differences and jealousies'.[87] In 1685 Charles II was succeeded by his brother, who became James VII of England and James II of Scotland. As a Catholic, he quickly lost the support of the Scottish Parliament as he began dismantling legal restrictions placed on Catholics.[88] A coup took place in 1688 when his wife produced a son, and James was thereafter exiled. His daughter Mary and her husband, William of Orange, were invited to take the English throne. The Scotland Parliament was forced to choose between an exiled Catholic or William and Mary. In February 1689 they voted for a Protestant succession, but another attempt to join England and Scotland through an act of Parliament failed. These events were followed by an uprising in 1689 and a massacre at Glencoe in 1692. In the 1690s 'Scotland experienced a level of collective misery and misfortune that was never approached again'.[89]

The college was divided; after 1684 the number of fellows dropped substantially and some of those left played little part in its activities; a draft pharmacopoeia had not been agreed by 1693. Disputes over medical philosophy were at the heart of professional differences. Whilst in 1618 delay in publication of the *LP* was largely due to differences between supporters of Paracelsian and Galenic medicine, in 1693 delay in publication of the *EP* was due to differences between supporters of Galenic medicine and those of a new approach to medicine, iatromechanics. This involved the medical application of physics, offering an explanation for medical practices using mechanical principles and attempting to explain physiological phenomena in mechanical terms. External events and arguments between proponents of the two schools of medicine exacted a heavy toll on the college; it took the election of Sir Archibald Stevenson as president in 1693 to restore order.[90] But his council was equally divided between Catholics and

Protestants and attempts at reform heralded a decade of discord. There were serious personal antipathies and antagonisms among the members based on both politics and religion, and there were factional disputes over the adoption of the 'new science.'

The pharmacopoeia was the most long-lasting of the college's many disputes, and in 1694 responsibility for it passed to Stevenson himself.[91] A succession of committees struggled to draw up an agreed version suitable for publication.[92] Sibbald was firmly resistant to all new ideas, especially iatromechanics.[93] Its leading exponent was Archibald Pitcairn, Stevenson's son-in-law and a staunch Catholic and Jacobite (supporter of James). Stevenson and Pitcairn considered Sibbald's galenicals and herbal remedies to be outdated, but any remedies suggested by them were rejected by Sibbald.[94] Finally, in 1699, a text that met with the college's approval was produced and the first edition of the *EP* was published nineteen years after work began.[95] But agreement on its contents had only been possible by a division within the college. Pitcairn, Stevenson, and the modernizers were suspended; reactionaries who supported Sibbald were quickly admitted to fellowship. Like the *LP* before it, the *EP* represented the victory of conservatism and tradition over innovation and change. It appeared too late to have any influence in Scotland's efforts at a colonial empire,[96] but Scottish colonialists later played important roles in the expansion of sugar plantations and slavery in the Caribbean and elsewhere.[97]

Although under its charter the college had the duty to 'examine and inspect the drugs and medicines sold,' the charter made no mention of a pharmacopoeia. There was no royal foreword mandating its use. The *EP* was 'official' only insofar as it was issued under the authority of the *RCP* of Edinburgh. But there was no mention of it in any act of Parliament; it was not 'statutory.' Its charter gave the college an important role in drug regulation, but this was separate and distinct from its pharmacopoeia. Compliance depended more on the perceived power of the physicians to damage an apothecary's reputation and business than on any statutory basis.

THE LONDON RESPONSE
TO THE *EDINBURGH PHARMACOPOEIA*

If the appearance of a 'Scottish' pharmacopoeia in 1699 presented any threat to the *LP* its compilers were in no hurry to respond. The current edition was that of 1677. The *EP* had discarded no more of the obsolete medicines based on Galenic principles than had the *LP*. Proposals were made to publish new editions in 1698 and 1704, but nothing was done. The RCP of London was then running its own dispensary and giving lectures, but Clark later noted that 'apart from the lectures little was done that had any connection with science'.[98] It was, however, actively involved in medicine supply: in 1700 it advised the Admiralty about a secret remedy for dysentery developed by William Cookworthy, and it declined to approve the remedy of a Dr Mannwaring because he would not reveal its composition.[99] The RCP finally agreed to a revision of the LP after Sir Hans Sloane (1660–1753) was elected its president in 1719. A committee was established to undertake the work, and the fourth edition was published in 1721.[100]

Its compilers were anxious to emphasize that its main purpose was to 'protect public safety', unlike the EP, whose main aim had been to 'protect the interests of the physicians against the apothecaries', although the means of protecting the public from harm was again by commanding apothecaries to follow instructions laid down by physicians. The king's proclamation in 1721 declared that 'nothing is more likely to be of fatal consequence to the health and lives of our subjects than the ill compounding or making up of medicines, to be administered to persons afflicted with sickness, contrary to the prescriptions of their physicians, besides that a gross deceit thereby would be put upon their patients'.[101] In emphasizing its role in public safety the new edition represented a shift in tone from previous ones. It was 'a work which will greatly tend to the publick good of our subjects, by preventing all deceits, differences, varieties, and uncertainties in making or compounding medicines'. Ignorance was no defence. 'Being persuaded that establishing the general use of the said book may tend to the prevention of such deceits, we require that apothecaries do not pretend ignorance of the pharmacopoeia'.[102]

As with all editions up to 1851, the 1721 edition was in Latin – except for the proclamation, which specified that it was to be official in 'any part of Our Kingdom of Great Britain, called England, Dominion of Wales, or Town of Berwick upon Tweed'.[103] There was no mention of overseas territories. It commanded that 'all ... apothecaries and others whose business it is to compound medicines ... not compound or make any medicine or medicinable receipt or prescription' that was included in the LP 'in any other manner ... than [that] set down by the said book'. If a medicine was mentioned in the LP it could only be supplied in the form specified therein. It represented a small but significant shift to a more rational approach to the selection of medicines.[104]

Some old remedies that derived their reputation from superstition or prejudice were omitted,[105] largely at the instigation of Sloane, who was re-elected president of the RCP every year until 1735. The revised catalogue of simples owed much to his knowledge of botany.[106]

Whilst the Edinburgh physicians published new editions of the EP about every twelve years or so, the London RCP proceeded more slowly. A revision committee was established in 1738, but the fifth edition of the LP was published only in 1746.[107] It contained many important revisions, and owed much to the efforts of Henry Pemberton, then Gresham Professor of Physic, described by Munk as 'one of the best chemists of the day'.[108] The committee spelled out the principles it used to decide what to add or delete, and its members were disparaging of the 'old masters' and critical of their predecessors, who had stuck with the old ways much longer than they should have.[109] They scorned 'the old practice of taking into account the four qualities of heating, cooling, drying and moistening, and modifying such attributes, which they say produced the most ridiculous farrago'.[110] Pemberton noted that 'every part of pharmacy has been over-run with superfluities', and he was particularly critical of 'that enormous composition, *antidotus Matthioli*, which contains more than one hundred simples and several of the most copious compositions'.[111] He declared, 'we have here endeavoured ... to retrench this excess and to furnish the shops with a sufficient number of elegant and simple medicines [that are] efficacious [and] well-tried'.[112]

It differed from all its predecessors in having nothing to do with the state of relations with the apothecaries. Clark noted that 'No motive seems to have been at work except the modernization and improvement of the recipes. Throughout this long period of gestation there were no overt hostilities between the two branches'.[113] This edition gave the first hint of better relations between them. Previously preparation of the LP had been the exclusive work of physicians, with apothecaries occasionally asked to comment. The first mention of 'cooperation' with the apothecaries appeared in 1785 when Sir George Baker was elected RCP president and initiated a revision of the LP. The Society of Apothecaries received an invitation to assist in order that it might be as 'correct and free from errors as possible, and all formulae should be such as can be easily prepared by the gentlemen of your Society'.[114] The cooperation apparent in the 1788 LP represented a move from the limited consultation of earlier editions and the afterthought of the first. But it was still far short of

Pharmacopoeias, Drug Regulation, and Empires

collaboration, and even further from the equal partnership that only came much later.

The 1788 edition contained fewer changes than that of 1746 but 'achieved more in the way of catching up with the progress of science.'[115] William Heberden drew attention to the nonsense of including ancient remedies consisting of large numbers of ingredients in a 1745 essay.[116] In excluding them they were ahead of many of their European colleagues; in the Netherlands *theriaca Andromachi* remained in the pharmacopoeia until the nineteenth century.[117] In Britain pharmaceutical texts increasingly incorporated scientific findings and deleted obsolete items, as Robert James put it in 1747, 'to prune away the branches of physic that bear no fruit.' He rejected 'the custom for writers of dispensatories to embarrass their compositions and for physicians to overload their prescriptions with a great number of superfluous ingredients.'[118]

New and useful articles were introduced, many from Britain's newly acquired colonies. Quassia, first imported for use by brewers, soon found a medicinal use. Castor oil was recommended as a purgative in 1764, although it had been used externally for many years; castor seeds were included with directions for preparing the oil.[119] Alkaloidal drugs were identified from the 1760s, and aconite, colchicum, stramonium, henbane, and belladonna were all included in the 1788 or 1809 editions of the *LP*. Calumba first became official in 1788. A pharmacopoeial version of a popular proprietary medicine, Dr James's Powder, was included.[120] The mercury thermometer had recently been introduced, allowing precise temperatures to be specified. Linnaeus's system of plant nomenclature was adopted, enabling plant drugs to be more accurately described. Foxglove was first included in the 1650 *LP*, but Withering's publication enabled a fuller description to be given in the *LP* of 1788.[121] The application of science became increasingly important to both the content and arrangement of the pharmacopoeia. When Grey compared the 1746 and 1788 editions of the *LP*, he noted that whilst the earlier text excelled in 'Galenic pharmacy', the later one excelled in 'chemical pharmacy'.[122]

A PHARMACOPOEIA FOR IRELAND

Physicians in Dublin followed the 1707 union between England and Scotland with concern. A college of physicians had been founded in Dublin in 1654, seventeen years before that of Edinburgh. Its royal

Pharmacopoeias for England, Scotland, and Ireland

charter, granted in 1667, was renewed in 1692, giving it authority over physicians, apothecaries, druggists, and others engaged in the sale of medicines.[123] The college was authorized to carry out inspections and to destroy faulty stock. Drug regulation was based on occupational control; the charter made no mention of a need for a pharmacopoeia for Dublin or the Kingdom of Ireland. Following the 1707 union of Scotland with England the Protestant Irish Parliament sought closer union between Ireland and England. But restrictions on its activities would have made it subservient to the English Parliament, and both the country and the college realized that English law might soon apply throughout Ireland.

The issue of a pharmacopoeia for Ireland was brought before the college in 1717, the choice being to adopt either the London or Edinburgh one or compile their own; to the latter end, in 1719 Duncan Cumming was asked to prepare a 'draft of the medicines that he thought proper for inclusion in a dispensatory.'[124] Little progress was made, however, and in 1721 a new edition of the LP was published. The college agreed 'to recommend to the Apothecaries of the City of Dublin the prescriptions of the last new *London Dispensatory* in making up their medicines.'[125] The resolution did not give it statutory authority in Ireland, and the apothecaries and surgeons viewed it as an attempt by the physicians to control pharmacy and create a monopoly.[126] The college members could not agree about adopting the LP and in 1726 a proposal was put forward to determine 'whether a new Dispensatory will be of use to this City and Kingdom.' It was unanimously agreed, and the fellows were asked to bring to the next meeting 'a list of the compositions in the … *London Dispensatory* that are proper to make part of the *Dublin Dispensatory*.'[127] It was to be an entirely medical work. But all attempts to compile one failed; it was impossible to reach consensus.

The next move came from the Irish Parliament, whose members were anxious to crack down on the supply of adulterated medicines by unqualified persons. In 1735 they passed 'an Act for preventing frauds and abuses in the making and vending of unsound, adulterated and bad drugs and medicines.' It authorized the college to inspect apothecaries' shops within a seven-mile radius of Dublin, and to destroy any medicines considered unfit for use. Drug regulation in Ireland now had a statutory basis. As in England, the apothecaries sought a charter incorporating them as a separate guild. The College of Physicians agreed, provided that the apothecaries were not given powers to determine the composition of medicines without its approval, and a charter was granted in 1745.[128] When the fifth edition of the *lp* was published in 1746 the college resolved to use it in future prescriptions.[129] The members appointed a committee to report any errors, and a Dublin edition was published in 1747.

The 1735 act failed to stop abuses, however, so in 1761 a new act was passed. This gave the college the power 'to frame and publish a code or pharmacopoeia containing a catalogue of drugs or simple medicines as they shall judge necessary.'[130] The *Dublin Pharmacopoeia (DP)* would have statutory force, unlike its English and Scottish counterparts. But the college made little attempt to compile one for another twenty-three years; political events at home and abroad – including the American War of Independence – left the physicians little opportunity to do so.[131] With the end of the war plans for a pharmacopoeia were revived in 1784. A committee was appointed 'to take the most speedy and effectual steps toward the preparation of a dispensatory, under the title of *Dublin Pharmacopoeia*, for the general use of this kingdom.'[132] Progress was again slow, and when in June 1788 a new edition of the *lp* was published the college agreed to use it as the basis of its own. By late 1788 the committee had reached 'as far as the article on *vina medicata*.' In January 1791 the college ordered that copies be printed and distributed. By 1794 the members were able to report that 'they had prepared and printed one hundred copies of a "specimen" which they had distributed to the Fellows and Licentiates of the College, to heads of College of Surgeons, to the Corporation of Apothecaries, and to Apothecaries Hall.'[133]

A new committee was appointed 'to revise its Latinity' and to report any alterations required. The cooperation of the College of Surgeons was sought in the preparation of 'such parts of the pharmacopoeia as relate to external applications.' The surgeons declined to cooperate. There were yet further delays; the fellows were engaged in an acrimonious internal dispute, and in 1801 Acts of Union united the Kingdom of Great Britain and the Kingdom of Ireland to create the United Kingdom. Union prompted renewed efforts to publish the *DP*. Changes were made to chemical nomenclature and weights and measures were standardized.

By May 1805 the *DP* was almost complete, and this second specimen was laid before the college in August 'for the perusal of Fellows and Licentiates.' Following further revision five hundred copies of the *DP* were printed and published in 1807 and dedicated to George III.[134]

Pharmacopoeias for England, Scotland, and Ireland   105

The committee reported that 'in the names and properties of ingredients for compound medicines' they had followed the *LP*, as the 1746 edition of this had 'been directed by our College to be the rule of compounding medicines in Ireland.'[135] Its proclamation included the following instruction: 'all and singular apothecaries and others whose business it is to compound medicines ... within this part of His Majesty's United Kingdom called Ireland ... immediately after the said *Dublin Pharmacopoeia* shall be printed and published, do not compound or make any medicine except ... by the special direction or prescription of some learned physician.'[136]

It applied to the whole of Ireland and its need was spelled out in the following terms: 'Medicines are prepared sometimes according to the London formulae, sometimes according to the Edinburgh, and not infrequently at the mere discretion of the Apothecary; some practitioners awaiting the further directions of the College continue to use the nomenclature of the pharmacopoeia of 1746; some adhere to the latter publication, and not a few prescribe according to one of the multiplied editions of the Edinburgh College.'[137]

THE THREE BRITISH PHARMACOPOEIAS

It had taken ninety years to publish a *DP*, but by the start of the nineteenth century separate pharmacopoeias were in use in England, Scotland, and Ireland. Of the three only the *DP* had statutory authority; the *LP* was authorized by royal decree; the *EP* by a royal college. Ireland had a pharmacopoeia that was not only official but statutory; any change would require legislation in the Irish Parliament.

Although the three pharmacopoeias had different origins and aims all were also expressions of local tradition and national identity.[138] The early nineteenth century saw a rapid shift from natural products to synthetically prepared chemicals. Major innovations took place in science, technology, and medicine, particularly in chemistry, botany, and physiology. Active constituents of botanical drugs were extracted and tested. Narcotine was extracted from opium in 1803; Sertürner extracted an impure form of morphine in 1805 and isolated it in 1816; and Pelletier and Caventou isolated quinine in 1820.[139] Isolation led quickly to their mass production; H.E. Merck began extracting morphine and other alkaloids on a commercial scale in 1826, and by 1831 morphine acetate was being manufactured by William Gregory.[140] The changing nature of materia medica impacted the professionalization of pharmacy. With the formalization of pharmacy education following the opening of the Pharmaceutical Society of Great Britain's school in 1842 pharmacy became increasingly scientific.[141]

The London RCP continued to exercise its authority in all pharmaceutical matters; in 1800 it refused to supply the Society of Apothecaries with a new formula for digitalis tincture on the grounds that there was no precedent.[142] In 1807 the current edition of the *LP* was that of 1788; the RCP gave its approval for a revision in September 1805. The work was delegated to a committee of fellows, who began work in January 1806, just as the Dublin physicians were making their final revisions.[143] The committee obtained 'the opinions of the profession at large, as well as of the individuals who attended the committee, respecting any changes which might be thought necessary.'[144] It later extended its consultation to 'every member of the College, to the Royal College of Surgeons, and Society of Apothecaries.' A new process of consultation with physicians, pharmacists, and others about the content of the pharmacopoeia was established. As a result 'they did accordingly receive numerous communications, which were arranged and considered under their proper heads.'[145]

Their next task was to 'establish certain general principles and then to consider and discuss the whole pharmacopoeia, article by article.' Its compilers 'derived great assistance from the recent pharmacopoeias edited by the Royal Colleges of Edinburgh and Dublin.'[146] Richard Powell acknowledged the work carried out by the Society of Apothecaries, 'who appointed a committee ... for the purpose of cooperating, in the use of their extensive laboratory, and in bringing to the test of that sort of experiment upon a large scale, which could alone render the suggestions of science practically useful.' Cooperation between the physicians and apothecaries had occurred previously, but the 1809 *LP* represented a significant expansion of consultation in revising the pharmacopoeia.[147] After 1809 the RCP relied less on the society for advice, despite the fact that its laboratory was a major manufacturer of medicinal preparations.[148] Pharmaceutical advice became more of a problem following passage of the 1815 Apothecaries Act, when most apothecaries became general medical practitioners. For the 1815 and 1824 editions there was only 'occasional consultations, for instance by Dr Babington, who had been an apothecary to St Bartholomew's Hospital.'[149]

After further revision, London followed Dublin's example by publishing a 'specimen', two hundred and fifty copies of which were printed in April 1808 and distributed to 'those persons whom they thought likely to afford assistance or information, although this group was limited to medical practitioners.[150] Sixty were returned with comments and suggestions, but some 'fell into improper hands' and their contents were subsequently published as unauthorized versions. A subcommittee prepared a second specimen, which was circulated among fellows resident in London, and a final draft incorporating items from both the *EP* and *DP* was approved by the RCP Council in March 1809. Its purpose was now 'to direct what simple medicinal substances ought to be found in the shops of apothecaries, and to describe such preparations or compositions of these, as cannot be made without length of time, yet are often wanted for immediate use'.[151] Its scope was now limited to items in regular use.

CONCLUSION

By the early nineteenth century three pharmacopoeias were in use in the United Kingdom, with substantial variation between each. Doctors going out to the colonies might have been trained in England, Scotland, or Ireland, and the items they prescribed might vary according to which pharmacopoeia they had used previously. The RCP considered how to respond to the changing political, scientific, and imperial landscapes. Immediately after publication of the 1809 *LP* it established a new revision committee. In 1810 it received recommendations from its censors who undertook the inspection of apothecaries' shops. They noted that 'the Scottish element among medical men practising in England grew', and that 'the anomaly of having independent standards for the two countries became more evident'. Clark records that, on 5 November 1813, 'for this or some other reason, it was moved that a committee should be appointed to consider the possibility of an imperial British pharmacopoeia'.[152] But the RCP motion was lost, although 'the idea persisted both inside and outside the College'.[153]

With all three pharmacopoeias in use across the empire, there could be no realistic prospect of an imperial British pharmacopoeia whilst all were official in some part of the United Kingdom. Publication of a single unified 'British' pharmacopoeia only became possible after passage of the 1858 Medical Act. However, before proceeding to that development, I first consider the use of official pharmacopoeias in the British Empire, and the emergence of 'colonial' pharmacopoeias.

5

The Emergence of Colonial Pharmacopoeias

The suggestion in 1813 for an imperial British pharmacopoeia was raised in a context of increasing awareness of Britain's imperial expansion and of the challenges of colonial administration. The Napoleonic Wars were nearing an end, and Britain would acquire new colonies following the 1815 Treaty of Paris. In India British territorial authority increased rapidly after the 1757 Battle of Plassey. From the early English settlements in North America and the Caribbean in the seventeenth century to the creation of colonies in Australia in the nineteenth, large numbers of British soldiers, sailors, and civilians travelled to distant lands to forge and develop the empire. Maintaining life and health was a constant battle; new ways of thinking about diseases and how to treat them were explored in both the metropole and the empire in the colonial crucible.

This chapter explores the role of medicines, pharmacopoeias, and drug regulation in the British Empire prior to the mid-nineteenth century. It considers which pharmacopoeias were used in British colonies during this period; what arrangements were in place to regulate the supply and use of drugs in the colonies; how these differed between settler colonies and ones with large Indigenous populations; and how the British authorities in both the colonies and the metropole responded to these situations. One response was the emergence of colonial pharmacopoeias, which served rather different purposes than metropolitan ones.

MEDICINES IN THE BRITISH EMPIRE

England's first attempt to colonize North America was in 1606, when James I granted a charter to a London corporation giving it the ownership of Virginia, which then included all the unoccupied territory

The Emergence of Colonial Pharmacopoeias

between Spanish settlements in Florida and French settlements in Canada. The first English colonists arrived in 1607, when ships containing two hundred and twenty-five men landed at Cape Henry, the so-called First Landing. Seven were practitioners of medicine; one was a physician, three were surgeons, and two were apothecaries; the seventh was a barber.[1] They quickly established a more defensible colony at Jamestown in May 1607. One more apothecary arrived in 1607, followed by another in 1608.[2] But the colony failed due to financial problems and conflict with the Indigenous population. Another attempt was made in 1620 with the arrival of the Pilgrims on the *Mayflower* and establishment of Plymouth Colony. Medicines were among their essential supplies, and it is possible they had with them a copy of the 1618 *London Pharmacopoeia* (LP).[3] The first apothecary in New England, David Thomson (1592–ca 1628) arrived in Piscataqua (Maine) in 1623.[4] 'The Great Migration' between 1629 and 1640 – when more than ten thousand English men, women, and children arrived – resulted in a rapid increase in population.[5] The Massachusetts Bay Colony was founded in 1630.[6] The new migrants included several physicians and surgeons and two apothecaries.

The transatlantic medicine trade grew rapidly as the population of the British North America colonies continued to rise. In 1650–51 it was around 55,000; by 1700–01 it had increased to 265,000; and by 1750–51 it had reached 1,206,000. By 1770–71 it had almost doubled to 2,283,000.[7] Apothecaries in London maintained close links with those who migrated to the colonies. Edward Cooke, master of the Society of Apothecaries in London, wrote to John Winthrop, the governor of Connecticut, introducing a Mr Birde in 1640. Winthrop lodged with his uncle, the apothecary Thomas Fones, who had been master from 1624 to 1626. Winthrop became one of the first manufacturers of medicines in North America, where his expertise and prescriptions were greatly valued.[8] The physician John Pott – who became governor of Virginia in 1628 – was also a qualified apothecary with several apprentices. Anthony Hinton, who became the society's master in 1675, had been a subscriber to the Virginia Company and shared responsibility for the medical care of the colonists, sponsoring physicians, surgeons, and apothecaries.[9] For much of the seventeenth century the trade was largely between apothecaries in London and physicians and apothecaries in the colonies. In 1677 Dr Daniel De Hart – a physician in New York – contacted the London apothecary Moses Rusden requesting that a box of 'the best and fresh medicines' be shipped to New York. Rusden sent a supply of twenty-six medicines.[10]

Pharmacopoeias published in Britain were widely consulted in North America and the West Indies in the late seventeenth century.[11] In 1690 Samuel Lee commented that Massachusetts practitioners 'use the *London Dispensatory* at pleasure or any other, tyed [*sic*] to none.'[12] In 1675 the surgeon William Locke submitted a request for medicines to the colony's administration. With only a few exceptions they were all listed in the 1650 LP. He gave instructions that they were not to be compounded in the colonies but imported from England.[13] Importing drugs yielded gross profits in the order of 250 per cent.[14] In Boston an American reprint of Culpeper's translation of the LP was published in 1720.[15] By the 1750s both the LP and the *Edinburgh Pharmacopoeia* (EP) were readily available in North America and 'widely used by colonial practitioners.'[16] They were viewed as useful reference works rather than as official standards, and included many items used routinely in colonial medicine such as Daffy's and Stoughton's Elixirs. Printed catalogues were supplied by wholesale druggists in England and distributed to customers in America through agents.[17]

Medical practitioners and apothecaries in the American colonies learned to make use of local materials,[18] although most relied on ordering supplies from England. A large number of merchant houses were involved. Most were general merchants who aimed to supply the full list of the requirements of their customers, obtaining any medicines requested from London apothecaries.[19] Renate Wilson noted that in the eighteenth century the import trade in medicines was conducted largely by smaller suppliers and firms.[20] Spier noted that those involved in supplying pre-revolutionary Virginia included John Norton and sons, Edward and Samuel Athawes, and Capel and Osgood Hanbury.[21] Thomas Corbyn at Holborn had direct dealings with Virginia. The firm of Robert Cary and Co. had been established early in the eighteenth century and included Washington and Jefferson among its customers. Each year Washington sent Cary a long list of items required for himself and his family, his household, and his plantations, and these would arrive in Virginia up to nine months later.[22] In about 1765 Timothy and Sylvanus Bevan at Plough Court, London, began to develop an export trade.[23] It was from Bevan that in 1765 Dr Morgan – the founder of America's first school of medicine – bought an assortment of medicines, which he took back with him to Philadelphia.[24]

The *lp* and *ep* were of little help with regard to recently introduced 'exotic' drugs. Newly imported items were subjected to limited physical examination. Zachary Dorner notes that in eighteenth-century Britain 'the loose regulation of medicines largely stemmed from the conditions of trade, rather than from concerns about their composition or application, as in other places.'[25] Little action was taken in the colonies. David Cowen found that before 1775 only two laws related to pharmacy or drugs in North America: the Virginia Act of 1736, which was specifically designed to regulate the activities of the apothecary, and the South Carolina Act of 1751, which placed restrictions on the apothecary as an adjunct to the regulation of slaves.[26] Only the Virginia Act made specific reference to pharmacopoeias: 'If the medicine administered be a Simple or Compound directed in the Dispensatories, the true Name thereof shall be expressed in the same Bill, together with the Quantities and Prices, in both Cases.' Anyone failing to do so would be 'nonsuited' – that is, the evidence they presented would be considered inadmissible. It was the first legal recognition of pharmacopoeias in North America.[27] But the American drug trade ground to a halt with the outbreak of hostilities in 1775.[28] Cowen found no further legislation until a federal statute in 1848 set standards of purity and strength by reference to American and European publications following publication of the *United States Pharmacopeia* in 1820. There had been no attempt to compile such a work during the colonial period.[29]

SUPPLYING MEDICINES FOR THE EMPIRE

Whilst it was the development of tobacco and cotton plantations that drove expansion in Virginia, it was the insatiable appetite for sugar that drove English colonization in the West Indies. As labour-intensive activities, all created a seemingly endless demand for slave labour. A Royal African Company founded in 1660 granted City of London merchants a monopoly over English trade along the west coast of Africa with the aim of searching for gold. A new charter in 1663 enabled the company to enter the slave trade, and it subsequently took over a fort on the Gold Coast from the East India Company.[30] As the empire expanded and involvement in the slave trade increased, so, too, did the trade in medicines.[31] Institutions became involved alongside individuals. The Society of Apothecaries began manufacturing and supplying medicines after 1660, when the royal apothecary, George Solby, became responsible for 'fitting medicaments for surgeons' chests to be used by the King's forces on land and sea'.[32] It was the start of an extensive and profitable business for the society. The Royal College of Physicians (RCP) began supplying medicines in 1675.[33] By 1690 it was supplying the army, but in 1691 problems arose with drugs sent to Ireland and the apothecaries stepped in to fill the gap. In 1692 the Navy Office was advised to obtain all its medicines from Apothecaries' Hall.[34]

During the Nine Years' War (1688–97) the number of sick soldiers overwhelmed the army's medical service in Ireland, and disease likewise disrupted campaigns in the Caribbean; in 1693 fever spread through the fleet.[35] The Admiralty considered whether it could secure more economic and reliable supplies of medicines elsewhere. But by the mid-1690s the RCP's bid to monopolize the army and navy business had come unstuck because of its allegiance to its pharmacopoeia. The RCP's medicine was still based on Galenic principles; Dorner notes that 'physicians prescribed complicated individualized treatments according to patients' constitutions and circumstances, whereas officials wanted simpler remedies, ones that would act like "specifics" [having the same effect on anybody anywhere suffering the same affliction]'. The RCP's approach 'did not fulfil the Admiralty's desire to more efficiently treat the diseases sailors suffered in a range of locations'.[36] Empire-building was incompatible with Galenic medicine.

The college refused to change its approach and lost the contract. It was quickly taken up by others, including the Society of Apothecaries, who were happy to supply specifics. Involvement in the drug trade had presented the RCP with a dilemma; through its pharmacopoeia it was in a position to influence the range of drugs used along with their supply, availability, and cost. The loss of the navy contract was much more than a financial setback; it was an attack on the Galenic principles underpinning its medical philosophy as embodied in the LP, despite the fact that rational scientific methods were well established by the mid-seventeenth century.[37] The college was nevertheless anxious to retain what trade it could. In 1704 Sir Thomas Millington was both its president and physician to the governor general of Jamaica. He proposed that the college's dispensary supply the West Indian expedition with drugs. The Society of Apothecaries protested as its members were contracted to supply the fleet. The expedition was eventually cancelled, but the queen declared that in future 'the Society should serve the Fleet with medicines and drugs

The Emergence of Colonial Pharmacopoeias

according to the proposals submitted.[38] It would be less tied to Galenic medicine and the LP than the college had been.

PHARMACOPOEIAS IN SETTLER COLONIES

In settler colonies such as the Canadian provinces British physicians and apothecaries took with them the pharmacopoeias and other texts that they had used in metropolitan practice. Large numbers of both groups migrated from Scotland, and in many places Edinburgh publications played a greater part in colonial practice than London ones. Drug regulation mainly relied on individual professional responsibility, with some authority exercised by professional associations but with no statutory control. The Quebec Act of 1788 was one of the first to regulate the practice of pharmacy in what later became Ontario. This made it an offence to sell or distribute medicines by retail or on prescription, or practise physic or surgery without a licence from the governor.[39] An act in 1791 extended the conditions of licence to include examination and approval by a board of surgeons. An 1815 act strengthened licensing arrangements for practitioners of physic and surgery throughout Ontario. The regulation of pharmacy and the control of medicines lay firmly in the hands of the physicians until the middle of the nineteenth century.[40] The doctors made several attempts to strengthen their legal control over the activities of apothecaries but without success; the apothecaries were strong enough to prevent the doctors depriving them of the possibility of self-regulation.

In Australia the early colonists were outnumbered by convicts transported from England. In Van Diemen's Land (Tasmania) convicts constituted over 70 per cent of the population in 1820, dropping to below 40 per cent in the late 1830s.[41] In New South Wales it was 46 per cent in 1828, dropping to below 20 per cent only in the early 1840s. Their health – along with the supply and regulation of drugs – was in the hands of ships' surgeons and government medical officers. The early settlers included no apothecaries. The first person in Sydney to be granted a certificate to practise as an apothecary and to compound and dispense medicines was an unqualified ex-convict, John Tawell.[42] Almost all the drugs used were imported from England. The Society of Apothecaries held a contract to supply the Moreton Bay Penal Settlement in Queensland from 1823. A convict pharmacopoeia was drawn up under the authority of the military commandant. It was a list of the drugs 'required for the use of the sick at the Settlement'. Only seventeen preparations were deemed necessary, including two pills, four tinctures, and three ointments or balms.[43]

Medicine supply and control in the Australian colonies was firmly in the hands of the medical profession until the mid-nineteenth century. Haines notes that 'colonial administrations did not appoint chemists to their institutions simply because there was no place for them in the arcane medical establishment'.[44] In 1840s Sydney, at least six doctors kept 'dispensing shops' for consultations, and many others owned pharmacies where they employed druggists to undertake the dispensing.[45] Doctors and druggists usually had with them the *London*, *Edinburgh*, and/or *Dublin Pharmacopoeias*, depending on where they had been trained, but they were used for reference purposes rather than as guides to quality and standards. There is little evidence of inspections of premises, of prosecutions for supplying bad medicines, or of any action being taken other than against unlicensed individuals. The situation only changed with the formation of the Victoria Pharmacy Board in 1857 and the passage of the Sale and Use of Poisons Act in 1876, by which time the first edition of the *British Pharmacopoeia* (BP) had been published in 1864, and the British Pharmacy and Poisons Act of 1868 had been passed.[46]

The LP and EP also became essential reference sources for practitioners in Europe and elsewhere. Cowen suggests that the spread and influence of British pharmacopoeias – particularly the LPs of 1746 and 1788 and the EP of 1756 – were due to 'British leadership in pharmaceutical reform'. They 'reflected the new advances in learning with the purging of errors, the addition of new and powerful drugs, and the lucid presentation of chemical procedures'.[47] However, the LP itself followed the pattern of other European pharmacopoeias; Paula de Vos noted that Felix Palacio's 1706 *Palastra pharmaceutica* was 'often identified with the emergence of chemical medicine in the late seventeenth century' and was 'an amalgamation of traditional Galenic pharmacy and chemical pharmacy, part of the "chemico-Galenic compromise" typical of many pharmacopoeias of the period'.[48] But practitioners in British colonies were usually more concerned with obtaining supplies of good medicines than with complying with a metropolitan pharmacopoeia. Drugs needed to be obtained as cheaply as possible, and use made of whatever was locally available. Testing of medicines was neither feasible nor necessary as the equipment needed for local manufacture and testing would have to be imported

The Emergence of Colonial Pharmacopoeias

from Britain. One solution would be to include local medicines in a colonial pharmacopoeia. It was an approach pursued by officers of the Indian Medical Service.

SUPPLYING MEDICINES
FOR THE INDIAN SUBCONTINENT

By the early nineteenth century Britain had had a presence in India for over two hundred years. The charter granted to the East India Company (EIC) gave it a monopoly on English trade with all countries east of the Cape of Good Hope and west of the Straits of Magellan, and it quickly established trade in India and the Far East.[49] British involvement in India grew steadily, with the company later establishing an army – initially to defend its trading interests, but increasingly to support its territorial expansion. Following the 1757 Battle of Plassey its authority embraced Bengal and its influence grew rapidly. Victory in the 1764 Battle of Buxar saw the EIC consolidate its power, and it soon began collecting tax revenues across Bengal, Bihar, and Orissa. By 1773 the company ruled large areas of the lower Ganges plain and expanded its territories around Bombay and Madras. Further wars led to it controlling large areas in the North, with the north-western territories annexed in 1801 and Delhi in 1803. Assam followed in 1828 and Sindh in 1843.[50]

The extensive scholarly literature on the history of medicine in British India has addressed a wide range of issues, including relations between British and Indian medical practitioners, the use of traditional medicines, and the emergence of the Indian pharmaceutical industry.[51] Whilst the EIC's policy was initially to import medicines from Britain, the situation changed after the Seven Years' War (1756–63), as the costs of maintaining the army and its associated health care grew rapidly.[52] Enormous strain was placed on the company's ordering system. It became increasingly difficult to maintain adequate and timely supplies of quality medicines from Britain. Alternative arrangements were explored. The government promoted the use of local remedies because of the high cost of importing drugs.[53] Following a rise in medicine spending the surgeon at Fort St George, Madras, suggested that a laboratory be established as it would 'institutionalize a higher degree of standardization in the preparation of the medicines consumed by company employees stationed abroad'.[54] Whilst it would provide for the manufacture of medicines locally, it required the employment of an apothecary and equipment. In order to assure consistency, the EIC followed the *LP* where possible. In 1797 its board noted 'the improvements made of late years in the Pharmacopoeia,' and surgeons increasingly asked for 'the materials for medical preparations instead of the preparations themselves.'[55] Copies were widely available in India, although what use was made of them is less certain.[56] The 1809 *LP* was translated into Hindustani in 1824 and published in Calcutta.[57]

In 1767 the directors rejected the proposal for a laboratory and granted a monopoly to the Society of Apothecaries for the supply of medicines to the Indian settlements. Had it been successful it would have lessened the EIC's dependence on London merchants and ensured a uniform standard in the production of medicines for its overseas employees.[58] During the 1770s and 1780s indigenous medical practitioners and their remedies were employed in EIC hospitals, and interest in indigenous plants grew among British medical officers. Botanical gardens were established for the growing of useful plants, including medicinal ones. By 1790 gardens had been established at Calcutta, Madras, Bombay, Darjeeling, and St Helena.[59] Plants grown included camphor, benzoin, indigo, cotton, sugar, and dates. Local production lessened the EIC's dependence on imported medicines and on its rivals (the Dutch, Spanish, Portuguese, and French had all established colonies in the region).[60] It also generated profit; the Spanish monopoly in cochineal production was undermined by growing the nopal plant and introducing cochineal insects. Botanical networks played a vital role; the Royal Botanic Gardens at Kew and others provided advice about a wide range of issues, including which plant medicines might be substituted for items included in the pharmacopoeia.[61]

Spending on medicines imported from Britain continued to grow rapidly and supply issues became severe. The virtues of many indigenous plants were recognized by EIC medical officers, and there was considerable scope for substituting them for imported medicines. Dorner notes that 'British medicines ... retained only tenuous supremacy over more local supplies' as scarcity took its toll.[62] Despite the fact that medicines sent by the Society of Apothecaries were frequently damaged in transit as a result of 'careless and injudicious' packaging they continued to supply the EIC army of around three hundred thousand men throughout the 1820s.[63] But by 1800 enthusiasm for local medicines was waning. Over the following decades the

The Emergence of Colonial Pharmacopoeias

EIC's medical officers 'deepened reliance on European medicines whilst also supporting a search for local substitutes and manufacturing capacity in India.'[64] Dorner found that both imported and locally made British medicines 'displaced country medicines in many once-hybrid spaces, and the roles of Indian medical practitioners in Company hospitals were reduced as part of a wider rejection of indigenous methods of health and hygiene.'[65] British medicines were then well established in the EIC's settlements across South Asia as its medical officers struggled with high levels of sickness and mortality among its soldiers and civilian staff.

In 1813 (the year an imperial British pharmacopoeia was proposed at the RCP) Whitelaw Ainslie (1767–1837), an EIC surgeon, published his *Materia Indica of Hindoostan*.[66] It was a collection of remedies that 'opened up the study of Indian botanical therapeutics to the English-speaking world.'[67] Ainslie's publication was the first of many concerned with the indigenous remedies of India. His purpose was to encourage their use by both British and Indian medical practitioners. He argued that suitable substitutes for British medicines were available locally, and that they should be used wherever possible. His book was a catalogue 'of such medicines of the British materia medica as are either the produce of Hindoostan, or brought to it from Asiatic countries, and are to be met with in the Bazaars of popular towns.' It was an 'eclectic collection of botanical and mineral therapeutic products found in the local markets.' Ainslie advocated the inclusion of Indian medicines in British pharmacopoeias, although Bhattacharya suggests that 'with its textual and epistemological certitude' his work can be seen as 'the beginning of the textual marginalization of indigenous drugs.'[68] Few would make the transition to official status.

A PHARMACOPOEIA FOR BENGAL

With continuing territorial expansion and further increases in the size of the army, the costs of imported medicines continued to rise at a worrying rate. The EIC was compelled to take action; in 1837 its Medical Board appointed a committee of materia medica to examine and report on the state of its dispensary, looking at the range, source, and cost of medicines then in use. The committee was asked to explore the possibility of making greater use of indigenous remedies, and to prepare a pharmacopoeia.[69] It included the company's apothecary-general, his deputy, the principal of the medical college, the assay

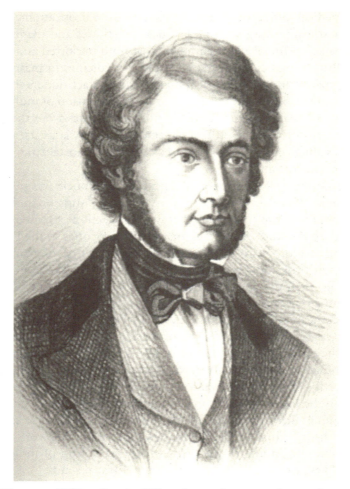

Figure 5.1 William Brooke O'Shaughnessy (1809–1889) around 1844.

master to the mint, the secretary to the Medical Board, and the professor of materia medica at Calcutta Medical College, William Brooke O'Shaughnessy (1809–1899) (figure 5.1). O'Shaughnessy was born in Ireland and joined the EIC in 1833, working as the opium agent's assistant before taking up his appointment at the medical school in 1835, where he began a programme of chemical and clinical experiments on drugs of Indian origin.[70]

It fell to O'Shaughnessy to assume the role of secretary. The committee reviewed the use of Western and Indigenous medicines in India,

The Emergence of Colonial Pharmacopoeias   119

along with the contents of the three British pharmacopoeias. Copies of the translation of the *LP* 1836 undertaken by the chemist Richard Phillips (1778–1851) were requested for use by the company's medical officers.[71] The committee reported in 1840, agreeing that none of the existing pharmacopoeias should be adopted for use in India. Instead they recommended that a pharmacopoeia for Bengal and North India be compiled, citing the unsuitability of many of the preparations in a hot climate, the unacceptability of certain items for some communities on religious grounds, and the expense involved in importing items from Britain; and that a careful examination of Indian medical remedies should be carried out.[72] O'Shaughnessy reported that 'the question of publication of the *Indian Pharmacopoeia* was also submitted to this Committee for their opinion.'[73] They considered such a pharmacopoeia to be both feasible and desirable as British expansion in India continued; Punjab, the North-West Frontier Province, and Kashmir were annexed after the Anglo-Sikh Wars of 1849–56.

Some months after publication of the report the EIC appointed a new committee to implement its recommendations. O'Shaughnessy was asked to relinquish much of his experimental research, which was progressing well, and devote himself to the task of compiling 'not only a Pharmacopoeia, but a Dispensatory of general materia medica.'[74] The first step was preparation of the dispensatory. O'Shaughnessy examined a large number of Indian drugs. Whilst some research was undertaken in London laboratories, the curtailing of the experiments in India meant that knowledge about some botanical drugs was limited. O'Shaughnessy based his dispensatory's content and layout on that of Edinburgh.[75] It began with an account of weights and measures, pharmaceutical operations, and the 'epitome of pharmaceutical chemistry', followed by brief accounts of botany and plant classification and the actions of several classes of drug. Last came a detailed account of the Indian materia medica 'chiefly compiled from the works of Roxburgh, Wallich, Ainslie, Wight and Arnold, Royle, Pereira, Lindley, Richard, and Fee, including the results of numerous special experiments'.[76] It was a guide for use by EIC officers and local practitioners. The *Bengal Dispensatory* was published in 1841, O'Shaughnessy noting that the committee had been appointed 'to examine and report upon ... the possibility of substituting indigenous remedies for some which are only procurable from other countries, at prices which place their use beyond the means of the mass of the community'.[77]

The dispensatory was 'published by order of government' in India. It was official but not statutory, as it had no force in law. It was judged to contain all the information needed for prescribing in the region. It was a pioneering work: David Cowen noted that 'in O'Shaughnessy's *Bengal Dispensatory* we have, perhaps, the first example of then modern modes of investigation brought to bear on the subject of indigenous drugs, the proximate chemical composition of a number of drugs investigated, and their physiological action determined.'[78]

With the dispensatory published, work could begin on the pharmacopoeia. Again, the work fell to O'Shaughnessy, and in 1844 the *Bengal Pharmacopoeia* was again 'published by order of government' in India.[79] It was a guide to the preparation of remedies used in medical practice in Bengal (figure 5.2). O'Shaughnessy was clear about its purpose; it was intended to achieve the formal recognition of indigenous medicines in national pharmacopoeias. 'The following pages are intended to supply a guide to the preparation of the remedies usually employed in medical practice in Bengal. The work embraces the few articles for which in this country we are still dependent on importation from Europe, and it includes a considerable number of remedies which, though long used by native practitioners, have not hitherto been formally recognised in pharmaceutical works of this description.'[80]

It was designed to provide 'a useful guide to the native medical student and practitioner, to the subordinate medical establishment of the Army Hospitals, and perhaps to the junior medical officers of the Bengal Presidency'. But its role was to be supplementary to British pharmacopoeias; it was to help them in an emergency 'to avail themselves of a good or tolerable substitute from the resources of the bazaar'.[81] As Jenner and Wallis point out, the EIC relied heavily on the bazaar, and its employees devoted much time and effort in 'appropriating substances from their indigenous contexts into the Western pharmacopoeia'.[82] Substances used in medicine were common items of trade, and many passed through bazaars on their way to European markets. Bhattacharya places the bazaar as the site of indigenous drug praxis, noting that praxis was 'key to explaining the emergence of the Indian Pharmacopoeia'.[83] The range of bazaar medicines was vast and included many drugs familiar to Europeans; some of those used in late eighteenth-century EIC medical establishments had been in use in Britain for years and were included in the LP.[84]

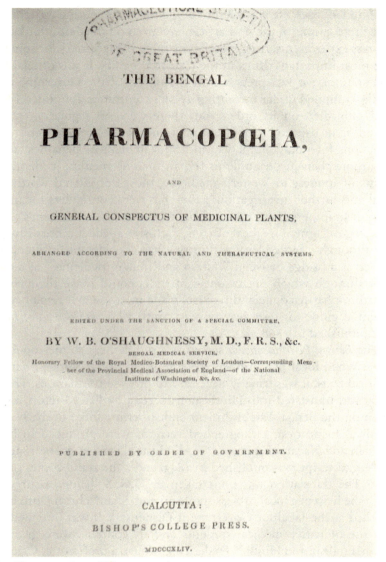

Figure 5.2 *Bengal Pharmacopoeia* 1844.

The *Bengal Pharmacopoeia* was laid out on the lines of the *EP* rather than the *LP*. O'Shaughnessy considered the *EP* to be 'the best pharmaceutical guide of all the European pharmacopoeias'.[85] But whilst methods for preparing tinctures, extracts, and mixtures were taken chiefly from the *EP*, a few were taken 'from that of the London or

Dublin Colleges'. He was keen to emphasize its scientific credentials: 'the preparations of the new articles are given on the data afforded by express experiments'. An appendix included bazaar prices for some of the most important drugs in the Calcutta market. It was official but not statutory; it was prepared on the orders of the Government of India, compiled under the authority of a committee appointed by it, and published on its orders. But there were no regulations commanding its use, no list of offences, no mechanism for inspection, no sanctions for non-compliance, and no statement of penalties. Yet it was more than just a guide to Indian materia medica; it identified items of interest to Western medicine, those considered worthy of trial and further investigation, items that were contenders for inclusion in an imperial pharmacopoeia. Inclusion enabled an item's ready use by government medical officers; exclusion made it more difficult. Yet although it lacked legal authority it had considerable influence; it served as a bridge between Western and Indian medicine – as a conduit through which practitioners in India could make their voices heard in pharmacopoeial discourse in the metropole. It remained an essential guide for over twenty years, until a *Pharmacopoeia of India* was published in 1868.

The *Bengal Pharmacopoeia* served as a supplement to metropolitan ones. When local practitioners were required to use British pharmaceutical texts, it was usually necessary to provide translations. The LP 1809 was translated into Hindustani in 1824 by Peter Breton, a surgeon on the Bengal Establishment and superintendent of the Native Medical Institution. Lithographed versions were produced in both Persian and Nagari characters.[86] A Hindustani version of the 1836 LP, in Nagari script, was published in 1843, and a thousand copies printed.[87] The translation was undertaken by G.G. Spilsbury, a surgeon, with the help of a local sub-assistant surgeon, Shamachrun Dutt; both worked at the Jabalpur Government Dispensary. It was intended for the use of native medical students and its contents were given in Latin, English, and Hindi.[88] Frederick J. Mouat, a professor at Calcutta Medical College, translated it into Persian and added an appendix giving the actions, uses, and doses of the LP 1836 preparations, publishing it in 1845.[89] Mouat explained that the majority of students came from the North-Western Provinces, and they had presented him with a petition 'requesting that a version might be prepared in a character intelligible to them'.[90] There was also a Bengali version of the LP in the form of Madhusudan Gupta's 1849 *Aushadh Kalpabali*.[91]

COLONIAL RESPONSES
TO PHARMACOPOEIAL DEVELOPMENTS

Elsewhere in the empire developments in Britain and India were followed with great interest. After 1807 three official pharmacopoeias were in use in the United Kingdom and across the empire. In an attempt to impose order an 1807 proclamation of the British governor in South Africa declared that the 1788 LP was to be used throughout the colony.[92] In Canada the activities of druggists and use of pharmacopoeias remained governed by the relevant clauses of the 1788 Quebec Act until at least 1860, but these were almost certainly not enforced.[93] All three pharmacopoeias were available in the colonies, but they were usually treated as guides rather than as standards to be complied with; all were produced by physicians, with minimal involvement by apothecaries or pharmacists; in the metropolitan context all were policed by colleges of physicians. Whether they were statutory or not made little difference in practice. Colleges were able to apply effective sanctions against erring apothecaries and keep them in line. Whilst at home drug regulation through professional bodies provided a degree of public protection against the worst excesses, the same was not true in the colonies.

With the 1844 publication of the *Bengal Pharmacopoeia* there were four official pharmacopoeias in use in the British Empire. The response of the metropolitan authorities changed in the early decades of the nineteenth century. Richard Powell's 1815 translation of the LP 1809 appeared after the RCP proposal for an imperial British pharmacopeia, of which he was a strong advocate. 'It is to be lamented,' he wrote, 'that a general Pharmacopoeia Britannica is not established, as one common dictionary, to which practitioners throughout the whole Empire may uniformly refer with confidence, and without the chance of mistake either in the name of an article or the mode of its preparation.'[94] He recognized the difficulties involved in producing such a volume, but noted that none 'would be insurmountable to men of sense and science, and I am persuaded that some future age will see the advantage and even necessity of the attempt.'[95] It was a statement of considerable prescience.

Revised editions of the three metropolitan pharmacopoeias continued to be compiled over the following decades. Despite rapid growth in chemical and pharmacological knowledge, the RCP exhibited extreme conservatism. Its 1824 LP had 'so few changes from the last that it was scarcely more than a reprint.[96] It closely resembled those of 1809 and 1815.[97] The 1815 'amended' *LP* had included a few tests for determining the purity of medicines, some simple chemical tests for acids, and specific gravities for several preparations.[98] Accurate chemical balances became available in 1823, although their cost meant that initially they were only used in laboratories.[99] These additions marked the start of the role of pharmacopoeias as tools for assessing the purity of medicines and detecting adulterants. Testing for adulteration highlighted the scale of the problem. Frederick Accum (1769–1838), a German pharmacist who worked in a London pharmacy, claimed in 1820 that 'nine tenths of the most potent drugs and chemical preparations used in pharmacy are vended in a sophisticated [i.e., adulterated] state.'[100] He particularly noted the iniquities of the drug-grinders and criticized the lack of pharmacopoeial standards, suggesting a number of simple purity tests.[101] Thereafter purity testing became a central feature of pharmacopoeias.

The London, Edinburgh, and Dublin physicians were fiercely protective of the distinctive nature of their pharmacopoeias. Before 1824 little effort was made to unify them; the practical difficulties of such an effort were great, but the political ones were greater. Pharmacopoeias were expressions of national identity and conveyed an equality of status between the three RCPS. The first move was made in London; following publication of the 1824 *LP* the RCP considered taking account of the needs of the other colleges. Furthermore, 'the rapid progress of the science of chemistry, and the recent introduction of various substances and preparations into medicinal use,' meant that it was already in need of revision. During RCP meetings in 1830 'ambitions were entertained that this might be the time for an Imperial Pharmacopoeia.'[102] They agreed to approach the other colleges. The Edinburgh physicians readily agreed. The Dublin college was then asked 'whether they would join with the London and Edinburgh Colleges in the formation of a general pharmacopoeia for the United Kingdom.' The Dublin fellows were equally divided but replied that 'though they wished to cooperate in any undertaking for the general convenience of the profession' they regretted that arrangements made regarding the last *Dublin Pharmacopoeia* prevented them from accepting the invitation.[103] The main obstacle was the large stock of unsold copies of the *DP* 1826 that would have to be written off.[104] An 1828 translation had been much more successful.

The Emergence of Colonial Pharmacopoeias

Despite the best efforts of the RCP even the more modest plan of a 'British' pharmacopoeia fell through.[105] Phillips reported that the London RCP had consulted with the fellows of both colleges, but 'on account of the great distances ... the task was found to be too difficult' and negotiations had to be abandoned.[106] Although 'Edinburgh was willing' no attempt was made to merge the LP with the EP. Relations between the Edinburgh and London physicians were strained. Macrae notes that the RCP 'remained determinedly elitist, whilst the Royal College of Edinburgh was more pragmatic in its commitment towards public service'.[107] For the Edinburgh physicians the problem was 'the exclusive spirit in which the London College of Physicians and the London Society of Apothecaries guarded the monopolies conferred upon them by their existing Charters'[108] Pharmacopoeial unity was delayed for over thirty years; in the 1840s the main focus of all three RCPs was medical reform.[109]

Following the failure to agree to work together the three colleges continued revising their own pharmacopoeias. London published the next LP in 1836. Special arrangements were made for practical experiments, and 'considerable help in chemistry was given by a Fellow of the Royal Society, Richard Phillips, who also wrote the English translation'. The chemical symbolism of Berzelius and Brande was added 'in compliance with the practice of some of the most eminent chemists'.[110] Phillips added identity tests for chemical medicines such as morphine, but his purity tests applied mainly to inorganic chemicals. Physical constants including freezing and boiling points were added. Other tests detected the presence of adulterants in animal charcoal, whilst honey was tested for the presence of starch.[111] But some of the 'defects' in the LP 1809 still appeared. Clark noted that 'the number of innovations was large, though not sufficient to satisfy everyone'.[112] The 1836 LP continued the shift from methods of preparation to methods of testing. The college no longer insisted that medicines be prepared exactly in the mode described in the LP, provided they met the tests for purity.[113] This direction had been the case since the first edition in 1618.

The 1836 LP illustrated the accelerating shift from natural to chemical remedies, from organoleptic to chemical testing, and from medical opinion to scientific evidence. But medicines of plant origin were still valued and new ones such as buchu added, as were natural product–based preparations such as compound rhubarb pills.[114] Experimental evidence became the main criteria for inclusion in the LP. Creosote and morphine both entered the *LP* in 1836. Creosote had been described in 1832 and found to have useful medicinal properties, particularly as a decongestant.[115] Morphine had been isolated from opium in 1805, and discussion took place on whether morphine should replace opium in the pharmacopoeia. Trials showed that there were distinct differences in their actions. In 1821 Magendie asserted that 'the variable effects of opium are due to the opposite principles of which it is composed.'[116] Orfila later concluded that opium extracts were more potent than the amount of morphine in them suggested; opium preparations were absorbed more slowly than pure alkaloids, so the effects took longer to appear. There had been previous proposals to include morphine in the *LP*, but it was only in 1836 that physicians felt they had sufficient evidence to do so.[117]

A LAST EDITION
OF THE *LONDON PHARMACOPOEIA*

In 1840 the RCP agreed that a new edition of the *LP* should be prepared. Work began in 1841, and it became the largest item of the college's business outside of medical reform, being completed only in 1850.[118] The tenth and final edition was published in 1851, still in Latin, despite the *DP* and *EP* both being in English. It was again prepared by Richard Phillips, who also produced an authorized translation. There were relatively few changes from the 1836 edition, although apothecaries' weights were replaced by avoirdupois, bringing it into line with the *DP*.[119] New remedies – including salts of morphine, atropine, and tannic acid – were added along with the first anaesthetic agents, chloroform and ether.[120] So, too, was cod liver oil, which had been used medicinally for many years.[121] Suggestions came from India and elsewhere for items to be included, but the RCP was less ready to accept new medicines of plant origin; despite the trials undertaken in India none of those listed in the *Bengal Pharmacopoeia* were included in the *LP* 1851. The RCP expected strong evidence that new medicines were as effective as items already included: it was rarely forthcoming. Yet they were also aware of the impact their inclusion might have on British trade with the colonies; metropolitan and colonial pharmacopoeias served different purposes.

Critics of the *LP* 1851 were quick to express the need for a single standard for medicines across the United Kingdom. Peter Squire

The Emergence of Colonial Pharmacopoeias   127

(1798–1884) had long called for standardization in the strength and composition of medicines ordered under the same names, and noted that with this revision the discrepancies had increased rather than diminished.[122] Theophilus Redwood (1806–1892), professor of pharmacy at the school run by the Pharmaceutical Society of Great Britain (PSGB), pointed out that changes to the system of weights and measures were unauthorized and that their use would be illegal.[123] Jonathan Pereira (1804–1853), professor of materia medica at the same institution, found a very large number of errors.[124] The *Pharmaceutical Journal* noted that pharmacists had no choice in its use. 'The medical practitioner, as is duty bound, procures a copy … With him it is optional whether he owes allegiance to the new Code or not … The chemist, according to law, has no choice. He must obey the pharmacopoeia.'[125] But it offered faint praise for the RCP's consultations with pharmacists: 'there is much less evidence of a disposition to puzzle and confuse the dispenser that there was in the [LP 1836] … it is obvious that the discussions that have taken place between medical men and chemists since the establishment of the Pharmaceutical Society have been attended with advantage.'[126]

Dublin published a third edition of the DP in 1850 and reprinted it in 1856. Edinburgh published a last edition of the EP in 1841. None of these made any concessions to the colonies. Yet the London RCP was fully engaged with empire; in the late eighteenth century it advised on medical appointments in North America and Jamaica.[127] Government departments invited its comments on drafts of Medical Acts for Jamaica, Tasmania, and Trinidad. They received reports about plague on warships in the Mediterranean in 1841, statistical reports from British Guiana in 1843, and inquiries about fever in Bermuda in 1844.[128] At the same time pharmacy leaders advocated greater involvement in the study of medicines arriving from the colonies.[129] Pereira proposed that the PSGB Council appoint 'a scientific committee for the promotion of pharmacological knowledge.' Its purpose would be the scientific investigation of materia medica: 'No country in the world possesses so many facilities for carrying on inquiries such as those to which I here allude as Great Britain. Her numerous and important colonies in all parts of the world, and her extensive commercial relations, particularly fit her for taking the lead in investigations of this kind … From her extensive possessions in different parts of the world, we draw a very large portion of the substances now used in medicine.'[130]

The PSGB Council agreed and immediately appointed a committee. Yet the extent to which the 'very large portion' was reflected in the pharmacopoeias was diminishing rather than increasing, as ever more chemical medicines were added. By establishing the committee, Pereira declared 'an opportunity would be obtained of bringing into notice the various medicinal substances produced in the different portions of this great empire'.[131] The *Bengal Pharmacopoeia* served the same purpose. Pereira supported a plea by Thomas Thomson for greater emphasis on medical botany and the study of indigenous drugs and advocated the substitution of exported medicines with colonial ones. 'Substances now unknown to, or little employed by us, might be brought into use, and in some instances ... the produce of our own colonies might be advantageously substituted for that of other countries'. The PSGB later inaugurated a British Pharmaceutical Conference, which became a key network for the exchange of information about plant medicines across the empire.[132]

CONCLUSION

The 1850s witnessed the ending of one era in British pharmacopoeial history and the beginning of another. Phillips died in 1851, Pereira in 1853, and John Ayrton Paris (1785–1856) – president of the RCP and a driving force behind the *LP* – died in 1856. In Britain medical reform culminated in the Medical Act of 1858, which mandated a newly created General Medical Council. This body would be legally required to 'cause to be published under their direction' the *British Pharmacopoeia*, which would henceforth supersede the *LP*, *EP*, and *DP*.

Elsewhere the world was undergoing rapid change. In India power transferred from the EIC to the British Crown after the 1857 'Rebellion'. Thereafter British India was ruled by a Government of India on the subcontinent appointed by a secretary of state for India in London. The proposal to prepare an imperial British pharmacopoeia was revived, receiving unexpected support from the United States. In 1855, Franklin Bache, professor of chemistry at Philadelphia, declared that the *United States Pharmacopoeia*, first published in 1820, 'could not be expected entirely to supersede the British Pharmacopoeias ... [and] include the whole of the materia medica and preparations of the British standards'. There would be many advantages for both English and American pharmacy by adopting a single pharmacopoeia for

The Emergence of Colonial Pharmacopoeias 129

the British Empire.[133] It was to herald subsequent American cooperation and influence in shaping the BP.

Over the course of the next twenty years the three British pharmacopoeias were unified, colonies and Dominions responded in different ways, colonial pharmacopoeias were suppressed by the metropolitan authorities, and a backlash from the colonies led ultimately to the 'imperialization' of the pharmacopoeia. I explore these themes in the next chapter.

6

One Empire, One Pharmacopoeia

For Great Britain the mid-nineteenth century was a period of rapidly expanding empire, developing colonies, increasing trade, medical reform, the professionalization of pharmacy, and emerging drug regulation, both at home and abroad. By the 1850s the long-running discussions about medical reform were coming to a conclusion.[1] Medical reform was the trigger for pharmacy reform and professionalization in Britain. In his history of the Pharmaceutical Society of Great Britain (PSGB) Holloway notes that 'of crucial importance in the initiation of the medical reform movement was the attempt to eliminate the competition of the chemist and druggist and to create a monopoly for the licensed practitioner.' Reform was also intended to 'increase the corporate power of the medical profession within society.'[2] Those powers were enshrined in legislation in the 1858 Medical Act.

When the PSGB was established in 1841 its founders saw pharmacists as a fourth force in the medical profession alongside physicians, surgeons, and general medical practitioners. Prior to passage of the 1852 Pharmacy Act – which provided pharmacy with its statutory foundation – the Select Committee of the House of Commons obtained evidence on laws relating to pharmacy in France, Germany, Sweden, and Mauritius. It found that those countries had a strict legal separation of medicine and pharmacy. Jacob Bell noted that 'physicians do not sell medicines and chemists do not prescribe ... In France the laws are so stringent that no person is permitted to give medical advice in the most trivial cases without possessing a qualification.' In Norway, Sweden, Denmark, Finland, Russia, and Germany 'not only are unqualified persons prohibited from practising in any department of the profession, but the number of regular practitioners is limited by law.'[3]

One Empire, One Pharmacopoeia

Whilst the 1852 act effectively sealed the separation of pharmacy from medicine in Britain,[4] the same was not true of the empire. In India and elsewhere doctors retained control of pharmacy and drug regulation. Bhattacharya notes that 'unlike in Western Europe and the United States, where pharmacists were professionalized in the nineteenth century and standardized their respective pharmacopoeias, there was no such process evident in colonial India.'[5] Although official the *Bengal Pharmacopoeia* had no statutory authority, and drug regulation barely existed in many parts of the empire.[6] But even in Britain there was no legal control over any substance, no matter how lethal. No substance was restricted to supply only on prescription; there was no need to declare the intended use of a poison, no need to keep records, and no penalties for inappropriate supply. The first attempt to regulate dangerous substances through legislation was the Arsenic Act of 1851, which placed restrictions on its retail sale.[7]

PHARMACOPOEIAS AND MEDICAL REFORM

The futures of the three metropolitan pharmacopoeias were closely tied to medical reform and to future relations between medical bodies operating in the United Kingdom. The 1858 Medical Act placed control of the practice of medicine in the hands of a new body, the General Council of Medical Education and Registration of the United Kingdom (the General Medical Council, or GMC). It also gave the GMC the task of producing a new publication to be known as the *British Pharmacopoeia* (BP), as well as a legal obligation to appoint a Pharmacopoeia Committee and to publish the pharmacopoeia.

When the GMC came into being on 1 October 1858 the balance of power in medicine shifted, with the dominance of the London Royal College of Physicians (RCP) 'decidedly reduced when its [sole] representative had to take his seat among the rest.'[8] The GMC had separate Branch Councils for England, Scotland, and Ireland. Although it was the first professional body to include members appointed by the state to oversee its day-to-day business, it was not an instrument for carrying out the will of the state. Official nominees were in the minority; the council consisted of nine representatives nominated by medical bodies (including the RCPS), eight nominated by universities, and six nominated by the Crown on the advice of the Privy

Council. The first two GMC presidents were surgeons. The Privy Council nominees included Robert Christison (1797–1882), an Edinburgh physician who had published a detailed commentary on the pharmacopoeias in 1848.[9]

Although the act gave the GMC the task of producing a single BP it did not give it the authority to supersede the existing ones. The GMC asked Parliament to grant the necessary powers. A second Medical Act in 1862 directed that the BP replace the three previous ones, but it made no reference to empire. It stated that 'the BP, when published, shall for all purposes be deemed to be substituted *throughout Great Britain and Ireland* for the several above-mentioned pharmacopoeias.'[10] One of the GMC's first acts was to establish a Pharmacopoeia Committee from among its members, all of whom were doctors. Alfred Garrod was appointed its secretary.[11] Whilst drawing on the experience of the London, Edinburgh, and Dublin RCPs in preparing pharmacopoeias, the committee consulted widely, including a broad range of both medical and pharmaceutical bodies, clearly recognizing the need for support from those with pharmaceutical expertise. In revising the *London Pharmacopoeia* (LP), the London RCP had previously requested the assistance of the PSGB, which had established its own Pharmacopoeia Committee.[12] In listing contributions made by pharmacists Jacob Bell concluded that 'these and other contributions served to show that there was not only the disposition but [also] the power to render valuable assistance in compiling the important work.'[13]

At its first meeting, held in November 1858, the GMC passed a resolution giving it 'power to communicate with the Pharmaceutical Society' for the purpose of requesting the latter's cooperation. Bell was delighted. He wrote, 'It could not have been otherwise than gratifying to the Pharmaceutical Society to find that it was thus placed in so prominent and honourable a position by the Medical Council in relation to the one subject on which it claimed to possess an amount of practical knowledge superior to that of medical men who were not engaged in pharmacy. It was the highest public recognition that could have been given by the most competent authority in the kingdom.'[14]

Peter Squire (1798–1884), who had been PSGB president in 1849–50 (and was again from 1861 to 1863),[15] assisted the committee with advice. Bell encouraged the society's members to submit items for inclusion in the new pharmacopoeia.[16] On 11 August 1858 the secretary of the Edinburgh RCP's Pharmaceutical Committee wrote to all

One Empire, One Pharmacopoeia 133

medical practitioners and chemists in Scotland asking for information about frequently used items not listed in the *Edinburgh Pharmacopoeia* (EP), any changes needed in EP processes, and any new processes that should be added.[17] Soon afterwards Scottish chemists received a request for the same information from the PSGB. It was eventually agreed that they should send their replies to the PSGB in London, which would forward their recommendations to both RCPS.[18]

Branch committees were established in London, Edinburgh, and Dublin. The London committee held 158 meetings, the Edinburgh one 108 meetings, and the Dublin one 141 meetings. Two conferences of delegates were held, one each in London and Edinburgh.[19] The PSGB was invited to appoint a member to serve on the London sub-committee.[20] The GMC also authorised its Pharmacopoeia Committee to appoint a chemist or chemists to carry out 'such chemical and pharmaceutical researches as may be found necessary' and to pay them 'such remuneration as the committee ... may think advisable.'[21] Many of those consulted had published the results of trials and experiments, both medical and pharmaceutical, and their views were frequently supplemented by chemical investigations carried out for the committee. Unlike earlier pharmacopoeias, the 1864 BP also 'drew on the experience of the newly established pharmaceutical associations, schools, and journals.'[22] Analysis and rationalization became the dominant 'way of knowing.'[23]

Reconciling the processes and descriptions of three pharmacopoeias was a formidable task.[24] At the start of their work representatives from England, Scotland, and Ireland agreed that 'an amalgamation of the whole into a *British Pharmacopoeia* was impossible without subjecting the prescribers and dispensers of medicine in all parts of the kingdom and colonies, to inconvenience for some time after the completion of the act of reform.'[25] Making it suitable for the whole empire necessitated first 'reconciling the varying usages in pharmacy and prescriptions of the people of three countries, hitherto in these respects separate and independent.'[26] Reconciling prescriptions and formulas was one challenge; agreeing which drugs and preparations should be added or deleted was another. The committee received proposals for new chemical medicines along with many suggestions from the colonies for the inclusion of drugs of plant origin. They had to consider which items included in the *Bengal Pharmacopoeia* should be incorporated into the BP. These were augmented by others listed in such publications as Edward John Waring's

(1819–1891) *Remarks on the Uses of Some of the Bazaar Medicines and Common Medical Plants of India*, published in 1859.[27]

The years between 1851 and 1864 – during which no new editions of metropolitan pharmacopoeias were published – saw great advances in medicine and science, chemistry, botany, physiology, and technology. Rapid progress was made in chemical analysis and testing methods, although in the late 1840s a new problem emerged as false and dubious tests were proposed.[28] Redwood examined various tests that had been proposed to detect adulterated balsam of copaiba, and concluded that the only satisfactory method for estimating its purity was 'to resolve it into its proximate constituents, and then to examine these separately with reference to their physical and chemical characteristics.'

The GMC's Pharmacopoeia Committee agreed to include more precise and quantitative tests in the BP.[29] Standardized weights and measures, and more precise and affordable balances, were essential if more accurate formulations were to be specified. The systematic application of microscopy enabled the accurate detection of adulteration in drugs, a cause pioneered by English physician Arthur Hill Hassall (1817–1894).[30] In his 1857 *Adulterations Detected* he made scant use of melting point or other constants, instead stressing microscopical observation. Microscopy made it possible to detect adulteration in many organic substances – such as medicinal plants – for which chemical tests were unavailable. John Abraham suggests that the microscope 'probably carried greater significance for the fight against adulteration than any other single instrument.'[31] Thomas Wakley, editor of *The Lancet*, invited Hassall to publish the reports of the microscopic examination of drugs in his journal between 1851 and 1854.[32] Hassall also advocated other methods, including distillation to determine the purity of cinnamon and clove oils, and the use of incineration to detect the presence of chalk in scammony and ipecacuanha.[33]

In Britain the campaign for government control of adulteration in food and drugs was taken up by several people, among them John Postgate.[34] A House of Commons parliamentary committee considered the adulteration of foods, drinks, and drugs in 1855–56. It heard a great deal of evidence, including that whilst plant medicines such as opium and scammony were widely adulterated, so, too, were chemical medicines such as chloroform.[35] Many called for legislation to tackle the problem. But the committee was reluctant to recommend action against the prevailing ideologies of laissez-faire and free trade. It opted instead to define the boundaries of 'honest competition'. 'The great difficulty of legislation on this subject', the committee declared, 'lies in putting an end to the liberty of fraud without affecting the freedom of commerce'.[36] It recommended that local authorities be empowered to appoint inspectors to examine any food or drug item for possible adulteration. It was enacted for foods in the Adulteration Act of 1860. Eight years later the 1868 Pharmacy Act extended the scope of this act to medicines.[37]

A 'BRITISH' PHARMACOPOEIA

The first edition of the BP was published in 1864 in English. It consisted of two parts, along with several appendices and an index. The first listed materia medica; the second, preparations and compounds. It included many medicinal plants listed in the earlier publications. Some new items commonly used in India did appear, but these were exceptions; for the first time there was an official monograph for *Cannabis Indica*.[38] But if the main parts reflected continuity with the past, the appendices indicated the future. Limited chemical tests for impurities and adulterants were included in the monographs. An appendix listed 'articles employed in the preparation of medicines', each of which had its own purity tests, whilst another listed 'articles employed in chemical analysis', along with the tests to which they related. These changes led to a greater focus on testing for drug adulteration.

The BP represented a seminal shift in the nature and purpose of pharmacopoeias in the United Kingdom. Whilst the *London, Edinburgh*, and *Dublin Pharmacopoeias* had been little more than lists of approved drugs and the preparations to be made from them, the BP was a book of standardized medicines and the tests used to assess their purity. When it came out, it was not popular with the medical profession in Britain. It no longer contained many of the preparations that doctors were used to prescribing and was found to be full of errors. The London RCP had not been able to control the book's compilation or content, and it raised objections to proposed changes to the system of weights and measures. Sir Thomas Watson, the RCP's president at the time, denounced the book as 'dangerous and not [to] be used'.[39] Shortly after it was published Squire issued his own supplement and commentary entitled *A Companion to the British Phar-*

macopoeia. It was to run to many editions, later edited by his son, before finally being amalgamated with Martindale's *Extra Pharmacopoeia*, first published in 1883.

Following its poor reception, work began immediately on a second edition, which was published in 1867. The work was carried out by a committee of five GMC members with Christison as chair and Richard Quain (1816–1898) – an Irish physician trained in London – as secretary.[40] This time they made use of the 1858 resolution and engaged the services of Robert Warington (1807–1867) – chemical operator at the Society of Apothecaries – and Theophilus Redwood (1806–1892) – professor of pharmacy at the PSGB's pharmacy school – as editors.[41] They followed a plan drawn up by Redwood.[42] The GMC fully acknowledged their contribution.[43] The errors and omissions that had prompted rapid revision of the 1864 edition were reviewed and changes made. The council reported that 'the important work of amalgamation having been effected, and national differences reconciled – in some cases at the cost of mutual concession – it has been thought desirable ... to submit the work to a general revision'.[44] In this edition 'some medicines not included in the former one have been introduced, some names ... have been changed, some processes have been altered, and descriptions have been modified'.[45] New laboratory equipment such as steam baths were mentioned in the 1867 BP for the first time.

The stated scope and purpose of the BP shifted again. The 1864 edition had emphasized its role as a 'national' pharmacopoeia, standardizing the range of drugs and preparations used in England, Scotland, and Ireland. Three years later the second edition had acquired imperial ambitions. The committee declared that it 'was intended to afford to the members of the medical profession and those engaged in the preparation of medicines *throughout the British Empire* one uniform standard and guide, whereby the nature and composition of substances to be used in medicine may be ascertained and determined. The Council have endeavoured to include in it all such remedies as the existing state of medical practice seemed to require'.[46] It was now a statement of standards; its foundation would be evidence-based practice; it would be comprehensive and include all items needed across the empire; and metropolitan doctors would determine what the empire needed. The second edition was rather more successful than the first and met with general approval in Britain.[47]

RECEPTION IN THE COLONIES

The *BP* 1867 received a mixed reception in the colonies. In the settler colonies of Canada, South Africa, Australia, and New Zealand pharmacy was undergoing professionalization, a process based largely on the British model.[48] Practitioners came together to form pharmaceutical societies, agreed arrangements for education and training, founded journals, and arranged conferences. They sought a legal foundation by seeking legislation in local parliaments, and many secured acts of Parliament, thereby establishing a system of drug regulation based on the British 1868 Pharmacy and Poisons Act. Colonies in Canada and elsewhere came together to form federations with their own parliaments passing their own laws. These were later given Dominion status by Britain and recognized as self-governing states. In Canada the physicians had made renewed efforts to control the pharmacists in the 1850s and '60s, but without success; the situation changed after Canadian Confederation in 1867. Pharmacists founded professional organizations to protect themselves from control by the doctors, and a new journal, the *Canadian Pharmaceutical Journal*, appeared in 1868. Legislation based on the British act followed; Pharmacy Acts were passed in Ontario (1871), Quebec (1875), and Nova Scotia (1876). Other Canadian provinces followed soon after.[49]

Attempts to regulate the pharmacy profession and to control the supply and use of drugs and poisons in other colonies usually only came after publication of both the 1867 *BP* and passage of the 1868 Pharmacy and Poisons Act in Britain. One by one colonies passed ordinances largely based on the 1868 act, although sometimes after several years' delay. Barbados passed a Pharmacy Ordinance in 1880, and Jamaica approved a Sale of Drugs and Poisons Ordinance in 1881.[50] In New Zealand a Sale of Food and Drugs Act was passed in 1887. In the Gold Coast a Drug and Poisons Ordinance was approved in 1892, but in Nigeria the Pharmacy and Poisons Ordinance was passed only in 1902. Circumstances were different in each colony; none more so than in India.

A PHARMACOPOEIA FOR INDIA

The start of the British Raj in 1858 represented a major turning point for the recognition of Indian medicinal plants by the British authorities.[51] The *Bengal Pharmacopoeia* was one of many texts that had been published on the materia medica of India since Whitelaw Ainslie's 1813 *Materia Indica of Hindoostan*. Others included two works by J.F. Royle published in 1847.[52] Royle had been commissioned by the Bengal medical board to compile a list of drugs available in bazaars that could be substituted for more expensive imported items; it contained over a thousand items. Later publications included Waring's *Remarks* (1859), Kanny Lall Dey's *Indigenous Drugs of India* (1867), and Dymock's *Vegetable Materia Medica* (1884).[53] By 1858 the *Bengal Pharmacopoeia* had been in use for fourteen years, but as it had no legal authority it provided no help in assuring the quality of the items listed. After 1857 European-style pharmacies sprang up, bringing with them a substantial expansion in the drug trade.[54] British pharmacists referenced the 1867 BP as a mark of quality for the drugs and formulations they supplied; for them BP endorsement was a useful selling point. But the 1868 Pharmacy and Poisons Act had no jurisdiction in India and, in the absence of enforcement and heavy penalties for noncompliance, adulteration and counterfeiting flourished.

Waring intended his 1859 *Remarks* to be widely used in remote areas of India. The last editions of the *London, Edinburgh*, and *Dublin Pharmacopoeias* made no reference to the *Bengal Pharmacopoeia*, which continued to be widely used in India. After the latter's publication in 1844 there was a lull in work on pharmacopoeias in India for two decades, largely as a result of the fluid political situation.[55] When the new BP arrived in 1864 the Bengal one remained in use, and pressure grew to revise it to make it suitable for the whole of India. But the BP was no better received in India and the colonies than it was in Britain. Although it contained a number of plant drugs, some of Indian origin, it did not include others commonly used in India. Their omission added to calls for a separate pharmacopoeia for India. The suggestion was made by Waring, then an assistant surgeon in the Indian Army.[56]

In 1864 Waring wrote to the undersecretary of state for India in London. He referred to the BP and to 'advances in the knowledge of medicinal resources of India since publication of the *Bengal Pharmacopoeia* in 1844'.[57] It was an ambitious proposal: 'With the view, firstly, of bringing in an official and succinct form to the notice of the Indian practitioner, those indigenous drugs which European experience has proved to be valuable in practice; and secondly, of assimilating the formulae of the old *Bengal Pharmacopoeia* with the standard now established by the Medical Council, I am induced to propose the publication of a work entitled the *Pharmacopoeia of India*, to be issued officially for use in all parts of our Indian possessions.'[58] Waring proposed that a committee be constituted for the purpose, and suggested that most of the work could be done in London. The main benefit of such a project would be to save the government money. 'That considerable pecuniary savings would eventually be effected by the publication of this work cannot, I think, be doubted; for if the Medical Officers in India were provided with an official guide to the more valuable indigenous drugs, they would receive a fair trial, and in time would supersede in many instances the more expensive European articles of the same class.'[59]

Waring's proposal received high-level support. Dr Shaw, principal inspector general of the Medical Department at Madras, felt that 'a work such as the proposed *Pharmacopoeia of India* would be of the greatest value to medical men in India.' Sir James Ranald Martin, the inspector general of hospitals, considered that 'India with its enormous medicinal resources should have its pharmacopoeias made up to the knowledge of the day.' But it also had its critics. J.R. Haines, professor of materia medica at Grant Medical College in Bombay, considered such an undertaking 'unnecessary in the light of the new BP'.[60]

The Government of India considered the various arguments for and against an Indian pharmacopoeia and eventually agreed to Waring's proposal.[61] Orders to commence work on the new pharmacopoeia were given in a letter from the India Office to Martin in 1865; it was formally commissioned by the secretary of state for India.[62] It was estimated that preparation of the work would 'not occupy a longer period than 18 months' and it was proposed that 'the first edition should consist of 2,000 copies.' Waring moved to London and began work, acting as its editor. The therapeutic claims of native vegetable remedies were carefully scrutinized by a committee chaired by Martin and including Sir William O'Shaughnessy Brooke, Thomas Thomson, Daniel Hanbury, and three other physicians. Its first meeting was held in March 1865 at the India Board Office in London.

Progress on the *Pharmacopoeia of India* (PI) was followed closely in India. In its very first issue in 1866 the *Indian Medical Gazette* reported that draft lists of Indian medicinal plants had been circulated 'amongst those from whom it is probable that information may be obtained … With a view to give the subject still wider publicity, and to invite general cooperation, they are now published in these columns.'[63] The *Gazette* considered it of great financial and commercial importance: '£20,000 are annually expended in the

140 Pharmacopoeias, Drug Regulation, and Empires

importation of European drugs to India, whilst the country contains effective substitutes, valuable even as simple native preparations, but which, properly prepared, might be obtained at little more than half the cost of European importation, and yield a considerable profit to speculators.[64]

The draft list divided medicinal plants into two groups. The first had four categories: those official in the *BP*; those official in the *Bengal Pharmacopoeia*; those 'not hitherto official in either of the pharmacopoeias, but which were proposed for introduction into the *Pharmacopoeia of India*'; and a fourth category listing articles 'about which there were doubts.' The second group included items 'the properties of which appeared deserving of further investigation.'[65] The committee examined all available works in English on Indian materia medica and received reports from medical officers and others across India. Preparation of the *PI* established the principle of consultation with practitioners in both the metropole and the colonies.

The model of drug regulation operating in India during the time of the East India Company (EIC) and in the early years of the Raj was that of consumer sovereignty. Yet the EIC's directors were clearly concerned about the quality and regulation of drugs used in India. Dorner notes that in 1766 'the apothecaries' laboratory offered the appearance of regulation and quality they had desired in the previous year's laboratory plan.'[66] Holloway made a distinction between 'the nationwide, individualistic, free-market model of the classical economists, and the local, popularist, communal model of the democratic radicals.'[67] The only controls over the quality of drugs was the judgements of EIC officials, officers of the Indian Medical Service, and individual consumers. The EIC relied heavily on the reputation of the Society of Apothecaries for quality and reliability, but any checks were limited to appearance, smell, and taste. Bad medicines could be rejected, and contracts cancelled, but there was little recourse to legal action in India.

SUBSTITUTION FOR THE BP IN INDIA

The *PI* was published in 1868 by the India Office, a year after the *BP*'s second edition (figure 6.1). It had been 'prepared under the authority of her Majesty's Secretary of State for India in Council' by Edward John Waring, who was 'assisted by a committee appointed for the purpose.'[68] It was an official committee, but the Government of India did

PHARMACOPŒIA OF INDIA,

PREPARED UNDER THE AUTHORITY OF

HER MAJESTY'S SECRETARY OF STATE FOR INDIA IN COUNCIL.

BY

EDWARD JOHN WARING, M.D.,

MEMBER OF THE ROYAL COLLEGE OF PHYSICIANS OF LONDON,
SURGEON IN HER MAJESTY'S INDIAN ARMY,

ASSISTED BY A COMMITTEE APPOINTED FOR THE PURPOSE.

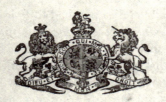

INDIA OFFICE:
1868.

LONDON:
W. H. ALLEN & CO., 13, WATERLOO PLACE,
PUBLISHERS TO THE INDIA OFFICE.

Figure 6.1 *Pharmacopoeia of India* 1868.

not give the pharmacopoeia statutory authority; there was no mandatory inspection of drugs, no list of offences, and no penalties specified for non-compliance. The *PI* was based on the *BP*, and 'while affording all the information contained in that work of practical use in India, would embody and combine with it such supplementary matter of special value in that country as should adapt it to meet the requirements of the Indian Medical Department.' It was to serve several purposes: 'In endeavouring to impart an educational character to the *Indian Pharmacopoeia*, the Committee ... have taken the surest mode of carrying into effect one of the primary objects of the work, namely, the introduction of the indigenous products of India into European practice in that country.'[69] It was effectively an official Indian supplement merged into the 1867 *BP*, although neither the *IP* nor the *BP* had statutory authority in India. Neither were enforceable, and the former did not have the endorsement of the GMC. Its educational and promotional aims were the same as those of other publications, including Waring's *Remarks* and Kanny Lall Dey's *Indigenous Drugs*.

This raises an important question: Why would the Government of India agree to an official pharmacopoeia for India that did not have statutory authority? It was undoubtedly a reflection of the influence held by senior medical officers and trade interests in India in promoting the use of indigenous products in Britain as well as India with the aim of having many added to the next edition of the *BP*. Previous texts on Indian materia medica had had little impact on the content of the *BP*; an official *Pharmacopoeia of India* compiled by a government committee and published in London might have more effect. Kanny Lall Dey considered that it 'signalized a new epoch in the establishing of the value of indigenous medicinal products. The more important were stamped with some measure of official recognition, a preliminary step to the ultimate adoption of several in the *BP*.'[70] But making it statutory would require inspection, enforcement, and prosecution; and the Government of India had no wish to get involved in policing medicines in the bazaars.

The final version of the *PI* divided articles into 'official' or 'non-official'. Official drugs were all those included in the *BP* 1867, plus forty products indigenous to India whose efficacy was, in the opinion of its authors, 'well established'. Non-official drugs were those possessing considerable activity but whose efficacy was not well established, along with some regularly used drugs considered of doubtful value. Materia medica were divided into vegetable, animal, and mineral, and here the *PI* differed from the *BP* by using a scientific classification rather than alphabetical order. Preparations were listed under each drug rather than in a separate section. Indian plants considered analogous to ones described in the *BP* were listed. Medicinal plants included in this volume but not the *BP* were a diverse group; several – including *Aconitum heterophyllum*, *Alstonia scholaris*, and *Plantago ispaghula* – featured in subsequent requests for inclusion in the *BP*.[71] Some were later used in Britain despite their lack of official status.

The Government of India considered the 1868 *PI* to 'contain all the information afforded by the *BP* 1867'.[72] It was widely distributed across India, the Bombay government alone distributing 250 copies, of which 159 went to civil officers and institutions. A fresh supply of 100 copies was ordered.[73] The *BP* was removed from use, and the *PI* alone was official in India after 1868.[74] Elsewhere in the empire the *BP* remained in use; in 1871 a Malagasy translation was published in Antananarivo, Madagascar.[75]

The *Pharmaceutical Journal* praised the content of the *IP* but was critical of the inclusion of a number of drugs it considered unimportant.[76] It also doubted the wisdom of including all the drugs of the *BP*, as 'certain of them, which were required to be used in a fresh state, were not available in India, and some would have undergone decomposition in the tropical climate'. But it did not believe that the answer lay in the production of an 'imperial pharmacopoeia'. Rather, it supported the inclusion of more indigenous drugs in existing pharmacopoeias: 'we cannot but believe that as our knowledge of these becomes more extended, many of them but little known at present, but of undoubted efficacy, will find their appropriate place in the British and other pharmacopoeias of Europe and America'.[77]

Among the submissions made to the committee in 1867 had been one from a native surgeon, Moodeen Sheriff (182?–1891), of the Triplicane Dispensary, Madras. Sheriff had submitted the names of indigenous plants included in the draft list in several Indian languages. In 1867 he was granted leave to complete the work, and it was agreed that the list should be included as an appendix in the *PI*.[78] But its printing was delayed, and it was decided that it should be published as a separate volume. When published in 1869 it was a substantial work of over three hundred pages, providing Indian synonyms for drugs and preparations included in the *PI*.[79] Names were given in English and fourteen other languages. Its sixteen indexes included one for each language, and listed all sources consulted during preparation.[80]

The supplement was more favourably received in India than the *PI* itself, about which the *Madras Monthly Journal of Medical Science* commented, 'We have all been somewhat disappointed with the work.'[81] The journal regarded it more as a handbook of materia medica than a pharmacopoeia.[82] Dr Waring had 'shirked one of the most difficult, and at the same time, most important parts of the work, when he transferred to Mr Moodeen Sheriff the execution of the portion that now appears as a supplement ... Overall, the Supplement has been prepared with great care, is highly creditable to its author, and will be of very great practical value in this country.'[83] The journal concluded that, 'But for its appearance, the *Pharmacopoeia of India* must, to a great extent, have remained a dead letter.'[84]

REVISING THE *PHARMACOPOEIA OF INDIA*

In 1868, as the *PI* was being published, a new Pharmacy and Poisons Act was passed in Britain; it linked the regulation of pharmacy with both the control of poisons and use of the *BP*. An Addendum to the *BP* published in 1874 made thirty-four additions and eleven corrections; it incorporated research by Redwood and Attfield, but added only one new medicinal plant – areca.[85] Section 15 of the Pharmacy and Poisons Act made it an offence to compound medicines included in the *BP* except in accordance with its formularies.[86] It later formed the basis of similar acts and ordinances across the empire.[87] But in India attempts by pharmaceutical chemists to secure a Pharmacy Act were unsuccessful.[88] In 1880 they petitioned the viceroy, pointing out that 'such an Act has been passed at home, and was subsequently extended to the colonies. Therefore, the undersigned beg that ... an Act entitled the "Pharmacy Act" be speedily brought into law.'[89] The petition failed; after the 1857 rebellion the government was wary of interfering with the practice of Ayurveda and Unani practitioners. A second attempt at securing a Pharmacy Act in 1894 also failed.[90] As a result there was no effective drug regulation in India before independence, and no pharmacopoeia had statutory authority. Drug rules under the 1940 Drugs Act were approved only in 1945, and a Pharmacy Act to regulate the profession of pharmacy was passed only in 1948.[91]

With the *IP* containing 'all the information afforded by the *BP* 1867' as the official pharmacopoeia in India, the India Office in 1876 established a committee under the chairmanship of Sir Joseph Fayrer

(1824–1907), the surgeon general in India, to advise on whether a revision should be undertaken, following a request from the military authorities.[92] Fayrer had returned to England in 1872 after his tenure in the Indian Medical Service, and was president of the India Office's Medical Board from 1874 to 1895.[93] He asked the government in Calcutta to consult with its provincial counterparts. The governments of Madras, Bombay, and the North-Western Provinces were in favour of revision and offered a number of suggestions for change. The Madras government considered that a revised edition should be restricted to Indian drugs and made as brief as possible.[94] The Bengal government was opposed to a new edition. Feyrer's report, published in January 1878, took a cautious approach and proposed conditional revision. 'While the BP should remain the authoritative guide to all medical officers in India so far as drugs not Indian are concerned, an *Indian Pharmacopoeia* should be prepared, carefully limited to drugs peculiar to India, and this ... should be compiled in India by committees of medical officers formed at each Presidency, all passing on their reports to a central committee which would sift, prepare, and print the material.'[95]

The new edition would be a collaborative effort by the Calcutta, Bombay, and Madras governments. But limiting it to drugs 'peculiar to India' would still result in a substantial volume. Feyrer concluded that the 1868 PI was sufficient for current needs, but that 'if a new edition was to be recommended it might take the form of an abridgement of Waring's [1868 edition] for regular use in every local dispensary, framed entirely on the model of the London pharmacopoeia.'[96] He noted that 'it was doubtful whether a new edition would repay the labour and expense involved in its publication', and he 'advocated an abridgement of the present long list of drugs, and greater care in the preparation of those approved.' His report was sent by the secretary of state for India (Viscount Cranbrook) to the governor general in India (Lord Lytton) in December 1879.[97]

Waring responded directly to the secretary of state in March 1880.[98] He suggested that a 'Materia Medica Indica' be compiled as a first stage in the revision of the PI. But the formation of a new government in Britain in 1880 resulted in a change of personnel in both London and India. The Marquis of Hartington became the new secretary of state and the Marquis of Ripon the new governor general. By then steps were already in train to revise the PI. In November 1880 Hartington acknowledged receipt of Ripon's predecessor's despatches relating to

146 Pharmacopoeias, Drug Regulation, and Empires

the proposed revision, in which Cranbrook had stated that – whilst the Medical Board at the India Office was in favour of the proposal – he would not sanction it unless the medical authorities in India agreed to the necessary additions and omissions.[99] In January 1881 Hartington concluded that a new edition was not needed. 'Taking all the evidence before us into consideration, we are of the opinion that neither a new edition of the [Indian] Pharmacopoeia, nor the issue of a *Materia Medica Indica* is at present wanted ... the *British Pharmacopoeia* should remain the authoritative guide to all Medical Officers in India.'[100]

EXTENDING THE AUTHORITY OF THE *BP*

Work began on a new edition of the *BP* immediately after publication of the 1874 addendum; it was undertaken by a committee of eight members of the GMC chaired by Quain.[101] This time, the text was edited by three joint editors: Professors Redwood, Attfield, and Bentley of the PSGB (figure 6.2).[102] Robert Bentley (1821–1893) was a pharmacist who later qualified as a doctor and became professor of botany at King's College London. The PSGB established its own Pharmacopoeia Committee, but the doctors were reluctant to engage with them. In a confidential note to the GMC in 1884 Quain wrote, 'It is said that in other countries pharmacists are placed on equal terms with medical men in preparing the pharmacopoeia. This statement is to some extent correct, but on the other hand there exists no such competent body in this country as the Medical Council to which the duty could be assigned; nor are the pharmacists of those countries quite analogous to our own.'[103] It was a view shared by Quain's medical colleagues, and it led eventually to the pharmacists withdrawing their support.

Further publications on medicinal plants by European and Indian practitioners appeared over the following years. George Barber published his *Pharmaceutical or Medico-Botanical Map of the World*, which listed nearly three hundred plant drugs and their origins, in 1870.[104] Flückiger and Hanbury's monumental *Pharmacographia* was published in 1874,[105] and Martindale and Westcott's *Extra Pharmacopoeia of Unofficial Drugs* in 1883.[106] A nine-volume work by George Watt listing around fourteen hundred plants used in India for medicinal purposes was displayed at the 1885 Calcutta Exhibition.[107] Between them they listed several thousand plants with claimed medicinal benefits.

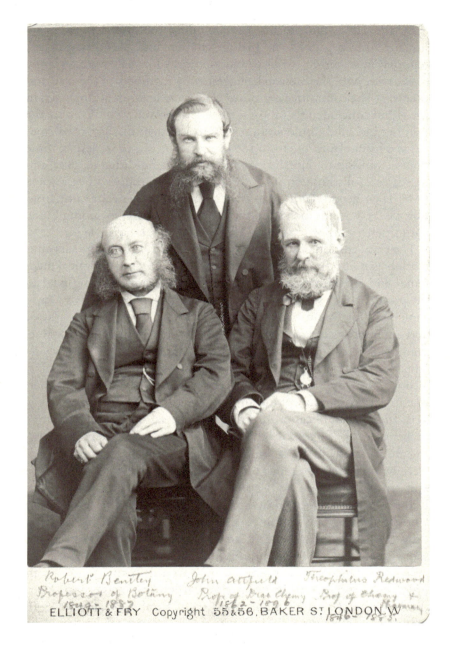

Figure 6.2 Robert Bentley (1821–1893), John Attfield (1835–1911), and Theophilus Redwood (1806–1892), ca 1881–87.

By the 1880s the process for compiling the *BP* was well established.[108] Investigations on the preparation and use of medicines reported in scientific, medical, and pharmacy journals were reviewed along with published research suggested by members of the GMC and others.[109] The committee examined claims made for items included in the *PI* but concluded that most were 'not of proven value'. Even so, the number included in the *BP* 1885 was greater than in 1867. Medicines derived from plants rose from 166 in 1867 to 175 in 1885, despite some notable omissions: digitalis from foxglove was not listed in 1885, and its African substitute, strophanthin, was only introduced in the 1898 *BP*.[110] Their geographical origins were diverse; 40 per cent came from Europe, 25 per cent each from the Americas and Asia including India, with smaller proportions from Africa and Australasia (table 6.1).

The third edition of the *BP* was published in 1885, eleven years after work began. It reflected the continuing ascendency of chemical medicines and chemical testing, with increasing attention being paid to the purity of drug substances and to the control of impurities.[111] Early limit tests for impurities indicated the future direction of national and international pharmacopoeias. New entries included cocaine, ergotine, and morphine, along with salicylic acid and sodium salicylate. New products of plant origin included menthol and thymol. It also included the first tablet – glyceryl trinitrate – and two hypodermic injections, apomorphine and ergotine.[112]

In India its publication prompted a reversal of the government's earlier direction to remove the *BP* 1867 from medical depots following publication of the *PI* in 1868.[113] The roles of pharmacopoeias were being reviewed against a rapidly changing world both at home and across the empire. British involvement in Africa increased greatly following the so-called Scramble for Africa and the 1884 Berlin Conference.[114] Many colonies and Dominions began introducing drug regulation measures. In Canada there was a real prospect that each province might begin compiling its own pharmacopoeia; to allow India to continue using its own would in this sense set an unfortunate precedent. In March 1886, following instructions from the secretary of state for India (the Earl of Kimberley), a new order made the *BP* 1885 the 'sole authority on all matters relating to pharmacy'. It also sanctioned its issue to all military hospitals in lieu of the *PI*.[115] The hegemony of the *BP* would be upheld; the *PI* would be discarded. There would be only one official pharmacopoeia in use across the empire.

Table 6.1
Plant medicines included in the *BP* 1885 by continent of origin

Region	Number (N = 175)	Per cent of total	Examples
Europe	70	40%	Elder flower, belladonna leaves, dandelion root, hemlock
Asia	44	25%	Asafetida, cardamom, kino, sumbul root, cannabis indica
Africa	15	9%	Acacia gum, calumba root, calabar bean, aloes, myrrh
Americas	44	25%	Jaborandi, senega root, cascarilla, sarsaparilla, cinchona, jalap
Australasia	2	1%	Sandalwood, eucalyptus leaves

Source: Adapted from Abena Dove Osseo-Asare, "Bioprospecting and Resistance: Transforming Poisoned Arrows into Strophantin Pills in Colonial Gold Coast," *Social History of Medicine* 21, no. 2 (2008): 271.

CONCLUSION

The order to make the *BP* 1885 the 'sole authority on all matters relating to pharmacy' was a significant moment in the shifting relationship between medicines, drug regulation, and pharmacopoeias, not only for India but also across the British Empire. The India Office in London had effectively overruled the Government of India. Despite the fact that a revised *Pharmacopoeia of India* would have facilitated substantial savings for the Indian Medical Service, only those included in the *BP* were to be official. Free trade trumped potential savings. Bhattacharya has described how 'as early as 1876, under an episodic tightening of budgets that the India Office in London enjoined on its administration in India, the Committee on the Supply of Drugs in India supported the publication of an *Indian Pharmacopoeia*.'[116]

Feyrer's inquiries had also exposed fundamental differences in the views of medical officers about the evidence required to justify the inclusion of new plant medicines in a pharmacopoeia. Some felt that no drug should be added without strong evidence; others felt that centuries of successful practical experience was sufficient justification.[117] Some were keen to see such substances in greater use in Britain: C.J.H. Warden, co-author of the 1890 *Pharmacographia Indica*, reminded the surgeon general that 'one of the primary objects of the compilation of the *Indian Pharmacopoeia* was the introduction of the indigenous products of the country into European practice.'[118] How the backlash from the colonies led ultimately to the 'imperialization' of the pharmacopoeia is the subject of the next chapter.

7

Towards an Imperial Pharmacopoeia

Across the world rapid changes were taking place not only in the size and nature of empires but also in science, technology, and medicine, in the drug trade, in the professionalization of pharmacy, and in the relationship between medicine and pharmacy. These issues had a significant impact on the attitude of governments and practitioners to the purpose and place of pharmacopoeias both at home and in the colonies. Medical officers in India resented the withdrawal of the *Pharmacopoeia of India* (PI) and its replacement by the 1885 edition of the *British Pharmacopoeia* (BP) as the 'sole authority on all matters relating to pharmacy'.[1] But they were not alone in questioning whether the BP alone could meet the disparate needs of practitioner across the empire. The response of the General Medical Council (GMC) was to undertake the 'imperialization' of the pharmacopoeia; the outcome was a limited *Indian and Colonial Addendum* (ICA) in 1900.

This chapter explores why the BP 1885 was imposed across the empire and why other pharmacopoeias were banned. It considers how it was received in the colonies, what action was taken as a result, and why in 1892 the decision was taken to imperialize the pharmacopoeia. It explores why a consultation process was used and how the Pharmacopoeia Committee collected the information needed. How were consultation processes adopted in different colonies? What was the extent of cooperation between doctors and pharmacists? How were the contributions of those with medical, pharmaceutical, and chemical expertise used in compiling the pharmacopoeia? And why was the outcome an ICA rather than an imperialized BP? This chapter examines these questions.

THE RISE OF DOMINION PHARMACOPOEIAS

Another change of government in London in July 1886 (from Liberal to Conservative) led to a change of personnel and a change of policy in the colonies. The new secretary of state for India (Viscount Cross) placed greater emphasis on promoting British trade and discouraging actions that would limit it. Most of the drugs used by the Indian Medical Service were imported from Britain or elsewhere, but at much higher prices than those available locally.[2] Although no longer official, the *PI* included many Indian plant drugs considered useful substitutes for imported ones, and continuing efforts were made by medical officers and others in India to have them included in the next *BP*, although some continued to lobby for the revision of the *PI*. In 1886 the issue was taken up with the governor general (the Earl of Dufferin), who conveyed their concerns to the GMC via the secretary of state for India (the Earl of Kimberley). The GMC assured Kimberley that Indian plant medicines previously included in the *PI* would be included in a planned addendum.[3]

The wish for a separate colonial pharmacopoeia was not confined to India. Doctors and pharmacists in Canada, South Africa, Australia, and New Zealand also showed interest in the possibility of producing their own, on similar lines to that in India. In Canada and South Africa pharmacopoeias of other nations were often used alongside the British one. Pharmacy professionalization had begun in Canada following Confederation in 1867 with the founding of pharmaceutical societies.[4] In 1878 the Nova Scotia Pharmaceutical Society approved a resolution accepting the *BP* as an official reference. 'The practice of pharmacy,' it declared, 'can only become uniform by an open and candid intercourse being kept up between the druggists of this Province.' This could be achieved 'by the adoption of one pharmacopoeia as a guide in the preparation of official medicines, as there is a division of opinion as to which pharmacopoeia is used by the profession.'[5] Variance would be permitted 'only in exceptional cases where sufficient authority has proved some other process more reliable to attain the same end.'[6] Publication of the 1885 *BP*, its imposition in India, and the removal of the *PI* prompted a robust response from pharmacists in Canada. Pharmacists in Quebec proposed the formation of an all-Dominion pharmaceutical association and publication of a 'Dominion pharmacopoeia.' Resolutions were put to their members by pharmaceutical societies in other provinces. In 1893 the Nova Scotia Pharmaceutical Society approved formation of a Dominion association for Canada and agreed that 'a pharmacopoeia for the Dominion would be advisable, and that the cooperation of the physicians and medical colleges should be secured to obtain a satisfactory compilation'.[7]

For the GMC the prospect of a Dominion pharmacopoeia was further evidence that the absence of a single pharmacopoeia would result in a free-for-all in which each colony compiled its own. The freedom of colonies to substitute local remedies for ones imported from Britain was a worrying prospect. Seriously limiting the export of British medicines to the colonies might damage the prospects of the rapidly developing pharmaceutical industry in Britain, particularly as the empire was fast expanding following the 1884 Berlin Conference, which ratified the 'Scramble for Africa', regulated European colonization and trade in Africa, and marked the start of the 'new imperialism' that continued until 1914.[8]

The BP 1885 was no better received by pharmacists in the United Kingdom than it was elsewhere; they did not consider that it reflected everyday practice. Several initiatives were taken to establish the extent to which official medicines were used in Britain. The Pharmacopoeia Committee of the Pharmaceutical Society of Great Britain (PSGB) asked pharmacists to rate them as 'frequently', 'seldom', or 'never' prescribed or sold, and to add any suggestions for additions and omissions to the BP. An analysis of ten thousand prescriptions dispensed in various parts of the United Kingdom during the first quarter of 1886 was published in *Chemist and Druggist* in April 1886.[9] An analysis of twelve thousand prescriptions dispensed in pharmacies in Aberdeen, Bournemouth, Carlyle, Cork, London, and Oxford was undertaken by William Martindale (1840–1902). Many BP preparations were 'never' or 'seldom' supplied, and even the list of 'frequently' used ones was relatively short.

The limitations of the BP 1885 received a great deal of attention in Britain. The late nineteenth century saw a rapid increase in the marketing and purchase of patent medicines.[10] These were increasingly prescribed by doctors, resulting in a drop in extemporaneous prescriptions presented at chemists' shops, including many BP formulations. At the 1885 British Pharmaceutical Conference, Thomas Greenish (the PSGB's president from 1880 to 1882), called for the production of a new, 'unofficial' formulary, which would list popular compounded medicines not included in the *BP*. Prescribers would write the name of a preparation made to a standard formula rather than write out the full list of ingredients. This would save the prescriber listing all the ingredients, and hopefully encourage doctors to prescribe fewer patent medicines, which were less profitable for chemists. The initiative took some years to materialize, but in 1901 the PSGB published an unofficial formulary in its *Yearbook of Pharmacy*. The *British Pharmaceutical Codex* followed in 1907.[11]

One of the arguments put forward in Canada for a Dominion pharmacopoeia was the rapid rise in the prescribing of proprietary medicines by doctors in the late nineteenth century. In 1896 the president of the Nova Scotia Pharmaceutical Society 'deplored the increase of proprietary articles which are daily dispensed'. He thought that 'druggists should show physicians that they are capable of preparing whatever is required from the crude drugs'.[12] The Dominion pharmacopoeia would be a list of simple and compounded medicines used across Canada. But unlike Greenish's 'unofficial' formulary in Britain – which would supplement the *BP* – in Canada it would replace it.

THE LEGAL STATUS OF THE *BP*

With the 1885 *BP* published and its use promoted throughout the empire, the Privy Council thought it prudent to obtain advice as to its legal status from the GMC's solicitor, Frederick Willis Farrar. Farrar gave his advice in a letter dated 4 February 1887:

> The legal authority of the *BP* seems to them [the GMC] a matter of such serious importance to the public and to the medical professional as to require the very gravest consideration ... It would seem that, while the *BP* has for three countries (England, Wales, and Scotland) been believed and intended to have full legal authority as the standard of drugs and compounded medicines and the like, in spite of Orders in Council and Acts of Parliament, it is only in Ireland that there is statutory penalty for infringing it. In England powers given by statutes of Henry VIII and Mary are obsolete, they only referred to London and seven miles around it ... Although the Pharmacy and Food Acts in some way may be

154   Pharmacopoeias, Drug Regulation, and Empires

said to support the pharmacopoeia, they only do so partially and indirectly. In Scotland there is apparently no penalty for infringing the pharmacopoeia.[13]

Farrar was in no doubt about the consequences of pharmacopoeias being official but not statutory. It was necessary, he concluded, that a pharmacopoeia not only be issued by an authorized body but also that infringements needed to be prosecutable in law. 'It is hardly possible to exaggerate the importance', he declared, 'of having [a] recognized standard authority for the purity and strength of drugs, extracts, etc, and for the correct proportions of compounded medicines. Without such a standard the public is open to frauds of the worst description followed by the most serious consequences, and the medical practitioner is helpless if the remedies he employs are uncertain in their purity and composition. Every other civilized nation has the standard authority in such matters – its own pharmacopoeia – the provisions of which it is penal to infringe.'[14]

Farrar's strongly worded advice about the legal status of the BP was considered by the GMC's Pharmacopoeia Committee in 1888. He advised that an amendment to the law should be sought declaring the BP to be the legal standard under the Food and Drugs Act for the drugs contained in it. The committee recommended to the full GMC that the necessary steps be taken. The GMC adopted the recommendation, but 'nothing came of it'. It entered the necessary but convoluted parliamentary processes and was eventually sidelined. Parliamentary Select Committees sitting in 1879 and again in 1894–96 considered similar suggestions, but the recommendations concerning the BP's legal status were never adopted, and the law was still unchanged in 1928.[15]

COLLABORATION AND COOPERATION

Having deferred consideration of new medicines and those in the Indian pharmacopoeias until after publication of the BP in 1885 – and having sought legal advice – the GMC's Pharmacopoeia Committee were in no hurry to begin work on an addendum. In 1889 they appointed a subcommittee and invited various medical authorities (but not those in India or the colonies), including the Royal Colleges, universities, and the Society of Apothecaries, to submit 'a list of such new medicines and compounds as possessed or appeared to possess well-recognized medicinal value and which had the general approval of the medical profession.[16] In all, 140 new items were proposed, of which the committee eventually selected 37 for inclusion in the addendum.[17]

The appointment of a subcommittee to look at new medicines represented a shift in the balance between medical and pharmaceutical contributions in compiling the pharmacopoeia. The GMC Pharmacopoeia Committee invited the two pharmaceutical societies (those of Great Britain and Ireland) 'to assist in preparing and defining any additions that might be recommended by the Committee and approved by the Council.'[18] But not for the first time it came very late in the day: 'the list of selected articles, after approval by the Council, was accordingly placed before these Societies.'[19] Nevertheless the PSGB appointed a special committee to look at it and make recommendations. It suggested the addition of a further four articles. The GMC Pharmacopoeia Committee noted 'with satisfaction the conjunction of medical and pharmaceutical work in the production of the present extension of the pharmacopoeia, a combination that cannot but be productive of future as well as immediate benefit both to medicine and to pharmacy.'[20] The GMC Council later conveyed its 'best thanks' to the PSGB 'for their very valuable assistance in the preparation of the Addendum.'[21]

In 1890 five thousand copies of the addendum were printed and distributed across the empire. It was no better received than the 1885 BP, with the most critical response coming from India. It was viewed as a 'British' addendum to a 'British' pharmacopoeia, with few concessions made to the needs of India or the rest of the empire. Medical officers in India were deeply disappointed yet again, having been promised that Indian plant medicines previously included in the PI would be included. Most of the new items accepted were chemical medicines – including acetanilide and phenacetin – although among them was an official version of a proprietary medicine, Seidlitz Powders, a patent for which had originally been granted in 1815.[22]

SUBSTITUTING BP DRUGS IN INDIA

The GMC's Pharmacopoeia Committee had again concluded that most of the plant medicines proposed were not of proven value. But in India investigations into plants with medicinal value continued, as did the suggestion of new items for inclusion in the pharmacopoeia. Guides to the use of Indian medicinal plants continued to be published as well. William Dymock, C.J.H. Warden, and David Hooper (quinologist to the Government of Madras) published the first of their three-volume *Pharmacographia Indica* in 1890.[23] Moodeen Sheriff's *Materia Medica of Madras* was published in 1891 after his death, following completion by Hooper.[24] A revision of Kanny Lall Dey's *Indigenous Drugs of India* was published in 1896.[25] Like Warden, Dey aimed to have as many Indian drugs as possible integrated into Western materia medica.[26]

Medical officers and others in India continued to press their case for Indian indigenous drugs to be made official and for the revision and reinstatement of the *PI*. On 12 November 1891 a letter with extensive supporting documentation was sent to the office of the Governor General listing items they wished to see added to the *BP*. It was forwarded to the India Office in London. It listed possible local substitutes and noted challenges presented by many *BP* formulations for tropical countries. 'Certain drugs described in the *BP* might, in the Indian Empire, be usefully substituted by drugs indigenous to India', it noted, and 'certain medicinal compounds employed there might be advantageously prepared according to altered or amended formulae.'[27] The India Office in turn forwarded the suggestions to the GMC,[28] at the same time clarifying the legal status of the *BP* 1885 in India: 'the Medical Act of 1858 has not been made applicable to India, but so far as the preparation of compound medicines is concerned, the formulae laid down in the *BP* are invariably followed by the Government Medical Stores Department as well as by private chemists and druggists'.[29]

THE REQUEST TO 'IMPERIALIZE' THE *BP*

With another change in government in Britain in August 1892 (from Conservative back to Liberal) and the return of the Earl of Kimberley as secretary of state for India (figure 7.1), medical officers in the subcontinent renewed their efforts. In November 1892 Kimberley – who opposed a separate pharmacopoeia for India – asked the GMC to investigate how the *BP* could be 'better fitted to the needs of India and the Colonies'.[30] It was a request that could not easily be ignored, and was the final push needed to 'imperialize the pharma-

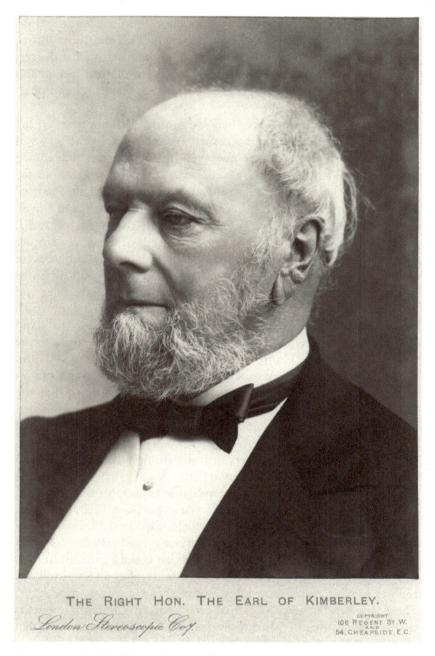

Figure 7.1 John Wodehouse, 1st Earl of Kimberley (1826–1902), ca 1897.

copoeia'. The GMC asked its Pharmacopoeia Committee 'to enter into correspondence, through the Privy Council, with the India Office and the Colonial Office, with a view to ascertaining to what degree, if any, the BP can be better fitted than at present to meet Indian and Colonial requirements as regards important natural drugs and pharmaceutical preparations'.[31]

By late 1893 the Pharmacopoeia Committee had approached the 'relevant authorities' throughout the empire to obtain the views of local experts so as to give the new volume an 'imperial character'.[32] Practitioners across the empire were invited to make suggestions for additions, deletions, alterations, and amendments. The Pharmacopoeia Committee agreed that when the fourth edition of the BP was published (in 1898) it should 'meet all the needs of India'. Indeed, the 'new volume' would serve the needs of the whole empire by making approved locally available materials 'official'. There were then seventy British dependencies administered in seven divisions (see table 0.1 in the introduction). They included Indian states and colonies in the African, Australasian, Eastern, Mediterranean, North American, and West Indian Divisions, along with the Falkland Islands. All were invited to submit comments and suggestions to the GMC Pharmacopoeia Committee. John Attfield again acted as editor. Some colonies responded quickly; suggestions from Hong Kong in 1894 were considered, accepted, and included in drafts for the fourth edition. But others undertook extensive internal consultations, and their comments continued to arrive well after the text had been finalized.

Whilst many medical officers in India supported the substitution of imported drugs with indigenous ones based on practical experience, others felt that the evidence available to support making them official was insufficient. In January 1894, the Government of India appointed a three-man committee, which in turn established provincial subcommittees to collect the information requested.[33] Its remit was to suggest drugs indigenous to India that could be substituted for drugs currently listed in the BP.[34] A few months later it submitted two reports making 'important contributions' to the planned BP 1898. These listed indigenous medicinal plants showing potential benefits that the government wished to see included, but excluded those that were simply local substitutes for ones already listed. In February 1894 it wrote to the principal of the Madras Medical College asking for assistance. The college appointed its own committee, consisting of the professor of materia medica, F.J. Crawford, and a lecturer in botany, R. Hollingsworth. These two presented their report to the Indian committee in June 1894, but by this time the latter had already submitted its reports to London and been disbanded.[35] Crawford and his colleagues sent their report containing a much longer list of Indian plant medicines – most of which were local substitutes for imported drugs – direct to the GMC's Pharmacopoeia Committee.

The matter was taken up by Kanny Lall Dey in December 1894. At the Indian Medical Congress in Calcutta he focused attention on the study of indigenous drugs, their systematic cultivation, and their increasing issue from medical depots.[36] Drug substitution occupied centre stage at the congress.[37] In response, the Government of India agreed 'rather reluctantly' in October 1895 to set up a Central Indigenous Drugs Committee (CIDC).[38] It was chaired by George King, superintendent at the Royal Botanical Garden in Calcutta; its secretary was G. Watt, the government's reporter on economic products. The other members were J.F.P. McConnel, professor of materia medica at Calcutta Medical School, C.J. Warden, medical storekeeper for Bengal, and Kanny Lall Dey, then professor of chemistry at the medical school.[39] They submitted their report to the Government of India in early 1897.[40] It specifically denounced the preparation of indigenous substitutes, and categorically rejected the idea of substituting local drugs for those included in the BP. They considered that 'the raw drug-materials that were obtained in India were impure and adulterated, rendering them unfit for chemical processing'. Furthermore, 'if such medicines – after the removal of adulteration with all pain and care – were locally produced, they would be, apart from doubtful efficacy, much more expensive than the imported drugs'.[41]

This was the official explanation for the suppression of substitution and the promotion of British imports. But there were many dissenting voices. J. Parker, medical storekeeper at Bombay, submitted a list of forty drugs 'which could act as proper substitutes for imported drugs, and which grew abundantly and cost little'.[42] Several drugs – including digitalis, hyoscyamus, jalap, and taraxacum – were already procured by the medical stores from Indian sources, and he saw no reason why indigenous drugs could not be similarly produced and supplied. Others opposed widespread testing of such drugs; J. Cleghorn, surgeon general of Bengal, considered that 'the work of investigations into the efficacy of the indigenous drugs [should] be left to individuals'.[43]

160 Pharmacopoeias, Drug Regulation, and Empires

Removal of the *PI* in 1885 had had a significant impact on the use of Indian plant medicines. Warden noted in disgust that few were available in government depots.[44] He had doubts about the sincerity of the government from the start of the committee's work. In his submission he declared that 'It is futile to compile pharmacopoeias if the Government remains unbending in its medical policy.'[45] This was the third time that 'the experiment of drug substitution' was being made, following publication of the *Bengal Pharmacopoeia* and the *IP*. Anil Kumar has noted that there was nothing new in the policy of rejecting drug substitution in 1901; the colonial government had been pursuing it for many years. 'Seeking proposals and rejecting them reflected not capriciousness, but a strategy to deny change in imperial preferences.'[46] In 1841 the government had asked the Medical Board to look into the possibility of manufacturing magnesia, sulphate of soda, and potash in India. All that was required was 'the use of improved technology as employed in England for the manufacture of common salt.' But the government declined to act, and 'the old practice of importation continued.'[47] A later request in 1880 to manufacture salicylates in India was also rejected.

The CIDC was intended to be a standing committee. Watt recommended setting up subordinate provincial committees, with the heads of medical colleges responsible for pooling information about indigenous drugs.[48] They would publish lists of proposed new drugs and those recommended for abolition.[49] But the provincial committees were not a success as a result of 'defects in the system.' By 1900 the CIDC had recommended their replacement 'by one or more selected physicians in important towns who would be required to give the various inquiries entrusted to them their special and personal consideration.'[50] Kumar concluded that 'nothing more than a fairly long-drawn-out debate emerged from the proceedings of this Committee.'[51]

PHARMACOPOEIAS AND ADDENDA

Work began on a fourth edition of the *BP* as soon as the 1890 addendum had been published. Sir Richard Quain, by then president of the GMC, was again appointed chair of its Pharmacopoeia Committee, Dr Nestor Tirard its secretary, and John Attfield was retained as editor. Attfield prepared annual reports with abstracts of research, opinion, and other material published by 'therapeutists, pharmacologists, pharmaceutical chemists and chemists and druggists, and scientific and analytical chemists, which might be of importance in any further revision.[52] Nine reports were produced between 1886 and 1894, with Attfield himself undertaking a range of experimental work. In 1895 the British Medical Association (BMA) surveyed its members, asking them to rate frequency of use of *BP* items as 'often', 'rarely', or 'never' used, and to suggest any additions or deletions. Nearly six thousand replies were received. Five of the top ten most frequently used items were of plant origin: these were pills of aloes and myrrh; strong ginger tincture; fresh orange tincture; syrup of poppies; and mustard paper.[53] The BMA set out its proposals in the *British Medical Journal*. It considered that the *BP* should include 'all such remedies as the existing state of medical practice requires'.[54] The PSGB was invited to convene a 'Committee of Reference in Pharmacy'. Its chair was Walter Hills, with its other members including William Martindale. In preparing the *BP* 1898 the GMC Pharmacopoeia Committee sat for thirty-five days – but so, too, did the equivalent committee within the PSGB, which submitted four reports. John Attfield attended the meetings of both. The GMC also received help and advice from sixteen United Kingdom medical bodies and referees in chemistry, botany, pharmacology, and therapeutics.[55]

The fourth edition of the *BP* was finally published in February 1898. Its content reflected continuing advances in science, with many new chemical medicines added, including cocaine, codeine, hyoscine, and lithium. Kaolin and liquid paraffin were added, as was a new biological product – dried thyroid. But the 1898 edition represented a radical departure from that of 1885; 187 drugs and preparations included in 1885 were deleted, as were all those that had been part of the 1890 addendum.[56] New chemical tests were added to monographs and appendices. A new section on 'tests for substances mentioned in the text of the pharmacopoeia' listed identity tests for inorganic elements and salts. It was now essentially a guide for assuring the quality and purity of medicines. Key users would be scientists in industry, university laboratories, and government testing facilities, rather than retail pharmacists.

It received mixed reactions across the empire. In Australia the *Brisbane Courier* noted that 'every medical and pharmaceutical journal has discussed the revision with reference to almost every preparation in its pages ... It may safely be said that more interest has been taken in this last issue of the pharmacopoeia than in all the previous issues put together."[57] It noted with satisfaction that 'some of the suggestions that emanated from Queensland have been adopted'. A bill was introduced to give the *BP* the necessary legal authority in Queensland; it would 'be regarded by the Legislature as purely formal and should be passed in the least possible time.'

But the request to make it 'better fitted to the needs of India and the Colonies' – along with the results of the consultations across the empire – had been put to one side. The GMC explained in the preface that it 'has in contemplation the early preparation of an Addendum, in which medicinal plants and other substances suggested for inclusion by Indian and Colonial authorities will be dealt with more fully than has now been possible.'[58] But some accommodation to the needs of the empire was made; it included 'a small number of alternative substances or preparations, the official recognition of which had been desired for local use', in an appendix.[59] Adjustments could be made as a result of 'prevailing high temperatures'. Some of the oil could be removed from lard; the amount of alcohol in liquid extracts could be increased to reduce the risk of fermentation; dried lemon peel could be used in place of fresh; and the amount of white beeswax used in suppositories to give the right consistency could be varied. But no substitutions of indigenous medicines for imported ones were approved.

THE *INDIAN AND COLONIAL ADDENDUM*

The 'early preparation of an Addendum' began in earnest as soon as the *BP* 1898 was published. The work was overseen by a renewed GMC Pharmacopoeia Committee chaired by Donald MacAlister,[60] with John Attfield continuing as editor. The *BP* 1898 had included almost none of the drugs suggested by the colonies, despite claims that it was 'already largely an Imperial British Pharmacopoeia'.[61] The addendum was 'designed to serve the needs of all the Divisions of the British Empire with locally available materials'.[62] Nine months after work began the Pharmacopoeia Committee finalized a draft, which was approved by the full GMC Council on 30 November 1898.[63] In December it was published in full in the *Pharmaceutical Journal*,[64] and by the end of January 1899 it had been circulated to medical and pharmaceutical authorities in Britain and all its overseas possessions.[65] It was very clear that a wide range of views existed concerning both the proposed *ICA* and the ultimate preparation of an imperial pharmacopoeia. In London imperialization was promoted enthusiastically by MacAlister and Attwood; their aim was to produce a volume that would meet the needs of the whole empire, and which would therefore be both inclusive and comprehensive.

Responses were received from almost every Dominion and colony, with submissions from India far exceeding those from elsewhere. Many doctors considered that such a volume should contain all the medicines used in daily practice, whilst others believed that it should include only items that had been fully investigated, and whose purity and identity could be tested. Others were more concerned with trade and export issues and felt that local substitutes for official British drugs should not be permitted. The GMC's Pharmacopoeia Committee noted that 'the interests of the provinces of India ... were centred in a special Committee [the CIDC] appointed by the Government of India in 1894' and in the subsequent report by Crawford and Hollingsworth.[66] The latter included suggestions relating to 'nearly all the drugs that now appear under "India" in the draft Addendum', along with a large number of suggestions for substitution.[67] The Pharmacopoeia Committee asked the Madras Medical College to conduct experiments with indigenous drugs and report directly to it, bypassing the CIDC in Calcutta. The college readily agreed, subject to approval by the secretary of state for India, which the GMC Pharmacopoeia Committee subsequently obtained.[68]

The governor general (Lord Curzon) advised the secretary of state (Lord Hamilton) that 'an explanation be given to the [GMC] Council of the measures that are being taken to obtain more complete and definite knowledge of the indigenous drugs of India.'[69] Crawford, this time assisted by Captain Donovan (Hollingsworth had retired) was invited to 'furnish contributions and assistance towards completion of the Indian Addendum to the British Pharmacopoeia.'[70] They were later joined by the government medical storekeeper, Lt-Col. H. St Clare Carruthers, described as 'a highly skilled enthusiast in all matters pertaining to the treatment of drugs and the production of efficient pharmaceutical preparations.'[71] Comments from GMC members were sent along with a request for specimens of the drugs. Crawford subsequently submitted 'a valuable Preliminary Report on the [draft] Addendum' in December 1899.[72] It was distributed to medical and pharmaceutical authorities in Britain, Ireland, India, and the colonies, and to the medical and pharmaceutical press. The GMC Pharmacopoeia Committee concluded that 'with the further help of the Madras Committee a satisfactory Indian Section of the Addendum can be compiled.'[73]

Most of the Indian plant medicines recommended by the Madras group were subsequently incorporated into the addendum. But their inclusion did not have the approval of the CIDC in India, having been made against its wishes.[74] The Pharmacopoeia Committee nevertheless recognized that the success of the addendum, and ultimately of the 'imperial pharmacopoeia', depended on the support of the CIDC: 'With the further assistance of the permanent Indigenous Drugs Committee sitting in Calcutta, there can be little doubt that the BP will sooner or later meet the medical requirements of every one of the fourteen Provinces of India.'[75] Other submissions included one from Surgeon General C. Sibthorpe stating that three medicinal plants were being investigated by the Indigenous Drugs Committee in Madras.[76] George Watt, secretary of the CIDC in Calcutta, sent voluminous but unofficial correspondence to London. His committee were keen to indicate 'the course they are adopting to secure much needed chemical, physiological, and therapeutic investigation of Indian indigenous drugs.'[77] Surgeon Major General (Ret'd) Bidie sent a long report on each of the drugs listed. Hooper contributed information on many drugs: he had been a strong supporter of the PI and was in favour of an imperial one.[78] 'Uniformity in the strength of medicines in every country is to be commended, and although it is premature to formulate a universal pharmacopoeia, the production of an imperial one will be an advance in the right direction.'[79] There was limited input from pharmaceutical practitioners. David Skinner Kemp, a long-standing resident of India who had established an English pharmacy in 1855,[80] sent notes on eleven of the drugs listed. Dr E.M. De Souza, a member of the council of the Burma branch of the BMA, writing also 'as a pharmacist of Rangoon', concluded that the BP 1898 'suffices for the requirements of the province.'[81]

RESPONSE TO THE
DRAFT COLONIAL ADDENDUM

Elsewhere in the empire much effort went into scrutinizing the draft addendum. In Canada 'medical and pharmaceutical interests in the Addendum of the eight provinces ... are centred in an influential

Committee sitting in Montreal.[82] It included the 'presidents of various medical and pharmaceutical societies and associations, professors of pharmacology, therapeutics, chemistry, botany and pharmacy, editors of journals, and other representative men'. Attfield corresponded directly with its president, Dr Adami. A draft report including thirty to forty drugs and preparations was circulated throughout the Dominion.[83] The report, along with 'voluminous suggestions' from Professor Morrison, was reproduced in the *Canadian Pharmaceutical Journal* and the British *Pharmaceutical Journal*.[84] The addendum was then expected to have separate sections for each Dominion or region. With Canadian practice heavily influenced by that in America the GMC Pharmacopoeia Committee announced that 'an endeavour will be made to secure ... harmony of treatment between the Canadian portion of the Addendum and the *United States Pharmacopoeia* of 1900'.[85]

The Canadian committee sent a list of thirty items that it proposed for official recognition in the BP. The GMC Pharmacopoeia Committee convened a special meeting to consider it three days later.[86] Items would be divided into two groups: those that would be restricted to North American colonies and be listed in a Canadian section of the addendum; and those that might 'find wider recognition in the text of the Pharmacopoeia itself'.[87] In April 1900 Adami reported that his committee accepted the principle of this division, but still 'desired to see a few of the articles of the second-class placed in the first or Addendum division'. A revised Canadian list was submitted and 'instructions were given to the Editor as to the preparations to be included for Canadian use'.[88] Pharmacy in Newfoundland – then a separate colony – largely followed that in Canada.[89] Dr Nutting Stuart Fraser wrote to the GMC Pharmacopoeia Committee stating his support for the Canadian response: 'As a private practitioner, there being no official channel through which to reply ... the BP of 1898 suffices for the requirements of the Colony, and as the climatic conditions and flora are practically those of the eight Canadian Provinces, the recommendations of the latter would be those of Newfoundland'.[90]

The West Indian colonies responded individually. The Montserrat medical officer noted that several plants mentioned grew wild in the islands, and he would welcome 'official recognition of those drugs'.[91] The secretary to the Medical Board of Trinidad and Tobago replied that many popular local remedies 'scarcely deserved official recognition. There were some highly regarded local drugs, but these 'had not been even cursorily examined pharmacologically', and their investigation would take far too long for their inclusion in the addendum. In British Guiana, the acting surgeon general consulted with medical and pharmaceutical bodies and concluded that 'the BP 1898 sufficed for the medical and pharmaceutical requirements of the colony', as did those from St Vincent, British Honduras, and Granada.[92] Medical authorities in Barbados had no suggestions, and the secretary of the BMA's Bermuda branch reported that the matter would be considered by its members. Contributions had previously been submitted by Jamaica and the Turks and Caicos Islands and been included in the BP 1898; no further additions were anticipated. Medical staff on St Lucia agreed that there were many plants growing there that possessed valuable medicinal properties, but 'they do not make any general recommendation for the official recommendation of any of them'.[93] By November 1899 the GMC Pharmacopoeia Committee had concluded that there was a high level of support for the 'broad principle of imperializing the pharmacopoeia'.[94]

Separate responses were received from medical authorities in the three Mediterranean colonies. In Malta, pharmacists had been obliged to adhere to the *London Pharmacopoeia* after 1854,[95] although the BP was adopted for use across the islands when it was published in 1864.[96] Local remedies were also used, and the chief government medical officer recommended inclusion in the BP of melon pumpkin seeds. These were, he assured the committee, 'an agreeable, safe, and certain taenifuge' (for expelling tapeworms).[97] He enclosed detailed botanical descriptions along with an account of their preparation and administration.[98] It was extensively used in Malta in preference to pomegranate bark and to kousso and male fern, both of which grew well in the colony. It was, he claimed, more easily taken than either.[99] The surgeon at the colonial hospital in Gibraltar had no additions to make but did report that some native remedies were derived from plants already listed in the BP 1885; however, the limited vegetation there was insufficient even to maintain a constant supply of local remedies.[100] The Cyprus authorities had no further suggestions.

THE AFRICAN RESPONSE

Medicinal plants from Africa had been included in the BP for many years before the GMC request. The British explorer Sir Harry Johnston noted that 'the forests of Africa ... teem with useful drugs, prominent among which may be cited the kola nut and the Strophanthus seeds'.[101] *Strophanthus* had been added to the BP in 1885. Johnston claimed that its introduction clearly indicated the potency of African plants.[102] From the 1880s drug companies collaborated with African scientists and healers in rural communities in Ghana, Madagascar, and South Africa to transform African medicinal plants into pharmaceuticals. Abena Dove Osseo-Asare has shown how traditional pharmacopoeias were part of the 'simultaneous and overlapping histories' between herbal medicine and pharmaceutical chemistry that 'cross geographic boundaries'.[103]

The draft addendum was sent to all British African colonies in early 1899. Lagos reported that 'the pharmacopoeia suffices at present for the medical needs of the colony', although 'arrangements have been made for district medical officers to report annually on native drugs ... Any useful discovery ... will be reported to the Medical Council'.[104] Basutoland replied that 'the BP of 1898 suffices for the medical and pharmaceutical requirements of this territory'. The colonial surgeon of Sierra Leone considered that the value of the addendum would be great but warned that 'the West Coast of Africa affords neither chemical, pharmaceutical, nor medical opportunities for the investigation of the powerful, the mildly diaphoretic, or the other native drugs'. St Helena expressed 'satisfaction with the BP of 1898 for all medical purposes'.[105]

In South Africa both official and unofficial communications were sent from Cape Colony. The secretary of the Colonial Medical Council in Cape Town reported that 'the question is now engaging earnest attention'.[106] The secretary of the BMA's Eastern Province branch noted that whilst the 1898 BP was considered to 'suffice for most present needs', many South African plants were known to have medicinal value. These were being investigated, locally and in England, with a view to future inclusion in the BP. They would await the final addendum before organizing 'committees for the investigation of certain enumerated indigenous plants of the South African Colonies'.[107] Dr Hewat of the Cape Medical Council suggested six drugs that he thought worthy of official recognition. The *South*

African Medical Journal published several contributions on the subject. The Natal Medical Council reported that sixty Zulu medicines had been sent from the protectorate to England for investigation, but the Transvaal Pharmacy Board noted that 'products indigenous to South Africa – though claiming certain medicinal virtues – had not been sufficiently established to warrant them being extended official recognition'.[108]

The call for comments received an equally enthusiastic response from medical officers in the Eastern colonies. In Ceylon, Dr Van Dort reviewed virtually every drug in the draft addendum.[109] Most were already in common use among the local population: 'With few exceptions the drugs are well known in this island, are of great repute, and largely used in native practice ... European practitioners testify to ... their fitness to supersede ... the various official European drugs for which they have been proposed as equivalents ... Nearly all are indigenous'.[110] In addition to those listed 'many other indigenous drugs have reputation in Ceylon'. He used three of them himself. Attfield requested that he 'obtain details concerning the best pharmaceutical forms of these or other Sinhalese or Tamil drugs used by the Vederales, or native doctors, and obtain any further general medical opinions from European practitioners that would be likely to be useful'.[111] The BMA's Ceylon branch asked its members for their opinions on the three drugs along with all those listed in the draft. They acknowledged 'the services rendered by the pharmacists who had prepared fluid extracts and tinctures of the drugs for the Committee'.[112]

There was often little expectation that items suggested would replace ones already in the BP. 'Even if the native drugs of proven efficacy are never likely to supersede the official drugs of the BP, the importance of being able to substitute the former for the latter in remote villages, where European drugs are not always available, or in dispensary practice as a measure of economy, does not seem to have been recognized hitherto in its proper light'.[113] They recognized 'the importance of a systematic and experimental study of native drugs from a strictly medical as well as commercial point of view'.[114] They proposed that a central research committee be created to assist the GMC in producing 'an Imperial Pharmacopoeia'.

The principal civil medical officer in Singapore reported 'the universal opinion to be that the BP of 1898 suffices for the medical and pharmaceutical requirements of this colony'.[115] Doctors and pharmacists received most of their texts from India.[116] A number of suggestions for additions had been sent from Hong Kong in 1894 following the earlier request; all were included in the BP 1898. Medical officers reviewing the drugs included in the draft addendum confirmed that – if they were all made official – the requirements of the colony would be fully met. So, too, did those in Labuan, Mauritius, and the Seychelles.[117]

In Australia the request for comments on the draft was relayed by the premier, George Turner.[118] Colonies reported separately, with both doctors and pharmacists consulted. The BMA's Victoria branch made recommendations in conjunction with representatives of pharmacy organizations. The list was compiled 'under medical advice and responsibility, but with the concurrence of authorities in pharmacy'.[119] It included items that had been proposed in 1894 but not accepted. They requested 'use of Botany Bay Kino in the Australasian parts of the Empire', as it 'had the same character and properties' of the official kino.[120] *Grindelia robusta* was recommended for inclusion by the Queensland authorities.[121] *Aconitum napellus*, cultivated in Victoria, corresponded to that in Britain, and fennel grown in Victoria was the same as the official one. The *Chemist and Druggist of Australasia* reprinted the Queensland and Victoria sections along with the preface, and investigated how often BP drugs and preparations were used in pharmacies. Paragraphs from the Addendum were also reprinted in the *Australasian Journal of Pharmacy*.[122]

The GMC Pharmacopoeia Committee commented on the relative importance to be attached to medical and pharmaceutical contributions. 'Pharmaceutical data, although valuable when considering whether or not to exclude an old drug, was of less value when the question related to the inclusion of a new drug'. They considered introduction to be 'a medical matter and necessarily antecedent to the general employment of the drug'. In New South Wales the Eastern Suburbs Medical Association strongly supported 'the proposed complete imperialization – sooner or later – of the BP on the lines now being followed'.[123] The New South Wales Pharmaceutical Society appointed a committee to review it.[124] The drugs used in the Australasian colonies were very similar to those used in Britain. The *Chemist and Druggist of Australasia* declared that 'One of the most striking features of the practice of pharmacy in Australia is the very small variation from the practice of the Old Country ... the climatic conditions do not differ very greatly'.[125] In South Australia the local

INDIAN AND COLONIAL ADDENDUM
TO THE
BRITISH PHARMACOPŒIA
1898

PUBLISHED UNDER THE DIRECTION OF

THE GENERAL COUNCIL OF
MEDICAL EDUCATION AND REGISTRATION
OF THE UNITED KINGDOM

PURSUANT TO THE ACTS
XXI & XXII VICTORIA CAP. XC (1858)
AND XXV & XXVI VICTORIA CAP. XCI (1862)

1900

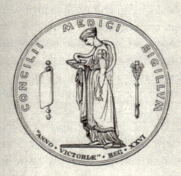

Printed and published for the Medical Council
BY
SPOTTISWOODE & CO. LTD., GRACECHURCH STREET, LONDON, ENGLAND
1900

Figure 7.2 *Indian and Colonial Addendum to the British Pharmacopoeia* 1898.

BMA branch and the pharmacy board both confirmed that the BP 1898 'suffices for the medical and pharmaceutical requirements of the province'. The Pharmaceutical Society of Tasmania 'cordially approved' the principle of an ICA 'as we can adapt it to our climatic and other requirements'. It offered to contribute to any fund set up to support research 'on colonial drugs having fairly good local reputation'.[126] The authorities in Western Australia had no suggestions.

In New Zealand medicinal plants had been cultivated for some time. In 1892 the *Lyttleton Times* had reported that the PSGB 'recently communicated with various Domain Boards on the Colony, urging the desirability of the cultivation of plants for medicinal purposes'.[127] The Auckland, Christchurch, and Dunedin boards expressed their willingness to cooperate, and the secretary of the Patea Domain Board agreed to provide information. Mr B.E. Armstrong sent the PSGB a list of over one hundred medicinal plants grown in the Christchurch Botanic Gardens; the draft addendum included some of them. It had been reviewed by 'the New Zealand Branch of the BMA, the Otago Pharmaceutical Association, and the New Zealand Pharmacy Board'.[128] The board referred it to the Central Pharmaceutical Association, as the matter of the addendum was outside its remit.

The most detailed response from Australasia came from the chief medical officer of the Fiji Islands. He strongly recommended the addition of *Piper methysticum*, or kava root (known locally as *yaqona*). Twelve pounds were sent to the GMC's office in London for examination. He also supported the inclusion of arachis oil, which had been 'used with satisfaction for the past ten years, in place of olive oil, at the hospital and other government institutions'.[129] The GMC Pharmacopoeia Committee noted that 'except British New Guinea, the ten Australasian colonies have all replied'.[130]

PUBLICATION OF THE *ICA*

By spring 1900 responses had been received from virtually every British colony. Attfield reported that by November 1899 'fifty-three of Her Majesty's seventy Dependencies had supported the broad principle of imperialization of the Pharmacopoeia', and by May 1900 'an additional fourteen have since expressed satisfaction with the already largely imperialized *British Pharmacopoeia* of 1898'.[131] Only New Guinea, the Bechuanaland Protectorate, and St Christopher and Nevis had failed to respond.[132]

Table 7.1
Drugs in the *Indian and Colonial Addendum* official in colonies besides India and Eastern Division

Latin name	Other name	India	Eastern colonies	Australasian	North American	West Indies	Mediterranean	African colonies
Agropyrum	*Agropyrum repens*	–	yes	yes	yes	–	–	–
Alstonia	*Alstonia scholaris*	yes	yes	yes	–	–	–	–
Arnica flores	*Arnica montana*	–	–	–	yes	–	–	–
Catechu nigrum	Black catechu	yes	yes	–	yes	–	–	–
Cucurbitae semina	Melon pumpkin seeds	–	–	–	–	–	yes	–
Datura folia	Datura leaves	yes	yes	–	–	yes	–	–
Datura semina	Datura seeds	yes	yes	–	–	no (leaves only)	–	–
Gossypii radicis cortex	Cotton root bark	yes	yes	–	yes	yes	–	–
Grindelia	*Grindelia aquarosa*	–	–	yes	yes	–	–	–
Hirudo Australis	5-striped leech	–	–	yes	–	–	–	–
Kavae rhizoma	*Piper methysticum*	–	–	yes	–	–	–	–
Kino ucalypi	Botany Bay kino	–	–	yes	–	–	–	–
Mylabris	*Mylabris phalerata*	yes	yes	–	–	–	–	yes
Oleum arachis	*Arachis hypogoea*	yes	yes	yes	–	–	–	yes
Oleum gaultheriae	Oil of wintergreen	–	–	–	yes	–	–	–
Oleum graminis citrati	Oil of lemongrass	yes	yes	–	–	yes	–	–
Oleum sesami	*Sesamum indicum*	yes	yes	–	yes	–	–	yes
Oliveri cortex	*Cinnamomum oliveri*	–	–	yes	–	–	–	–
Turpethum	*Ipomoea turpethum*	yes	yes	–	yes	–	–	–
Viburnum	Black haw	–	–	–	yes	–	–	–
	TOTAL	10	11	8	9	3	1	3

Source: Adapted from *Indian and Colonial Addendum to the British Pharmacopoeia 1898* (London: General Council of Medical Education and Registration of the United Kingdom, 1900), 1–56.

The *Indian and Colonial Addendum* to the BP 1898 was finally published on 30 November 1900; it contained fifty-nine pages (figure 7.2).[133] Of the hundreds of items suggested, fifty-four drugs and sixty-five preparations – all but one of which were made from newly recognized drugs – were made official.[134] The original plan to group items under Indian, Australasian, Eastern, and Canadian sections – where those listed in one section would be official in that section but not others – was considered unworkable. The addendum listed items alphabetically, each medicine and preparation including a statement as to where it was 'official'. Thus, dried arnica flowers were official only in North American colonies, and arachis oil only in India and the African, Eastern, and Australasian colonies. Most were made official only for India and the Eastern colonies. Only 20 were made official for other colonies, and only 9 of them were not official for India and the Eastern colonies (table 7.1). For most colonies it provided few new 'official' medicines; whilst North America gained 9 and Australasia 8, West Indian and African colonies gained only 3 each, and the Mediterranean colonies just 1.

In India the addendum made 'official' oil of wintergreen, melon pumpkin seeds, and other items which were not normally available in India. But this was a tiny proportion of the plant medicines used in India either in indigenous practice or as substitutes for Western medicines.[135] Rachel Berger has pointed out that the 1895 Indigenous Drugs Committee had privileged a few useful Indian drugs, whilst ignoring the knowledge system of Ayervedic medicine. The addendum 'presented medically useful components of Indian agriculture as something that Europeans had stumbled upon, of which Indians had been unaware'.[136] Nandini Bhattacharya has since argued that the inclusion of over fifty Indian drugs suggested that 'while Ayurvedic drugs were incorporated within the BP, their usage by western practitioners was tolerated within limits'.[137] Not all were Indian substitutes for Western medicines; some were novel contributions to Western medicine and pharmacy.

Although official the BP and its addenda were not usually statutory. The extent to which they were complied with depended on the existence of local laws and their enforcement. In India the repeated failure to pass a local version of the British Pharmacy and Poisons Act of 1868 meant that there was no effective drug regulation anywhere. Legislative priorities lay elsewhere, although some laws did have a bearing on the medicines trade. The intentional adulteration of a drug or the sale of a drug 'not of the nature, quality or substance demanded by the purchaser' could be prosecuted under certain sections of the Indian Penal Code; an Opium Act in 1878 dealt with poppy cultivation and the manufacture, import, export, sale, and possession of opium; the Indian Merchandise Marks Act of 1889 provided a check on misbranding, false marketing, and trade description; and the Sea Customs Act of 1878 prohibited goods with false descriptions from being brought into India. The latter act, along with an Indian Tariff Act of 1894, provided for the levying of import and export duties on a wide range of goods including drugs, chemicals, and medicines.[138] Yet there was widespread flouting of the rules; enforcement was weak and prosecutions few. Pharmacopoeias that were official but not statutory stood little chance of being fully complied with, since it was very unlikely that anyone not complying with the BP or its addenda would find themselves in court.

CONCLUSION

The need to review the large number of suggestions that had been generated by the consultation exercise meant that the 1898 BP itself was not the 'imperial pharmacopoeia' originally intended. The decision to publish an addendum in 1900 was a pragmatic response, but the efficacy of many of the drugs included was not subjected to the rigorous testing that some demanded. They were included largely because medical officers in India and elsewhere had endorsed their virtues, and the GMC Pharmacopoeia Committee was committed to the production of an imperial pharmacopoeia. Consensus among the imperial medical community was prioritized to keep the project alive. But the competing forces of science, trade, politics, and custom had been resolved to few people's satisfaction.

Important issues including religious sensibilities had been overlooked. Hog's lard was included as an ingredient in some preparations; others included beef suet. In March 1901 six copies of the addendum were sent to the Government of India.[139] A week later they were to be withdrawn, as the presence of lard had been noted. Army regulations forbade the use of hog's lard and beef suet in the manufacture of ointments, as pork products were forbidden to Muslims, and the cow was sacred to Hindus.[140] Mutton suet from sheep was specified as a substitute. A *Government of India Edition* of the addendum was published in 1901, incorporating the necessary changes.[141]

Towards an Imperial Pharmacopoeia 175

Arachis or sesame oil could be used instead of olive oil in making soap, and adjustments were made to the compositions of various plasters and ointments.[142] With the amendments agreed, 3,500 copies were printed and dispatched in March 1902.[143] But the issue of substitution of medicines with local alternatives had barely been addressed. The arguments would resurface when items included in the addendum needed to be incorporated into the main body of the *BP*.

8

From Colonial Addendum to Imperial Pharmacopoeia

At the start of the twentieth century medicines and their preparations were official by virtue of their inclusion in the *British Pharmacopoeia* (BP) 1898, its 1900 *Indian and Colonial Addendum* (ICA), or the 1901 *Government of India Edition*. They received a mixed reaction in Dominions and colonies, and compliance was usually poor as this depended on the passage and implementation of relevant legislation locally. Yet the early 1900s saw the passage of drug legislation in many countries; dominant models of drug regulation were shifting from consumer sovereignty to bureaucratic regulation at the national level. At the same time engagement with all parts of the empire by the Pharmacopoeia Committee of the General Medical Council (GMC) in compiling the pharmacopoeia had raised expectations; disappointment with it led several Dominions to prepare their own publications.

This chapter explores developments between publication of the ICA in 1901 and the appointment of a committee of inquiry in 1925 to review all aspects of the pharmacopoeia, including its role in the empire. It was a period that saw the publication of a pharmacopoeia 'suitable for the whole empire' in 1914 – an effort that was, however, interrupted by the First World War. It also witnessed further change in the size and nature of the empire, with rising autonomy in the Dominions and the rise of independence movements elsewhere. It saw growing professionalization of pharmacy in many colonies, major advances in Western medicine (including the discovery of new medicinal substances), the marginalization of plant medicines, the rise of drug regulation embedded in legislation, and the final transition of the pharmacopoeia to a legal standard for the quality and purity of medicines.

From Colonial Addendum to Imperial Pharmacopoeia 177

The chapter considers why the ICA was not well received in India or the Dominions, as well as the actions taken in response to its publication. It describes the efforts made to revise the ICA and explores how the BP and its addenda came to be replaced with a single pharmacopoeia 'suitable for the whole empire'. It asks what impact the outbreak of war had on its use and what the implications were for the future of the BP. It describes, finally, post-war plans for its revision, before examining what led pharmacists to withdraw from work on the pharmacopoeia and to the calls for a committee of inquiry in 1925.

RECEPTION OF THE
ADDENDUM IN THE EMPIRE

The 1901 *Government of India Edition* of the addendum was not well received in India, despite a small number of positive reviews in Indian medical journals.[1] Bhattacharya notes that British officials largely dismissed it as either academic or of purely historical interest.[2] Of the large number of Indian plant medicines originally suggested, only a small proportion had been made official. Yet knowledge and experience with indigenous Indian medicines was extensive.[3] Doctors in India again complained that medicines that could be used as substitutes for items in the BP had not been included in the ICA; the *Indian Medical Gazette* noted that many of the drugs that could be obtained from local markets (the bazaar medicines) were 'in every way efficient substitutes for the better-known drugs of the BP'.[4]

As well as complaints about the limited attention paid to views of indigenous practitioners, there were also criticisms of the consultation process and about the importance that had been attached to British trade and exports. An editorial in the *Indian Medical Gazette* noted that the official Central Indigenous Drugs Committee had not been consulted and that the drugs eventually included had not been approved by it.[5] In 1899 the *Chemist and Druggist* noted that the committee had been appointed by the Indian government to report on native medicines and hoped that it 'might have something that would assist the compilers of the Addendum'. So far 'practically no useful end appears to have been served by the committee'.[6] It was a view shared by many in India, where there were widely differing opinions about the value of native medicines. Western-trained doctors usually demanded evidence based on scientific investigations, but the Indian

178   Pharmacopoeias, Drug Regulation, and Empires

chemist P.C. Ray noted that 'the efficacy of these drugs has been proved beyond doubt by their universal use in the households of Bengal.'[7]

Anil Kumar has noted the central position of trade in discussions about substitution, with 'the colonial interest in India serving as exporter of raw materials and importer of finished products' operating 'quite handsomely in the chemical and pharmaceutical sector.'[8] In the twentieth century India became one of the largest markets for finished products of the chemical industry – particularly medicines – although they made up a diminishing proportion of total trade. Drugs were obtained from wholesale druggists and manufacturers and delivered to a central depot from where they were distributed. As a contemporary observer noted, 'the system is a remnant of bygone days, when there were no wholesale druggists in India, and all drugs had to be obtained from England.'[9] By 1900 a number of wholesale drug firms existed and drug contracts could have been put out to tender.[10] Official channels could be bypassed; medical officers were allowed to purchase small quantities of 'special' remedies locally, and hospital budgets had an allocation for bazaar medicines.[11]

Disappointment with the *ICA* was shared by doctors and pharmacists in the Dominions; many considered that it offered little of relevance to them. Most items they had suggested for inclusion had been rejected. Several Dominions concluded that the time had come to develop their own publications. Pharmacists in Australia had noted Greenish's proposal in 1885 to produce a separate formulary containing items not listed in the *BP*. When a copy of the unofficial formulary compiled by the Pharmaceutical Society of Great Britain (*PSGB*) (included in its 1901 *Yearbook of Pharmacy*) reached Australia, the Dominion decided to publish its own. The initiative was taken by Harry Shillinglaw, secretary of the Victoria Pharmaceutical Society.[12] He was confident that a book of formulas for non-official preparations in general use would 'meet with general approval.'[13] Under his direction an *Australian Pharmaceutical Formulary* (*APF*) was published in 1902; its purpose was 'to counteract the increasing practice by medical men of ordering proprietary articles, the composition and strength of which are alike unknown to the prescriber and dispenser.'

The first edition consisted of twenty-seven pages and included syrups, liquors, mixtures, wines, elixirs, emulsions, and essences. Formulas were largely copied from the *PSGB*'s *Yearbook of Pharmacy*.[14] The *APF* contained no pills, ointments, powders, pastes, pessaries, or plasters – only liquid medicines. A short addendum suggested by the South Australian Pharmaceutical Society contained a liniment and throat spray. Medical practitioners and chemists were asked to avoid the use of 'fancy or coined names which are patented or copyright of any particular firm, such as *Tabloid* for tablet, *Lanoline* for wool fat, *Hazeline* for witch hazel, *Vaseline* for petroleum jelly? Prescribers were asked to mark their prescription APF. The publication was an immediate success. However, the APF did not have the desired effect of reducing the level at which doctors prescribed proprietary medicines.

In March 1904 Sydney chemists appealed directly to doctors through the pages of the *Australian Medical Gazette*. The doctors agreed to sign prescriptions and not simply initial them, to help prevent forgeries. Prescriptions would not use undisclosed private recipes or be written in code; and no prescriptions would be written for proprietary medicines, as this would result in loss of practice for the doctor and loss of business for the chemist.[15] Wherever possible doctors would prescribe either official preparations, those listed in the BP, or non-official items listed in the APF. In the event, very little changed. It was easier to prescribe proprietary products, and there was no noticeable increase in the use of official medicines. In early twentieth-century Australia the BP played little part in prescribing, although pharmacy apprentices still needed to be familiar with its contents in order to pass the PSGB's examinations. As in Britain manufacturers complied with pharmacopoeial standards as a means of demonstrating the quality of their products. Pharmacists often struggled to keep up with the pace of scientific developments. Greg Haines noted of their leaders in Britain that 'Greenish and those who followed him did not appreciate the nature of the revolution which had just begun in science, medicine and pharmaceutical manufacturing.'[16] It was as true of pharmacists across the empire as it was of those in Britain. An enlarged second edition of the APF was published in 1911 with the expanded title *Australasian Pharmaceutical Formulary* under the authority of 'the Combined Pharmaceutical Societies of Australia.'[17]

In New Zealand the BP was viewed as 'the pharmacy Bible' and served as an essential reference in pharmacies alongside other British texts. Pharmacists made constant reference to it to ensure 'that the many preparations made by the pharmacist were uniform in composition and appropriate in presentation.'[18] But it also served as a convenient instrument for controlling the costs of drugs and limiting access to more expensive medicines. In the early 1900s the contract between local Friendly Societies – which provided free medical services to members – and New Zealand pharmacists covered BP items only. Unlisted items were chargeable – an issue that often caused embarrassment when patients did not understand the terms of the contract and were asked to pay.[19]

Canadian pharmacists were disappointed to find that only nine additional items had been made official for North America in the ICA. Although the BP was widely used in Canada, so, too, were the official pharmacopoeias of the United States and France.[20] Pharmacists followed publication of the 1901 British *Yearbook of Pharmacy* and the 1902 *Australian Pharmaceutical Formulary* with interest. The Ontario College of Pharmacy (OCP) established a committee to 'obtain all possible information in regard to unofficial formulae, with the object and intention of compiling a small book of formulae to be authorized and adopted by OCP.'[21] It was sent to all members of both the OCP and the College of Physicians and Surgeons. The first edition of the *Compendium of Canadian Formulary* was published in 1905, comprised twenty-four pages, and listed sixty-eight formulas. A second edition in 1908 was more widely distributed and was adopted as 'an official book of formulas for the Dominion of Canada.' Further editions appeared in 1910, 1915, and 1921. Its copyright was acquired by the Canadian Pharmaceutical Association in 1929 and a sixth edition published in 1933. But its three sections were not of equal status; whilst two were 'official', the third was an 'unofficial compendium of formulas.'[22]

As elsewhere, Canada saw an explosion in the use of patent medicines. At the start of the twentieth century the Canadian Parliament appointed a committee to inquire into the industry. It found that the market included hundreds of secret formula medicines, many of which contained drugs such as cocaine, opium, strychnine, arsenic, and other equally dangerous ones, whilst many were simply alcoholic beverages sold under the guise of medicine.[23] The result was passage of the Proprietary or Patent Medicine Act in 1908. It originally applied only to internal medicines but was later extended to include secret formula preparations for external use.[24] The act defined patent medicines mainly by their absence from official texts; they were items 'the name, composition, or definition of which is not to be found in the BP, the *Codex Medicamentarius* of France, the *United States Pharmacopoeia*, or any pharmacopoeia approved by the Minister, the Canadian Formulary, the National Formulary of the USA ... and approved

From Colonial Addendum to Imperial Pharmacopoeia 181

by the Minister.'[25] They were, however, exempt if the true formula or list of medicinal ingredients was printed on it in a conspicuous manner.

In Newfoundland – as in the other Dominions – British pharmacy texts, including pharmacopoeias, were a vital resource for apprentices, as courses were usually self-taught. Translations and commentaries on the pharmacopoeia were usually of much greater value than the BP itself. Other British texts in use included Alfield's *Chemistry* and *The Art of Dispensing*, although American textbooks were also used, especially Remington's *Science and Practice of Pharmacy*, first published in 1886.[26] The ICA had little impact in the West Indies; only three additional items were made official.[27]

RECEPTION IN THE METROPOLE

The ICA received a half-hearted reception in the metropolitan medical and pharmaceutical press. *The Lancet* considered that it might play a part in welding together the colonies and dependencies by supplying information relating to the modifications of treatment that were frequently necessitated by local conditions.[28] The inclusion of Indian and colonial drugs in an addendum failed to have the impact that inclusion in the main body of the BP would have had. Proponents of imperialization had expected that the addendum would not only include most items used throughout the empire but would also promote their use in Britain. In this it was unsuccessful. David Hooper observed that the drugs and preparations included failed to establish a position in British medicine.[29] Publication also failed to have a unifying effect in British pharmacy practice, given that the BP and ICA excluded a large number of drugs and preparations then in regular use, along with many new dosage forms. This led to a demand for supplementary texts, and several followed hot on the heels of the official publications. The first was Edmund White and John Humphrey's 724-page *Pharmacopedia: A Commentary on the British Pharmacopoeia, 1898*, published in 1901. This made only a brief reference to the ICA, pointing out that certain formulas in the *Government of India Edition* differed from those in the original, and providing detailed notes on each item.[30]

In 1904 William Chattaway at the Society of Apothecaries published a *Digest of Researches and Criticisms Bearing on the Revision of the British Pharmacopoeia 1898*, prepared by direction of the GMC.[31] Chattaway collected and abstracted the published criticisms, research, and suggestions he thought likely to be useful for its revision, most of which were published between 1899 and 1902. Criticisms related mainly to the composition and assay of drugs and galenicals; ones dealing with the botanical features of drugs were remarkably few. He looked particularly for suggestions for the improvement in the manufacture and preservation of official preparations.[32] He proposed the inclusion of refractive index and other physical and optical constants as test methods for oils;[33] optical rotation had first appeared as a purity test in the *United States Pharmacopoeia* in 1890.[34] Chattaway's report was approved in November 1903; both refractive index and optical rotation were subsequently included in the BP.

In the same month the PSGB's Council agreed to produce a more extensive reference work that would include formulas for items not included in pharmacopoeias.[35] In 1907 it launched the *British Pharmaceutical Codex: An Imperial Dispensatory for the Use of Medical Practitioners and Pharmacists* (the BPC) under the authority of its council. This had a broader scope than the BP as it covered all drugs, medicines, and excipients in common use throughout the British Empire.[36] It included dosage forms not listed in the BP such as tablets, capsules, and cachets, along with drugs and medicines listed in the pharmacopoeias of France, Germany, and the United States. It provided an alternative form of official recognition by being published by a pharmaceutical body with statutory recognition rather than having the legal status of the BP. It was aimed at a pharmaceutical rather than a medical audience. The BPC subsequently provided an official home for many plant medicines listed in the *Pharmacopoeia of India* that never found a place in the BP or its appendices.

The dominant model of drug regulation in the metropole transitioned within the occupational control model from medical to pharmaceutical control underpinned by legislation. Whilst the 1868 Pharmacy and Poisons Act had provided some control over a small number of poisons, a new Pharmacy Act in 1908 gave pharmacists additional responsibilities, requiring the purchaser of opiates to be known to the seller, and stipulating that an entry be made in the Poisons Register. But it placed no control over the manufacture or possession of narcotics, and both opium and cocaine were freely available in unregulated quantities without prescription.[37] The task of policing the act was given to the PSGB, although the only real protection against abuse was the professional discretion of the pharmacist.[38] International concerns about the control of addictive substances led to a series of conferences culminating in the 1912

From Colonial Addendum to Imperial Pharmacopoeia 183

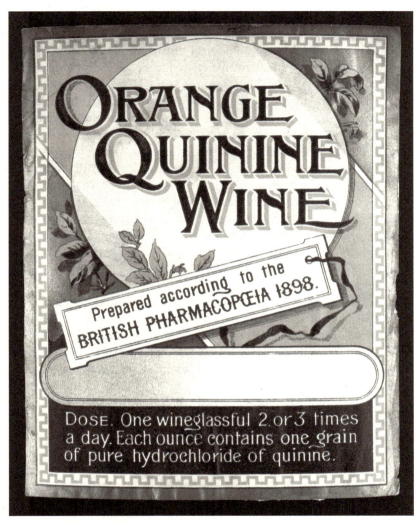

Figure 8.1 Orange quinine wine, prepared according to the *British Pharmacopoeia* 1898.

International Opium Convention at The Hague. Legislation in Britain and its empire was delayed until after the First World War.

Despite its lack of a statutory basis the BP continued to be used in the courts as a guide to the purity of drugs listed within it.[39] Proprietary products directed at the public were advertised as being 'prepared according to the British Pharmacopoeia 1898' (figure 8.1) But by the start of the twentieth century physical and chemical testing was not possible for some drugs then being considered for inclusion; attention moved to the physiological testing of biological materials. In 1909 a pharmaceutical company in Liverpool began submitting drugs to the physiological laboratories at the University of Liverpool for testing.[40] The activity of digoxin, squill, and strophanthus was tested using isolated mammalian hearts; ergot was tested using isolated rabbit uteruses following the description of the test by Moor in 1902.[41] By 1906 the extent of testing required by the BP led to serious concern among retail pharmacists in Britain. They considered that the methods then required such specialized techniques and equipment that the manufacture of galenicals would become the sole province of manufacturing or wholesale companies, diminishing the role of community pharmacists and undermining their businesses.[42] An editorial in the *Pharmaceutical Journal* opposed physiological testing but acknowledged that such methods might have a place 'where galenicals were difficult to make uniform'.[43]

Medicines were an obvious target for states looking for a ready source of revenue. In Britain a stamp duty was first imposed on proprietary or quack medicines in 1783; the tax lasted until 1941.[44] Pharmacopoeias played an important part in debates around the tax from an early date and continued to do so into the twentieth century. Chemists and druggists sought to minimize the range of medicines to which the tax applied, whilst the Board of Customs and Excise sought to minimize exceptions. A Medicine Stamp Act in 1802 had introduced an enlarged schedule of articles that were dutiable.[45] Following a campaign by a London surgeon, William Chamberlaine, provision was made to exclude remedies described as 'known, admitted and approved' from liability to the tax when sold by a qualified surgeon, apothecary, chemist, or druggist.[46] After 1904 the board exempted items where a statement appeared confirming that the medicine had been prepared in accordance with a formula in the BP 'or other well-known and recognized books of reference' by including letters such as BP or BPC.[47]

'Other well-known references' were not defined, and new books of formulas were quickly produced. *Chemist and Druggist* published *Pharmaceutical Formulae* containing nearly seven hundred mixtures for coughs, diarrhoea, and neuralgia.[48] The *Pharmaceutical Journal* began publishing a formulary in which chemists could have the formula of their own particular medicine included, and then claim exemption from the tax if it was widely advertised.[49] By the end of the year the board had told its officers which books were to be considered 'well-known and recognized' for the purpose of tax liability. They included not only the *BP* but also the new *Chemist and Druggist* and *Pharmaceutical Journal* publications. Medicine stamp duty was later considered in 1937 by a Parliamentary Select Committee, which recommended that it should be retained but recast in fresh legislation.[50] After wide discussion the revenue authorities concluded that it should be abolished. In 1938 they recommended that the chancellor of the exchequer 'abandon the duty altogether', which he duly did.[51]

INTERNATIONAL AGREEMENTS

With the 1898 *BP* and its addenda in force across the empire, the GMC considered its next steps. In addition to commissioning White and Humphrey's *Pharmacopedia*,[52] it invited the two pharmaceutical societies to 'cooperate in the necessary enquiries and investigations'. The evidence gathered was considered by a joint conference, which agreed the 'researches necessary with a view to the preparation of the next pharmacopoeia'.[53] Studies were carried out by a chemist, Norman Collie, FRS, and by Henry Greenish (son of Thomas) at the PSGB. Professor Dunstan at Imperial College carried out work on arsenic tests; and Attfield and Chattaway prepared 'digests of researches' in 1900 and 1902.

The compilers of pharmacopoeias increasingly had to take account of international agreements on their standardization. In September 1902 an international conference was held in Brussels 'to consider what steps should be taken to obviate the risks that arise from divergencies in the composition and strength of dangerous medicines as laid down in the various national pharmacopoeias'.[54] It was attended by representatives from the United States, the Government of India, Britain, and seventeen other European governments. Whilst agreeing to the general recommendations, the British government reserved 'the right of introducing into the stipulations ... such modifications in details as the progress of medical and pharmaceutical science may render necessary', and also the right 'of denouncing it with reference to each of the British Colonies or Possessions separately'.[55] Its impact on the next edition of the *BP* would be minimal.

In October 1904 the GMC's Pharmacopoeia Committee considered what was needed to enlarge and improve the *ICA*. A new round of consultations was instigated with practitioners across the empire, again facilitated through the India and Colonial Offices. They were asked what additions, deletions, and other modifications were necessary in revising the *ICA*,[56] although the aim remained the 'ultimate production of a complete Imperial Pharmacopoeia.'[57] In India the request was considered by the Central Indigenous Drugs Committee, but its position remained unchanged; none of the Indian drugs listed had yet 'had that long and careful trial which they thought the drugs should have before judgement is passed on them.'[58] As support for the *ICA* evaporated, support for revision of the *Pharmacopoeia of India* grew stronger.[59] The GMC Pharmacopoeia Committee continued work on revising the *BP* itself. In 1905 it established separate Committees of Reference in Pharmacy, Chemistry, Botany, and several other subjects. In 1906 the Committee of Reference in Pharmacy presented a detailed report on the published criticisms of the 1898 *BP*, with recommendations for changes.[60] A second report a year later recommended general principles that should be adopted in revising the pharmacopoeia. It was followed by one on changes necessary to give effect to the 1906 international agreement,[61] and a progress report on revision work undertaken to date.[62]

In May 1907 the Pharmacopoeia Committee 'decided that the time had come to invite the various medical authorities to furnish their suggestions for a revised pharmacopoeia.'[63] Consultation was carried out on similar lines to previous ones; the three Royal Colleges and other medical bodies in Britain – along with those in the colonies – were asked to comment. A great many reports were received from 'British medical bodies and government authorities outside the United Kingdom, with suggestions for the better adaptation of the *BP* to their local requirements.'[64] In 1908 the Committee of Reference in Pharmacy submitted a report on the frequency with which medicines – both official and non-official – were prescribed in Britain, based on an analysis of 48,000 prescriptions dispensed by pharmacists. By October 1908 it had also submitted two reports listing pharmaceutical revisions required. Some limited laboratory research was also undertaken.

With all the information gathered, the results were tabulated and decisions about the future scope and content of the *BP* and its *ICA* could be made. In October 1909, after careful consideration, the committee made a fundamental decision. The contents of the 1900 addendum – 'or such part as after due revision might be retained' – would be incorporated into the next pharmacopoeia.[65] There would be a single 'imperial pharmacopoeia' and no separate, updated, *Indian and*

Colonial Addendum. The Committee of Reference in Pharmacy submitted further reports on revisions required in 1910 and 1911. Professor Tirard attended an international conference in Paris in 1910 to discuss greater collaboration on developing methods and standards of analysis for food and drugs. The resolutions agreed 'appeared to have a bearing on the analytical portion of the BP' and were referred to the GMC's Pharmacopoeia Committee for consideration. The conflicting aims of imperializing the pharmacopoeia by including plant medicines from the colonies that had not been subjected to detailed testing, and emphasizing its role in setting standards, would be difficult to reconcile.

By 1911 the material gathered was vast, and the Pharmacopoeia Committee began the task of preparing the final text. Professors Tirard and Greenish were appointed as joint editors for the new edition, and Committees of Reference in Chemistry and Botany were appointed 'to give expert assistance in technical matters'. First drafts were ready by June 1912, and work continued throughout 1913. Technical papers by experts on aspects of the BP's contents were submitted, and the Committee of Reference in Pharmacy presented supplementary reports on arsenic tests and ointments.[66] By early 1914 work was complete, and on 13 July 1914 the full GMC Council signed off on the fifth edition of the BP.[67] Two weeks later war broke out; by 4 August it had spread to engulf Germany, France, and Britain, along with their colonial empires. Publication of the BP was postponed to 31 December 1914.

A PHARMACOPOEIA
'SUITABLE FOR THE WHOLE EMPIRE'

The GMC considered that by 'inclusion in the text of such articles as have stood the test of experience' it had now produced a BP 'suitable for the whole Empire'.[68] But it was not a merger of the BP 1898 and its addenda. Although some items included in the ICA were retained, 168 drugs or preparations listed in the BP or the ICA were deleted; most of the deletions were plant medicines indigenous to the colonies.[69] Most of those requested by India were excluded,[70] although some – including berberis, betel, and butea seeds – were retained. Of the 44 new items, almost all were chemical medicines – including adrenaline, barbitone, hexamine, methyl salicylate, and resorcinol.[71] Their monographs included chemical tests for identity and purity; the same was not true of plant medicines, some of which were official for only a short time; *Aristolochia* was included in the 1900 ICA but excluded from the 1914 BP because of concerns about its safety and efficacy. Sumbul root was included in the BP 1864 but deleted from that of 1898 because of limited use.

Most of the BP's appendices were concerned with testing and materials used for testing. Directions for determining specific gravity appeared for the first time.[72] Others described the processes of percolation, re-percolation, and maceration, and how to make lamellae and lozenges. Some accommodation to the needs of empire was made. An appendix described 'alternative processes sanctioned for use in tropical, sub-tropical, and other parts of the British Empire.'[73] It listed bases that could be used in place of ones specified in the BP to improve consistency or avoid fermentation, or where an item was unavailable (dried lemon peel could be used in place of fresh for example). Instructions were usually colony- or region-specific and items were included with conditions. Thus 'in India, and in the Eastern, African, Australasian, and North American Divisions of the Empire, Arachis oil or Sesami Oil – but no other oil or fat – may be employed in making the official liniments, plasters, ointments, and soaps for which Olive Oil is directed to be used.'[74] Likewise 'in India and the Eastern Divisions of the Empire, Butea Gum may be employed in making the official preparations for which Kino ... is used.'[75]

In Britain, the new BP had been eagerly anticipated. *Chemist and Druggist* reported that it would include 'certain special drugs and variations in galenicals suited for India and the overseas Dependencies.' Discontinuing the addendum emphasized 'the imperial character of the work.'[76] But balancing the many conflicting demands – of empire, international agreements, and scientific progress – was near impossible. *Chemist and Druggist* noted that the principal galenical changes arose from the international agreement, showing that the GMC had endeavoured to conform, but had 'signally failed to make the potent preparations the same in strength as they are [in] Continental Pharmacopoeias.'[77] It was also criticized for not sufficiently reflecting scientific progress. One reviewer concluded that 'the work ... cannot be taken as an index of the progress of this branch of medical science during the past few years.'[78]

In the colonies publication of the new BP was announced in government gazettes. The notice in Hong Kong helpfully included a list 'of some of the important alterations, together with some notes by the

From Colonial Addendum to Imperial Pharmacopoeia 189

Society of Apothecaries', reprinted from the *Pharmaceutical Journal*. There were 'notable alterations in potency', and 'notable changes in nomenclature'.[79] It noted that 'Vinum Xericum' (sherry) 'has now to conform to much stricter tests', a remark that was 'common to many of the drugs and preparations of this pharmacopoeia'.[80] Substances originally introduced under trade names were now listed in the BP, including acetyl salicylic acid, barbitone, and diamorphine. The greater emphasis on chemical medicines and analytical methods was noted, along with the efforts made to adapt the BP to the needs of tropical colonies.[81]

IMPACT OF FIRST WORLD WAR

If the 'imperial British pharmacopoeia' was finally realized in 1914, its influence was short-lived. For the duration of the war Dominions and colonies had little choice but to depend on what was available locally. Anuradha Roy noted that the war brought into focus the 'importance of a country like India being able to supply its own wants. One of the vital requirements of India was drugs'.[82] Anil Kumar observed that 'for the first time it was officially accepted by the Government [of India] that most of the drugs approved by the BP were native to India and exported in large quantities, only to be re-imported in the form of finished medicines'.[83] The government at last considered it not unreasonable that these drugs should be made into medicines where they grew. Private cultivation of medicinal plants was encouraged.[84] It resulted in increased recognition of the value of an Indian pharmacopoeia and the beginning of a new approach to drug manufacture in India.[85]

Compliance with the BP became challenging as attacks on allied shipping led to severe shortages. By late 1914 suggestions for amendments were appearing in the pharmaceutical press. Many of the new chemical medicines were known by German brand names. In December *Chemist and Druggist* published a list of English products that could be substituted for German specialties and that could – it suggested – be sent to all doctors.[86] A table listed BP items imported from Germany and their British equivalents (table 8.1). The war witnessed a rapid expansion of Britain's pharmaceutical manufacturing capacity, one of the largest beneficiaries being Burroughs Wellcome (BW). Arsphenamine, the only effective treatment for syphilis, was marketed as Salvarsan by Hoechst in Germany but was not listed in the BP. In

Table 8.1
Alternatives to products of German origin in BP 1914

German name	Chemical name	BP name
Aspirin	Acetyl salicylic acid	*Acidum acetyl-salicylicum*
Veronal	Diethyl barbituric acid	*Bartitonum*
Betacutaine lactate	Benzamine lactate	*Benzaminae lactas*
Chloralamide	Chloral formamide	*Chloral formamidum*
Heroin hydrochloride	Diacetyl morphine hydrochloride	*Diamorphine hydrochloridum*
Urotropine	Hexamethylene tetramine	*Hexamina*
Diuretin	Theobromine and sodium salicylate	Theobrominae et sodii salicylas

Source: "German specialities," *Chemist and Druggist* 85 no. 1822 (1914): 88.

September 1914 BW applied for the suspension of patents protecting Salvarsan and Neosalvarsan.[87] The company produced its own versions of both, followed by substitutes for other German imports including phenacetin, salicylic acid, and quinine.[88]

With expiry of the patent on aspirin in 1915 BW promoted its Tabloid Aspirin, although it faced increased competition from other companies.[89] The result was a proliferation of unbranded products of variable quality. Some firms used inferior chemicals that did not conform to BP standards or met only minimal requirements. Instances were reported of substitution of the active ingredient with French chalk, sugar, or other diluents.[90] A batch confiscated in North America was found to contain mainly talc and starch and very little salicylic acid.[91] BW's agents were told to emphasize that Tabloid products 'conformed to a standard higher than that of the BP.'[92] Its sales increased by over a quarter to more than £1 million in 1918 whilst its net profits almost doubled.[93] By 1917 Jesse Boot in Nottingham was manufacturing vast quantities of aspirin, phenacetin, and atropine (all BP products) for government, domestic, and overseas buyers. He claimed that he would soon be able to supply the entire British demand for phenacetin.[94] He later obtained permission to adopt the methods given in patents for Bayer's Adalin and Casella's Flavine.[95]

In July 1917 the GMC's Pharmacopoeia Committee withdrew a large number of preparations from the BP because of shortages of sugar and glycerol.[96] Only three official mixtures survived – chalk,

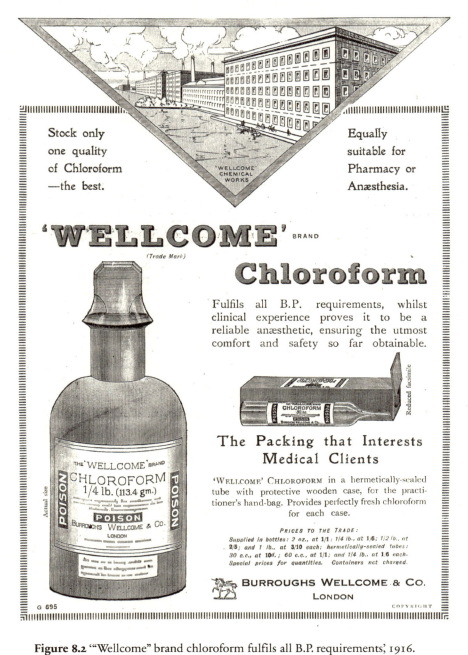

Figure 8.2 '"Wellcome" brand chloroform fulfils all B.P. requirements,' 1916.

compound iron, and castor oil – and only six of the twenty-three official syrups and three of the official lozenges remained. Further amendments were made in 1918, when monographs for a number of products were withdrawn.[97] These allowed the substitution of olive oil with arachis or sesame oil in all parts of the empire – not just those listed in the appendix. Some standards were suspended; an inferior commercial grade of castor oil was allowed to be used in place of the castor oil sanctioned by the BP.

The BP was invoked as the benchmark of quality in discussions around replacing German chemical medicines across the empire. Claiming that drugs met BP requirements became an important feature in their promotion to doctors and pharmacists (figure 8.2). In September 1915 the federal attorney general of Australia declared himself satisfied that 'a sample of aspirin made in Australia was purer than the German product'.[98] He granted a licence to Shmith and Nicholas to manufacture it 'despite the fact that Aspirin was a German trademark.' The conditions of licence would 'ensure that the drug shall comply strictly with the requirements of the BP, and that the conditions of manufacture and price ... shall be satisfactory'.[99] Following tests, the medical profession could be reassured that the Shmith and Nicholas product 'contains no free salicylic acid, and that in all respects complies with the requirements of the BP'. Yet considerable stocks of the German product remained in stores across Australia. The public were asked to not purchase it 'both from patriotic and prudent motives'.[100] But use of the name continued; the *Australasian Journal of Pharmacy* protested that 'Aspirin is a German proprietary name and conveyed no meaning, while Acetyl-salicylum B.P. is a substance of a definite chemical nature, its characters and properties being clearly defined in the Pharmacopoeia'.[101] Alternatives to other German medicines were added to the APF.

Other colonies made similar arrangements. The Transvaal Pharmaceutical Society circulated the non-proprietary names of German medicines so that suitable substitutes could be used. Doctors were asked to substitute sodium for potassium in their prescriptions, as most potassium was imported from Germany. It also encouraged its government to forbid the medicinal use of glycerine 'unless required for preparations of medicines whose formulae were given in the BP'; the glycerine saved 'would release a large supply for the purpose of munitions'.[102] The government did not implement the proposal because of guaranteed supplies from the United States, but the long

From Colonial Addendum to Imperial Pharmacopoeia

list of shortages resulted in soaring prices for many items, including aspirin, Epsom salts, phenacetin, and hexamine.[103] Patients were asked to return empty bottles to suppliers because of glass shortages.[104]

DOCTORS, PHARMACISTS, AND PHARMACOPOEIAS

With the end of the war and improving supplies the legal status of the full text of the BP was reinstated on 30 April 1919.[105] But if the GMC thought that pharmacists would again be willing to assist in preparing a new edition of the pharmacopoeia they were sadly mistaken. The work involved in preparing the 1914 BP had placed a heavy strain on the relationship between the doctors and the pharmacists; the latter felt that pharmacists undertook all the pharmaceutical work whilst doctors took all the credit. All work relating to pharmaceutical preparations – including the development of detailed methods of preparation and the setting of specifications for characteristics and tests – was delegated by the GMC's Pharmacopoeia Committee to the equivalent body of the PSGB. In his evidence to the Macmillan Committee in 1925 Henry Greenish stated that he 'did not know that there was a member of the GMC that was expert in any of those subjects.' He attended their meetings but had no vote. The Committee of Reference in Pharmacy held 105 meetings of about three hours each between 1895 and 1914, with some members travelling from Scotland and receiving no fees or travelling expenses; in contrast, the GMC Pharmacopoeia Committee held a one-hour meeting every six months.[106] The pharmacists had had enough. Yet the doctors rightly pointed out that the legal responsibility for the contents was theirs, and they saw no reason to change. Their position had been spelled out in 1892: 'For the presence of medical and pharmaceutical practitioners on one and the same committee would involve much waste of pharmaceutical time, and, in the present or immediately prospective relations of medical men to chemists and druggists in this country, would probably be found to be impracticable.'[107]

Some attempts were made to ease relations between the two groups. Dr Leech, chairman of the GMC Pharmacopoeia Committee between 1898 and 1900, had instituted regular pharmacopoeia conferences between that committee and representatives of the two pharmaceutical societies. These recommended what research should be carried out by the PSGB's laboratory, although the pharmacists were treated as junior partners. At the British Pharmaceutical Conference meeting in 1910 the president, Francis Ransom, drew attention to the different ways in which the production of national pharmacopoeias was organized in Britain and other countries: 'In nearly every other instance the national pharmacopoeias were revised by commissions on which the pharmacists as well as the medical men were represented ... A more direct recognition of pharmacists in future revisions would be found to embody more fully the results of pharmaceutical research in our national pharmacopoeia'.[108]

Long before work began on revising the BP 1914 the pharmacists had made the doctors fully aware of their feelings about the lack of support and recognition. But each time their pleas and warnings went unheeded. The secretary of the GMC's Pharmacopoeia Committee, Sir Nestor Tirard, later reflected that even before the 1914 BP had been issued the committee had been told by the Pharmaceutical Society that 'under no circumstances would the same facilities be given to us, or the same personnel be allowed to be employed'.[109] Yet the GMC was in no position to carry out the work without pharmaceutical assistance. The result was stalemate; it could only be resolved at a higher level.

MEDICINES AND STATE REVENUES

The post-war need to raise revenue led many colonial governments to revisit the issue of medicine stamp duty. Pharmacopoeial drugs became tools in negotiations, with BP products often exempt from tax. In South Africa the duty became the focus of efforts leading to the formation of a federated national pharmaceutical society. It had been imposed for a short while in the Cape in 1908.[110] The federal government planned to reintroduce it in 1923 – against considerable opposition – with pharmacy representatives lobbying the minister of finance about its implementation. Cape pharmacists concluded that the commissioner of revenue 'intended to push this tax to its limit – indeed, beyond the bounds intended by the Government'.[111] The commissioner argued that labels on items such as cod liver oil indicating their contents, dosage, and intended use were in fact 'cures' and therefore subject to tax. The pharmacists decided to test the issue in the courts.[112]

The list of medicines that would be subject to tax included 1,100 patent and other medicines; use of terms such as 'throat lozenge', 'toothache drops', or 'headache powder' would render the medicine liable to tax. Yet proprietary remedies including Woodward's Gripe

Water and Elliman's Embrocation were exempt. Other anomalies included the taxing of Dutch medicines bearing a bilingual label, whilst those bearing a label only in Dutch were exempt.[113] This angered pharmacists since 'known, admitted and approved' remedies in English – equivalent to the Dutch ones – were not.[114] Over the following months further concessions were agreed. But the editor of *African Chemist and Druggist* pointed out that many of these were mentioned in the BP or BPC and should have been exempt from the tax in the first place.[115] These and others not advertised to the public were later exempted.[116] In the Transvaal the minister agreed to about half the changes, but pharmacists nonetheless continued to seek repeal of the tax. They and those in the Orange Free State agreed to apply stamps to all taxable items, and the Transvaal Pharmaceutical Society urged its members 'not to use the tax as a means of cutting prices'. It was repealed shortly afterwards following a change of government.[117]

The taxing of medicines was also an issue in trade between Britain and India, which included small quantities of patent medicines made in India and exported to Britain. In 1899 British manufacturers complained that stamp duty was not applied to imported medicines, but no action was taken as exports to India greatly exceeded imports.[118] To raise revenue after the war the Government of India appointed a Taxation Committee, which recommended taxing patent and proprietary medicines – whether of local or overseas origin – but not pharmacopoeial ones.[119] Manufacturers, wholesalers, and the retail trade strongly opposed the tax, but the government proceeded anyway.[120] The import duty payable on all items of foreign origin was then 30 per cent, and manufacturers lobbied for its abolition. The issue was subsequently considered by the Drugs Enquiry Committee in 1930; it recommended that every patent or proprietary medicine with a 'secret formula' – whether Indian or imported – should be registered, as they were in Canada under its Proprietary or Patent Medicine Act. False, misleading, or exaggerated claims were prohibited. Imported medicines – but not those manufactured in India – were to carry an additional tax of 20 per cent over and above the existing customs duties.[121] This put a high premium on British medicines.

Agreement was later reached in 1932 at the Imperial Economic Conference in Ottawa to give British exports to India an advantage.[122] A preferential tariff rate of 10 per cent was agreed on a range of products including drugs and medicines.[123] The proportion of the Indian drug trade held by Britain gradually reduced as imports from

Germany, Japan, and the United States increased.[124] Finished patent medicines were usually the most profitable, but large quantities of crude drugs were also imported for use by retail pharmacists, government health facilities, and by the emerging Indian drug industry.[125] Vegetable extracts, powders, pills, pastilles, and ointments were imported on a vast scale, as were morphine and opium preparations and quinine salts extracted from cinchona bark. Many drugs were imported into India and then re-exported; there was a large re-export trade in camphor, originally imported from Japan, Formosa, Hong Kong, and China.[126]

INDIA AND INDIGENOUS MEDICINES

The importance of indigenous medicines to India had been highlighted by wartime shortages. But doubts remained about the efficacy of many of them, and in response to continuing demands the Madras Government commissioned a report on their efficacy in 1921. It was conducted by M.V. Koman, a physician at Madras General Hospital.[127] It was written after extensive consultation with hakims (practitioners of Unani-tibb) and vaids (Ayurvedic practitioners) and was entirely dismissive of almost all indigenous drugs then used in India. The superintendent at Madras General Hospital reported that patients refused to be treated with indigenous drugs and that admissions fell as a result of the trials he was conducting. Koman was unable to find anything either from practitioners or the available texts that provided any useful knowledge or treatment that was not already known to Western medical practitioners: 'in vain have I attempted to find any drug or medicine whose reputed marvellous properties are shrouded in mystery or are not already known'.[128]

Koman's report was picked up by *Chemist and Druggist* in London. It noted that whilst 'it has been constantly urged in Indian medical journals and in pamphlets and other publications that the forests of India are rich in botanicals of medical value ... it was now clear to all that – barring a few commonly used bazaar drugs – unwarranted claims have been made on behalf of the indigenous materia medica, and of the systems of medicine'.[129] For the GMC's Pharmacopoeia Committee, Koman's report provided confirmation of its decision not to include drugs listed in either the *ICA* or the *BP* 1914, and it marked the end of any substantial presence for plant medicines in Western pharmacopoeias. In India demands for the reinstatement of the *Pharmacopoeia of India* continued, and the colonial government came under intense pressure to set up an inquiry into the cultivation, production, import, marketing, and sale of drugs. The Drugs Enquiry Committee was instituted in 1929 and reported in 1931.[130]

CONCLUSION

The BP 1914 represented the ultimate fulfilment of the project to create a British imperial pharmacopoeia. In striking a balance between conflicting roles – as a benchmark of standards for medicines and guide to tests for purity and identity, or a publication 'suitable for the whole empire' by including all drugs and preparations in common use – the GMC's Pharmacopoeia Committee had little choice but to emphasize the former. But it was as much a political as a scientific product; it represented a fusion of disparate metropolitan and colonial interests and opinions, from medicine, pharmacy, and science, to diplomacy, education, and trade. Its geographical range was vast. In emphasizing the importance of both the drug trade and the BP Mann referred to 'the divisions of the British Empire which were to be dosed with the contents of the BP at the time of the outbreak of World War I'.[131] In some ways the 1914 BP was innovative; for example, it was the first to give directions for determining melting points and boiling points.[132] But it also had limitations; biological tests were not included, even for preparations for which it was acknowledged they might be useful.[133]

By the mid-1920s the GMC Pharmacopoeia Committee was confronted with many difficulties. It could not proceed without the cooperation of the pharmacists; international agreements mounted up; and wartime experience had altered patterns of drug use in many colonies. Advances in medical, chemical, and biological sciences had continued apace. Few plant medicines merited places in the pharmacopoeia, despite their continuing role in medical practice in many colonies. But if the Koman Report effectively signalled the end of attempts to imperialize the pharmacopoeia, it also marked the start of its decolonization. Colonies ceased to be beholden to a metropolitan pharmacopoeia and were able to develop their own. Was a pharmacopoeia 'suitable for the whole empire' still necessary or even possible? Only a review of all aspects of the pharmacopoeia would resolve the impasse. In 1925 the government agreed to commission one.

9

A Committee of Inquiry

Whilst the First World War had put the imperial pharmacopoeia project on hold, the return of peace highlighted the challenges of such a project. In Britain the relationship between doctors at the General Medical Council (GMC) and pharmacists at the Pharmaceutical Society of Great Britain (PSGB) had broken down; in India calls for an Indian pharmacopoeia grew ever louder; practitioners in the Dominions came increasingly to rely on their own formularies; and in many colonies greater reliance on Indigenous medicines during wartime had become normalized. Diversity of practice across the empire was increasing rather than decreasing. Colonies passed new legislation on drug regulation, but the status of the *British Pharmacopoeia* (BP) varied. Control of both pharmacopoeial and non-pharmacopoeial medicines became increasingly subject to international agreements rather than imperial ones.

In Britain a Select Committee on Patent Medicine had been convened in 1914 to consider the advertising and sale of patent and proprietary medicines in the light of two reports on 'secret remedies' by the British Medical Association (BMA) in 1909 and 1912.[1] It concluded that drug regulation in Britain lagged behind that elsewhere: 'The existing law is chaotic and has proved inoperative, and ... successful prosecution for fraud in the advertisement and sale of secret remedies is fraught with the greatest difficulty', although the committee added that 'the Public Prosecutor has perhaps not sufficiently tested the powers of the existing law in respect to such cases'. But 'in British Dominions and foreign countries severe legal restrictions exist, and ... there is a tendency still further to strengthen the law against these articles'.[2] Yet the use of pharmacopoeias remained largely outside the law. Post-war legislation in the metropole included a Dangerous

Drugs Act in 1920, which controlled the sale and supply of narcotic drugs,[3] as well as a Therapeutic Substances Act in 1925 regulating the sale and supply of medicines that could not be assessed by chemical means such as vaccines and sera.

The relationship between pharmacopoeias and drug regulation, the role of doctors and pharmacists in their preparation, and their legal status in the empire, converged in the 1920s when the GMC indicated that it was making plans for the next edition of the *BP*. This chapter considers why a committee of inquiry (in fact a subcommittee of the Committee of Civil Research established in 1925) was required to resolve the dispute between the doctors and the pharmacists, and why its remit extended to the whole empire. It draws on the extensive evidence considered by the subcommittee, which asked fundamental questions about the legal status of pharmacopoeias and whether a change in the law was required; whether the *BP* should continue to be 'suitable for the whole empire'; and whether colonies should be able to publish their own. The subcommittee asked what roles doctors and pharmacists should play in the pharmacopoeia's compilation, and what part the empire should play. The answers to these questions would determine the nature and role of the *BP* for decades.

THE REQUEST FROM THE GMC

Although the trigger for the inquiry was the dispute between the doctors and the pharmacists over the role of the two professions in compiling the pharmacopoeia, the pharmacists were not alone in being unhappy with existing arrangements; medical school teachers – a powerful group within the medical community – complained that the GMC ignored expert advice, and wrote to the Medical Research Council about their concerns. 'We understand that a new edition of the *BP* is being prepared by a committee of the GMC. The GMC is not appointed for this purpose mainly and contains among its members few or no experts in materia medica or therapeutics', the letter stated. It conceded that the GMC's Pharmacopoeia Committee had 'generally consulted experts in the past in preparing new editions' but argued that such advice was ignored and that the pharmacopoeia was edited on 'fundamentally wrong principles'.[4] It was a damning indictment of both the workings of the Pharmacopoeia Committee and its arrogance in ignoring the advice offered by outside experts. Readers of the *BP* were led to believe that it was compiled by consensus after taking full account of the best available advice. This was clearly not the case.

The PSGB prepared its response in advance of an approach from the GMC seeking its assistance in preparing the next edition. On 4 November 1925 the PSGB Council resolved that, if a letter inviting its cooperation was received without an invitation to the society to appoint nominees to the Pharmacopoeia Committee, it should be declined.[5] The council then set up a subcommittee to communicate its views to the Privy Council.[6] The anticipated letter arrived two days later. It was signed by Sir Donald MacAlister, by then both chair of the Pharmacopoeia Committee and president of the GMC itself.[7] He had anticipated potential difficulties with the PSGB, and his letter proposed the setting up of two subcommittees reporting to the GMC's Pharmacopoeia Committee. One would deal with medical matters, whilst the other – to be called the Pharmaceutical Advisory Committee – would include three members nominated by the PSGB's Council. It would 'advise on all general pharmaceutical questions submitted to it'. The letter concluded, however, with the statement that the GMC had the legal responsibility for the contents of the pharmacopoeia, and it therefore 'reserves its freedom with regard to the final adoption of the reports, proposals, advice, and suggestions which may be submitted'.[8] It would not be constrained by any advice offered, whether by pharmacists or anyone else.

The PSGB's response was measured but emphatic. Its president, Philip Rowsell, regretted that the modifications suggested 'were not satisfactory'.[9] He enclosed a copy of a letter dated the same day from Sir William Glyn-Jones, the PSGB's secretary, to the lord president of the Privy Council, expressing the PSGB Council's profound dissatisfaction with the conditions governing production of the BP. It was highly critical of the GMC's decisions regarding the pharmacopoeia: 'the intervals between the editions are too long ... In some respects each edition is out of date when it is first published'; and it claimed that 'the work performed in its preparation is adequate in neither quantity nor quality'.[10] The PSGB made it clear that at the very least there should be a pharmacist member on the GMC Pharmacopoeia Committee. After the GMC claimed that there were 'legal difficulties' in arranging for the PSGB to be formally represented the society took legal advice and promptly declared 'that there is no legal obstacle to prevent the granting of the representation for which they ask'.[11] It also informed the GMC of the actions it had asked the Privy Council to consider, specifically the setting up of a departmental committee or 'some other means of inquiry' in order to 'secure the preparation of future editions upon a basis which will result in a pharmacopoeia satisfactory to users – medical and pharmaceutical – throughout the British Empire'.[12]

The Privy Council took up the matter with the GMC, who referred it to its Pharmacopoeia Committee. The committee acted swiftly, calling for a conference to be held on 23 February 1926 and chaired by Sir Donald MacAlister. Some twenty-three delegates from various medical, pharmaceutical, and scientific bodies attended. Many were extremely critical of both the way in which the BP was produced and its current content. The PSGB presented legal opinion questioning the GMC's view that it was a legal necessity for the committee responsible for producing the BP to be entirely medical.[13] The pharmacists argued that if their cooperation was indispensable – as it was conceded to be – then their position should be recognized by giving them a right of participation in the work not just as advisers but as equal partners.[14] The GMC listened to the views expressed and considered its next move. At its meeting on 2 June 1926 it agreed that an independent committee of inquiry should be established. It wrote to the lord president of the Privy Council formally asking him to set up such a committee. No mention was made of the similar request that had been submitted to the Privy Council by the PSGB Council six months earlier.[15]

A CABINET COMMITTEE

The formal mechanism then in place for such an inquiry was for the Privy Council to refer the matter to the Committee of Civil Research. This had been established in June 1925 as a Cabinet committee in a 'dramatic attempt to bring expert scientific attention to critical practical problems during the economic crises of the inter-war years'.[16] It's subcommittees considered problems outside the remit of a single government department. On 29 July 1926 the committee reported the appointment of a subcommittee asked 'to make inquiries, to collect information, to receive evidence, and to make recommendations on the question whether it is desirable to make any – and if so what – alterations in the existing law or practice relating to the preparation or publication of the *British Pharmacopoeia*, and to its adaptation to the requirements of the British Empire'.[17]

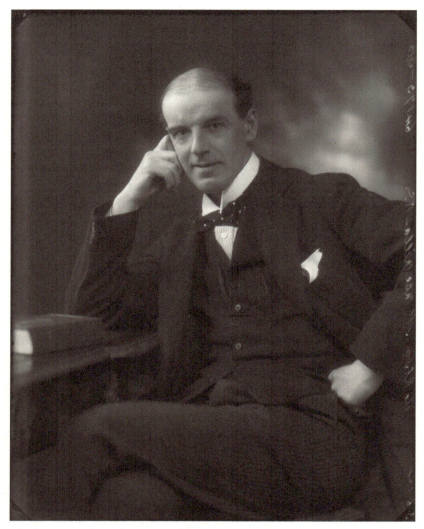

Figure 9.1 Hugh Pattison Macmillan, KC (1873–1952) in 1924.

The subcommittee would be chaired by Hugh Pattison Macmillan, KC, a lawyer who had been appointed lord advocate in Scotland and a member of the Privy Council in 1924 (figure 9.1). It had only five other members. Three were doctors – the president of the GMC (MacAlister); an eminent physician (Lord Dawson); and a representative of the BMA (Dr H.G. Dain). The others were a pharmacologist (Dr, later Sir, Henry Dale), and a past president of the PSGB, Edmund

White. Mr A.F. Hemming, assistant secretary to the Committee of Civil Research, acted as its secretary.

The subcommittee consulted widely, probed deeply, and finally submitted its report in May 1928. The *Report of the Sub-committee on the British Pharmacopoeia of the Committee of Civil Research* (the Macmillan Report) filled fifty-seven pages, a significant proportion of which were devoted to the legal status of the *BP* in Britain, its Dominions, and colonies, and to its adaptation to the needs of the empire.[18] The subcommittee's search for evidence was not limited to Britain and its empire, however; through the Foreign Office it obtained information about the methods employed in the preparation of the national pharmacopoeias of the United States, Germany, France, Holland, Sweden, Italy, Austria, Belgium, Norway, and Switzerland. Between 3 December 1926 and 8 April 1927 some twenty-one witnesses gave evidence in person.[19] The subcommittee heard a catalogue of criticisms about every aspect of the pharmacopoeia, but especially its content, purpose, and method of compilation.

The subcommittee received extensive written evidence from medical, pharmaceutical, and scientific bodies in the metropole, almost all of which was highly critical of both the existing arrangements for its compilation and the relevance of its current content.[20] Many important drugs (mainly chemical) had not yet been added; many older drugs in regular use were excluded; its contents lagged far behind best medical practice in the metropole; it was considered inferior to the pharmacopoeias of other countries, especially that of the United States; many of the standards included were inadequate in order to guarantee effectiveness; some of the standards were so poor as to be potentially dangerous; and there were no standards at all for biological products.[21] The *BP* played little part in the everyday practice of metropolitan practitioners. Several medical witnesses reported that they consulted it to check the officially recognized drugs that they needed to teach their students, but that they otherwise did not use it themselves. For information about drugs in circulation they referred to other handbooks such as Martindale's *Extra Pharmacopoeia* or Squire's *Companion to the British Pharmacopoeia*.[22] Its use was largely limited to pharmacists making up prescriptions for *BP* preparations, and to manufacturers making and selling *BP* products.

Dominion governments were asked to solicit opinions from medical and pharmaceutical bodies, including whether they had 'any suggestions to offer regarding their representation on any body that might be created for the purpose of undertaking future revisions of the BP'.[23] The BMA also asked its branches in the countries concerned to make inquiries of its members. The subcommittee received 'expressions of professional opinion' from Canada, Australia, and South Africa. In the case of India, it noted that 'we have derived our information chiefly through branches of the [British Medical] Association there'.[24] There was widespread engagement with the questions put, including whether drugs used only in colonies should be integrated into the BP, included as an appendix, or published as an addendum, and whether colonial supplements should be allowed, as well as the extent of empire representation on metropolitan committees. Evidence received from governments, medical and pharmaceutical bodies, and individuals was extensive and wide-ranging.[25]

PURPOSE AND LEGAL STATUS

The shifting nature of official pharmacopoeias over time was fully recognized by the subcommittee. Early pharmacopoeias were 'little more than descriptive lists of medicines in use by the profession, and their compilation was generally the work of medical men'. By contrast a modern pharmacopoeia 'must contain not only a carefully scrutinized list of current drugs of repute, but also authoritative standards whereby the purity and efficacy of these drugs may be tested'.[26] The subcommittee concluded that many of the criticisms of the BP were the result of misconceptions about its purpose: 'It is not designed to be a manual of therapeutics to be consulted by the physician in his daily practice. For the physician its function is that of a guarantee that when he prescribes a drug mentioned in the BP, he can rely on his patient obtaining an article of the quality and character therein defined. To the dispenser ... it is actually a manual of practice. He must dispense according to the standard of the BP any medicament contained in it which is mentioned in the prescription'.[27] It was, then, both a medical and pharmaceutical publication.

The subcommittee examined the legal basis of the BP in Britain and the empire in great detail. It noted that in 1858 three pharmacopoeias were in use and that their legal status varied; but 'there has been no subsequent legislation dealing generally with the legal status of the BP'.[28] When it was published in 1864 the legal position of the BP differed materially in England, Scotland, and Ireland. Its official nature was enshrined in law in the 1858 Medical Act, which required the

GMC to 'cause [such a publication] to be published'; but its statutory nature only extended to its production, not to its compliance in practice. Once published its legal position was less clear. The subcommittee did find references to it 'in a number of enactments which confer statutory recognition upon it for certain purposes'. Thus the 1868 Pharmacy Act provided that 'any person ... who shall compound any medicines of the *British Pharmacopoeia* except according to the formularies of the said pharmacopoeia shall, for every such offence, be liable to pay a penalty or sum of five pounds'. Similar provisions were included in Pharmacy Acts in Ireland (1875) and Northern Ireland (1925). Responsibility for policing it resided with the PSGB. The 1868 act had been used as the basis for ordinances and legislation across the empire.[29] But the subcommittee could find 'no instance of its enforcement' anywhere in Britain's overseas possessions. Its terms were 'so indefinite as to render it of little or no use'.[30]

In the metropole 'the most important modern legislation relating to the purity of medicaments is contained in the 1875 Food and Drugs Act'. Public analysts used the pharmacopoeia as 'an unofficial book of standards which has been accepted by the High Court to test whether a particular drug is of the nature, substance and quality demanded'.[31] Yet it had no legal status. 'The policy of the legislature', the subcommittee noted, 'has been not to enact or adopt any standards of quality as regards drugs, but in general terms to require under penalties that "no person shall sell to the prejudice of the purchaser any ... drug which is not of the nature, substance and quality of the article demanded by such purchaser."'[32] The acts' purpose had not been to establish standards for the quality of drugs. The BP was not mentioned in them, but the Courts decided that if a drug listed in it was supplied by a chemist and druggist but was not of the standard required, then an offence had been committed.

The working of the Food and Drug Act was reviewed by a Parliamentary Select Committee in 1878–79. It noted that the court of reference for all disputed cases of analysis was the Department of Inland Revenue's laboratory. Its head, James Bell, declared that making the BP the official standard under the acts would be 'very difficult to carry out', since 'in the preparation of many compounds you cannot in practice get the article of the exact composition laid down in the BP'.[33] To do so would mean prosecution for the slightest deviation from the pharmacopoeia. Although his view ultimately prevailed it was opposed by government officials who pressed for sections of the 1868

206 Pharmacopoeias, Drug Regulation, and Empires

Pharmacy Act to be incorporated in food and drugs legislation.[34] The subcommittee noted that the standards laid down in the BP were not absolute; several items had non-medicinal uses, so the purchaser's intended purpose had to be taken into account. They suggested that different standards might be appropriate for some articles. Sherry was included, but 'the housewife who purchases what is euphemistically called cooking sherry from her grocer is certainly not thinking of the BP ... The truth is', the subcommittee concluded, 'that the BP is not primarily designed to serve the purposes of a prosecutor under the Food and Drugs Act ... It affords a useful and reliable general standard for the articles it includes, but it has not always the precision necessary to found a prosecution.'[35]

The legal foundation of the BP was slight and highly fragmented. Responsibility for ensuring its production fell to the GMC under the 1858 Medical Act; that for ensuring that the drugs listed were supplied only in the form of its preparations to the PSGB, under the 1868 Pharmacy Act; but that for ensuring medicine quality remained outside the legal framework – although for drugs listed in it, BP standards were usually accepted by the courts under the 1875 Food and Drugs Act. The reason for the government's failure to make the BP statutory was its adherence to a laissez-faire policy. Finding a clear definition of drug adulteration eluded the authorities. Although the 1875 act gave a vague definition of 'drug' it had avoided the term 'adulteration' altogether.[36] Early efforts to do so had stressed 'deleterious' rather than 'fraudulent' adulteration, with the focus being on the intent and knowledge of the manufacturer and vendor and the expectations of the purchaser. For preparations not listed in the BP no standard existed.[37]

LEGAL STATUS OF *BP* ACROSS THE EMPIRE

The BP's legal position in the metropole was replicated across much of the empire. Macmillan did 'not profess to have been able to ascertain the state of the law in every part of the Empire outside the United Kingdom', but had nonetheless been able to 'gather together a sufficiently representative collection of enactments'; the situations in Canada, Australia, South Africa, and New Zealand were considered. The subcommittee found considerable variation. The Canadian legislature had gone much further than had the British government in conferring full statutory authority. The 1920 Dominion Food and

Drug Act stipulated that 'Every drug shall be deemed to be adulterated within the meaning of this Act if its strength, quality, or purity falls below the professed standard under which it is sold: or if – when offered or exposed for sale under or by a name recognized in the latest edition of the BP [or several other publications] – it differs from the standard of strength, quality, or purity laid down therein'.[38] Where a drug was judged by an authority other than the BP, it would still 'be deemed to be adulterated unless it conforms to the standard of strength, quality, and purity for such drugs as these are defined by the latest edition of the BP'.

Canadian provinces passed their own acts giving the BP legal status. Ontario's 1914 Pharmacy Act stated that 'unless the label distinctly shows that the compound is prepared according to another formula, every compound named in the BP shall be prepared according to the formula directed in the latest edition ... '.[39] But it would operate only 'until the College of Physicians and Surgeons of Ontario selects another standard'. Manitoba gave the BP legal status through amendments to its 1914 Pharmaceutical Act. It was similar to the Ontario one, although any changes to formulas would be decided by pharmacists alone. 'All compounds mentioned in the BP shall be prepared according to the formula directed in the latest edition ... unless the [Pharmaceutical] Association shall select another standard, or unless the label distinctly shows that the compound is prepared according to another formula'.[40] The subcommittee noted pointedly that 'the selection of the standard is confided in Ontario to a medical body, and in Manitoba to a pharmaceutical body'.[41]

In Australia, legal recognition of the BP was provided for in state rather than Commonwealth legislation, although the 1906 Commonwealth Trade Descriptions Act covered medicines and medicinal preparations. The governor of Victoria reported that 'each state at present, under state laws, has full power and control over the pharmacopoeia within state boundaries, i.e., BP standards may be altered or modified under the various Health Acts; and the BP requires to be adopted formally by each state under the Medical Acts'.[42] Arrangements for inspection, offences, prosecution, and penalties were spelled out in regulations. The BP was one of several references cited; for items not named in the regulations the instruction was to 'set out the name most commonly applied to the substance in the English language in the pharmacopoeias of Great Britain and the United States of America, or in the *British Pharmaceutical Codex*, or other recognized authority.'[43] But this related to *bp* nomenclature, not to standards of purity.

The *bp* received full statutory recognition in Victoria and Queensland. In Victoria a 1915 Medical Act stated that the *bp* 1914 'shall be the pharmacopoeia in force in Victoria as a uniform guide and standard in the preparation of medicines ... together with the true weights and measures of which they are to be prepared and mixed.' It also allowed for any future edition to be 'substituted for the *bp* theretofore in force.' A Victoria Health Act in 1915 adopted parts of the United Kingdom's 1875 Food and Drugs Act and authorized the fixing of standards by regulation. Similar arrangements were enacted in Queensland through a specific British Pharmacopoeia Adopting Act in 1898. In South Australia regulations were made under the 1908 Food and Drugs Act, which held that drugs listed in the *bp* must 'conform with descriptions and tests prescribed for them in the said pharmacopoeia.' The act authorized the substitution of olive or arachis oil by cottonseed oil and the use of Australian wine: 'In a preparation where wine is used as specified in the standard, it shall not be deemed to be adulterated in so far as it is compounded with wine ... of Australian origin', provided it contained at least 28 per cent proof spirit.[44]

Western Australia enacted legislation about the labelling of drugs through its Food and Drug Acts 1913–14. In New South Wales, the *bp* was referenced in the 1908 Pure Food Act; any drug sold under a name included in the *bp* but did not comply with the relevant *bp* description and tests would 'be deemed to be a drug which is not of the substance of the drug demanded by the purchaser.' New South Wales gave authority to the *bp* in pharmacy education. Its 1921 Pharmacy Regulations required that 'every candidate must be able to recognize the various articles enumerated by the *bp*, and explain the processes by which they are preserved; also to describe the composition of such as are compounded and give the proportion of the active ingredients.' The subcommittee noted that 'a regulation similar to this is understood to be in force in other parts of the Empire.'[45]

In South Africa the *bp* was adopted as a legal standard in the Cape of Good Hope, Orange River Colony, the Transvaal, and Natal. In the Cape the 1899 Medical and Pharmacy Act Amendment Act required that 'all chemists and druggists shall prepare their medicines according to the *bp* unless otherwise directed.' But provision was made for local variation; the governor was authorized 'to determine what edition of the *bp* shall be used', and to agree 'such alterations in the preparations mentioned therein as may be found necessary to meet the special climatic conditions of this Colony'. Similar arrangements applied in the Orange Free State and the Transvaal, but Natal went further; its 1899 act required 'the standard of strength and purity of all drugs prescribed by a medical practitioner to be that of the BP'. In New Zealand, the word 'drug' was defined in the 1908 Pharmacy Act as 'any medicine or compound included in the BP'. Under the 1908 Food and Drugs Act the governor was empowered to make regulations prescribing 'the standard by strength, weight, quality, or quantity of any drug or of any ingredient or component part thereof'.[46]

Dominions had considerable discretion in adapting metropolitan regulations to local circumstances. The governor general of Canada confirmed that 'under the Food and Drugs Act of Canada, the Proprietary or Patent Medicine Act, and other Acts, the BP becomes the primary authority for the purity of drugs, and consequently, not only all physicians and pharmacists, but also all persons in Canada, are affected by any changes made in the pharmacopoeia'.[47] The subcommittee noted that, for the Dominions, 'in effect, an alteration in the Pharmacopoeia amounts to an alteration of their law'.[48]

MEDICINES LEGISLATION IN INDIA

Although drug regulation in India was largely non-existent before the First World War, some legislation was passed afterwards. A Poisons Act in 1919 regulated the importation, possession, and sale of poisons by the issue of licences to vendors.[49] Legislation was passed to authorize the inspection of premises. The 1924 Cantonment Act empowered authorities to enter any shop or place and seize any article of medicine found to be adulterated, or that differed from what it was presented as being.[50] But this arrangement related mainly to European enclaves; no attempt was made to regulate the quality of drugs sold at bazaars, where most drug transactions took place. The British authorities avoided interference in traditional and established practices as this was likely to cause unrest. There was in any case a porous interface between indigenous and European practice, and many drugs moved freely between the two.[51] Medical officers had little interest in drug regulation, despite concerns over adulteration. Most were more concerned with which items they were able to use than with standardizing their quality. They saw the contents of pharmacopoeias more as 'descriptive lists of medicines in use by the profession' than as sets of 'standards whereby the purity and efficacy of drugs may be tested'.[52] Demands for a separate Indian pharmacopoeia continued.

The subcommittee reviewed the legal status of the *Bengal Pharmacopoeia* and *Pharmacopoeia of India*, as well as that of the BP and the *Indian and Colonial Addendum*. In 1891 the India Office had told the GMC that although the 1858 Medical Act had not been made applicable to India, 'as far as the preparation of compound medicines is concerned, the formulae laid down in the BP are invariably followed by the Government Medical Stores Department, as well as by private chemists and druggists'.[53] But dissatisfaction with the BP was as strong in India as it was in Britain. The BMA's Bombay branch largely agreed with proposals submitted in London. There was strong support for keeping drugs used in India separate from the main text. For future editions it was recommended that a local committee of experts – both pharmacological and pharmaceutical – be appointed by the Government of India to investigate and prepare a list of Indian indigenous drugs 'used successfully in common practice in India'. Such drugs should be included in a separate volume or addendum.[54] The Hyderabad branch of the BMA also wished to see preparations used in different parts of India – and in other parts of the empire – included in a separate volume. It claimed that doing so would reduce the size of the main volume and allow the list of additional drugs to be more readily amended.[55] As Bhattacharya notes, demands for an Indian pharmacopoeia persisted throughout the late nineteenth and early twentieth centuries in the subcontinent – demands that had substantial political and economic consequences.[56]

EVIDENCE FROM CANADA

Canada submitted extensive evidence. Separate submissions were made by the Canadian Medical Association (CMA) and the Canadian Pharmaceutical Association (CPA), together with a joint memorandum from both bodies to the Canadian minister of health, and further information provided by the Canadian branch of the BMA. A joint committee of the CMA and the CPA had been convened in 1925.[57] The CMA confirmed that the BP had become the standard of purity, quality, and nomenclature in Canada, and was incorporated in various Dominion and provincial acts. However, it drew attention to a consequence of the introduction into the 1914 BP of items considered suitable only for some parts of the empire. The result had been that 'pharmacists and physicians and students are ... required to familiarize themselves with many drugs which they will never have occasion to use'. Moreover, 'drugs intended for use elsewhere in the Empire as a substitute for others well known and commonly used in Canada are thus rendered available as ingredients of proprietary mixtures'. They were then 'liable to become the source of fraudulent misrepresentation by enabling the proprietor to advertise that the drug is a new and important remedy recently introduced in the BP'.[58]

The CPA was highly critical of the existing revision body, particularly its lack of imperial representation. In order to 'have an effective voice in the preparation of future editions' it pressed for direct Canadian representation on 'any body which may be created for the purpose'. This could be achieved, it was suggested, by the CMA and the CPA each appointing two or three representatives to serve on the revision committee, which could appoint specialist subcommittees to carry out the detailed work. Canada could be represented on these by corresponding members. The association thought that any part of the empire wishing to do so should be free to issue addenda containing drugs of local application for use in its own territory. Finally, it felt that a permanent pharmacopoeia secretariat should be established.[59]

The CPA's recommendations closely followed those of the CMA, although these went further by suggesting that each Dominion should establish a standing committee to deal with revision, and that each should be in correspondence with the proposed central committee in Britain to which they would send recommendations. The standing committee should include representatives appointed by the CPA, the CMA, and the Government of Canada. In a joint memorandum the two associations made a further suggestion: 'if the BP is to be an Imperial Pharmacopoeia' it was desirable that 'its preparation should be entrusted to a body summoned ... by the Privy Council which should be representative of the physicians, pharmacists, and Governments of each of the constituent parts of the Empire'. This would be a very large body, and it should 'work through sub-committees and a permanent staff, very much on the lines adopted in the preparation of the US [pharmacopoeia]'. The BP should not include drugs of only local application, and each Dominion should be free to publish addenda containing 'such drugs as are peculiar to their territories, or such modifications of preparations as are necessitated by the character of the climate'.[60] They also urged the dominion minister to give official recognition to the Canadian committee appointed to suggest amendments.

The Dominion Council of Health fully supported the proposals. 'Canada should have representation upon the Committee of Revision,' it declared. But the differences in the views of doctors and pharmacists were noted with concern by the subcommittee, which attempted to establish whether a unified Canadian approach might be possible. If it was difficult to obtain consensus within one Dominion, it would be much more so to achieve it between several. The subcommittee approached the Canadian government, but without success: 'we have on two occasions invoked the assistance of the Dominions Office, in the hope that the Canadian Government would be able to appoint an authoritative representative to discuss with us the best means of adapting the BP to Canadian requirements. Unfortunately, the Canadian Government has not found it possible to assist us in this way.'[61] It did not bode well for a future imperial pharmacopoeia.

EVIDENCE FROM AUSTRALIA

In Australia the Commonwealth government consulted interested parties and concluded that the appointment of an Australian representative on the revision committee was unnecessary. It requested, however, that the chief medical officer, Dr C.L. Park, 'be associated with the revision committee to present any suggestions already communicated from Australia, and that any questions likely to have special interest for Australia should be referred to him before the revision was completed.' The subcommittee welcomed the suggestion. Park declared that direct representation was impracticable owing to the distance and expense involved, but that Australian participation in the process was nevertheless essential. The matter could be adequately dealt with by the revision committee communicating directly with committees established in each state. The high commissioner would act as a link between the revision committee and the minister of health, who was in touch with all matters affecting health as well as 'the general activities of other bodies such as the pharmacists.' The minister could arrange for a corresponding body to be established in each state.[62] Views would be collated and presented to the revision committee by the chief medical officer.

Park supported a permanent secretariat responsible for revising the BP. Between editions, it should 'follow the progress of the science and art of pharmacy, collect material and criticisms, and in other ways keep abreast of the times'. New editions should be published at ten-year intervals. He noted that Australia was not a significant drug-producing country; although parts were tropical in climate, they differed from similar regions in that 'they contained no large Indigenous population'. But the Commonwealth government considered that 'locally produced substances of equivalent therapeutic value to drugs produced in other part of the world' should be given pharmacopoeial recognition – at least for use in Australia. It also called for the policy of inserting notes at the end of particular monographs in the BP 1914 authorizing the use of alternative drugs in specified areas to be developed.[63]

The issue of substitution of BP items with locally available ones was a concern across much of the empire. Park noted that cases might arise where a local drug – similar but not equivalent to one in the BP – might prove efficacious, and he suggested that standards for these should be included in separate monographs authorizing their use in Australia or other parts of the empire and published in a separate appendix rather than in the main text. Park also considered it essential that 'close attention be given to the possibility of reducing the cost of substances and preparations included in the BP'. Substances requiring biological tests would not pose a problem for Australia; if included, the Serum Institute at Melbourne would be able to carry out the tests required.[64]

Separate evidence was submitted by each of the Australian states and the BMA's Federal Committee, which felt that 'the BP should be the sole pharmacopoeia for the whole Empire'. In 'collecting information for use in compiling future issues', the GMC should communicate with 'organized bodies in the Dominions and Colonies (e.g., the British Medical Association and Pharmaceutical Councils)', along with the chief medical officers of Australia and New Zealand. They were in favour of including 'all local drugs deemed proper for admission' and proposed the publication of an annual supplement.[65] Most state governments thought it unnecessary to be directly represented on the revision committee, although Victoria felt that it was 'of vital importance to the people of the Commonwealth … that Australia should be represented'. New South Wales had a list of 'suggested alterations and amendments' that it would submit in due course; Queensland considered amendments it had already submitted 'sufficient to meet its requirements'. South Australia had no observations to make.

214 Pharmacopoeias, Drug Regulation, and Empires

Pharmacists in Australia were well informed about the PSGB's concerns regarding the role of pharmacists in revising the BP. When the Queensland Pharmacy Board was consulted by its government it 'strongly pressed for adequate recognition of pharmacists in assisting in the preparation of the BP'. Likewise, when the Government of Tasmania consulted its pharmacy board, it supported the views expressed in the letter from the PSGB to the Privy Council regarding the role of pharmacists in preparing the BP.[66] It concluded that 'if effect is given to these representations, the wishes of pharmacists generally in the Colony, will ... be adequately met'.

EVIDENCE FROM OTHER COLONIES

The Union of South Africa government was satisfied with existing arrangements and did not seek direct representation on the revision committee. However, if the system was to be changed, it would recommend that 'prior to each revision of the BP, a committee be appointed in South Africa to correspond with the revising body in Great Britain'. This should include representatives of the Department of Public Health, the Union Medical Council, and the Union Pharmacy Board, the federal councils of the professional associations, universities with medical faculties, and 'any other bodies that might be interested'. Such a committee would be of value even if it were 'only on a small scale both as to personnel and scope of duty'. The government strongly supported the decision taken in 1914 'that drugs officially recognized on the recommendation of the Dominions and Colonies should be included in the main text of the BP'. It deplored the suggestion that 'local drugs should be relegated to a separate Addenda'.[67]

The Federal Council of the South African Medical Association raised concerns about the BP's statutory position. It noted that it was based on the independent recognition of the BP in each of the provinces of the union; local variations could be authorized on the advice of provincial medical councils and pharmacy boards. Draft legislation that would replace these with a single medical board and a single pharmacy board for the whole union was before the Union Parliament. This consolidation would, the council suggested, 'be of great advantage to the Union in submitting its views when the BP is under revision'.[68]

Not all colonial bodies wished to be involved in revising the BP. The New Zealand government indicated that it had no desire for New

Zealand to be directly represented. Similar replies were received from the Governments of Newfoundland and Southern Rhodesia, the governor of the latter colony replying that 'my Ministers ... do not consider that a committee set up in Southern Rhodesia could help in the revision of the BP.'[69] He suggested instead that the Medical Council of Southern Rhodesia could act as a corresponding body. The Government of the Irish Free State – established in 1922 – replied that it did not intend to press for special representation on the revision committee. The Pharmaceutical Society of Ireland had previously indicated that it wished to be represented, but later agreed that 'in view of the political changes since the last edition of the BP such representation would not need to be so large as on previous occasions.'[70]

THE RECOMMENDATIONS OF THE SUBCOMMITTEE ON THE *BRITISH PHARMACOPOEIA*

Having considered all the evidence the subcommittee prepared its report. It made eight recommendations, some in several parts. It concluded that 'it is not necessary or desirable to make any alterations in the existing law relating to the preparation or publication of the BP', but that radical change was needed with regard to how this was done. The GMC would continue to have the legal duty of publishing it, but it was given the task of 'selecting persons to form a new body to be designated "the British Pharmacopoeia Commission."'[71] This was to consist of four persons appointed by the GMC; three appointed jointly by the councils of the PSGB, the Pharmaceutical Society of Ireland, and the Pharmaceutical Society of Northern Ireland; and two persons nominated by the Medical Research Council. A Selection Committee would be appointed to identify who should sit on it. Pharmacists would at last have a say in the decision-making process of the pharmacopoeia. In his evidence to the subcommittee Henry Greenish had indicated that there should be a ratio of one medical to three non-medical members of the commission. But doctors would still form a majority of the Selection Committee; however, although its chair would be a doctor appointed from among the GMC representatives, the chair of the Pharmacopoeia Commission itself would be selected from among its members.

The subcommittee recommended that the number of commission members should not be prescribed, and that it 'should have power from time to time to select additional persons for permanent or temporary membership, including representatives of India or the Dominions.[72] But in suggesting more prominent roles for India and the Dominions in revising the BP the subcommittee was also limiting the role of smaller colonies. In the event, no representatives of India or the Dominions were ever given either permanent or temporary membership of the commission itself; only in-country arrangements were made to advise that body. The subcommittee recommended that the BP contain only standard drugs in general use throughout the empire. Where it was 'desired in any part of the Empire to sanction the use of particular local drugs, or alternate preparations not included in the BP', this should be left to the governments concerned by the issue of local supplements or addenda. The GMC should request that the Dominion and Indian governments 'set up responsible and representative committees, to cooperate with the Pharmacopoeia Commission in the revision of the BP', if they desired and were willing to take part in the work.[73] Local substitution was sanctioned, and colonial authorities would be able to 'make official' any medicine by including it in a supplement or addendum.

CONCLUSION

The Macmillan Report represented the first systematic attempt to review the methods and practices adopted by other countries – including France, Germany, Holland, Italy, Belgium, and the United States – in the preparation of pharmacopoeias. By the early twentieth century considerable harmonization had taken place in the approaches used following international meetings such as the 1902 International Conference on the Unification of the Formulae of Powerful Medicaments held in Brussels.[74] The subcommittee had gathered together information from across the empire that had not been available to the GMC. In so doing it had exposed enormous variations; in Britain pharmacopoeial standards and drug regulation operated in parallel but separately; drug regulation was achieved through piecemeal legislation; and the BP had little statutory force. But the subcommittee saw no reason for change; the BP was not designed to serve the needs of prosecutors. Issues concerned with compliance with BP requirements – inspection, prosecution, and penalties – were matters for drug legislation. Some Dominions linked the BP directly with drug regulation in legislation, but in most parts of the empire the official and statutory natures of the pharmacopoeia were separate and distinct.

Publication of the Macmillan Report was a watershed moment in the history of pharmacopoeias in Britain and its empire. It redefined their meanings and functions, recognized that these change over time, and clarified their role in drug regulatory processes. The BP would be a set of standards for selected drugs; it would be at once a medical and a pharmaceutical text; it would cease to be both comprehensive and inclusive and would 'contain only standard drugs in general use throughout the Empire'.[75] The colonies would be free to select whatever drugs they wished and to publish their own addenda or supplements. As a means of unifying pharmacy practice, of standardizing the range of drugs, and of regulating how they were used across the empire, the 'British imperial pharmacopoeia' clearly had severe limitations.

The Macmillan Report was formally submitted to the government on 12 March 1928 and presented to Parliament the following May. The recommendations were agreed unaltered, and the report was published immediately by His Majesty's Stationery Office. Once the new Pharmacopoeia Commission had been appointed, work could begin on revising the BP for the whole empire.

10

Decolonizing the Pharmacopoeia

With the recommendations of the Macmillan Report accepted, the future purpose, scope, and shape of the *British Pharmacopoeia* (*BP*) in the metropole and empire were settled. There would be no change in its legal status, pharmacists and others would be equal partners with doctors, and Dominions and colonies would be free to publish their own supplements or addenda. The arrangements it set in motion remained in place for the next forty years, a period of immense change, not least in the relationship between Britain and its colonies. Under the Balfour Declaration in 1926 Dominions were recognized as 'autonomous communities within the British Empire, equal in status, in no way subordinate one to another in any aspect of their domestic or external affairs, though united by a common allegiance to the Crown and freely associated as members of the British Commonwealth of Nations.'[1] The 1931 Statute of Westminster confirmed their full legislative independence; it 'set the seal on the new conception of Dominion nationhood by renouncing the Imperial Parliament's right to legislate for the Dominions unless at their explicit request.'[2] Dominion status was henceforth accorded to Canada, Australia, New Zealand, Newfoundland, South Africa, and the Irish Free State. But for India 'the years from the outbreak of the First World War to independence were among the most turbulent in its history.'[3]

This chapter examines the changing relationship between pharmacopoeias, drug regulation, and empire between 1928 and 1968 in the light of rapidly changing political and economic environments in which major developments in science and medicine were also taking place. The continuing rise of a research-based pharmaceutical industry led to discoveries in medical science and the introduction of ever more new chemical medicines.[4] The steady transition from plant-

Decolonizing the Pharmacopoeia 219

based to chemical and biological medicines necessitated developments in drug regulation, with the creation of new legally defined categories of medicine including dangerous drugs and therapeutic substances. This chapter explores the extent to which the empire continued to be consulted in the compilation of the *BP*; the methods used to engage colonial practitioners in its preparation; the influence that medical and pharmaceutical practice beyond the empire had on its content; and the actions taken by newly independent states with regard to pharmacopoeias and drug regulation. The 1968 *BP* was the last to be published by the General Medical Council (GMC); the chapter concludes by examining what led to responsibility for it being moved from a Pharmacopoeia Commission to a Medicines Commission reporting directly to government.

APPOINTMENT OF A
PHARMACOPOEIA COMMISSION

With the recommendations accepted, a British Pharmacopoeia Commission (henceforth the BP Commission) was duly appointed as a permanent body with a permanent secretary. Its first chairman was Arthur Beddard, a retired physician and lecturer in pharmacology at Guy's Hospital, London. It had six other members from a variety of backgrounds: F.R. Fraser, a professor of medicine; J.A. Gunn, a professor of pharmacology; J.H. Dunn, the director of the pharmacology laboratory of the Pharmaceutical Society of Great Britain (PSGB); and H.G. Greenish, a professor of pharmaceutics. The final two members were T. Tickle, a public analyst, and R.R. Bennett, a pharmacist. One contemporary observer noted that 'for the first time in this country we had a Pharmacopoeial Commission which was fully representative of all interested professions, and pharmacy was amongst them.'[5] The GMC continued to appoint its own Pharmacopoeia Committee, but its role was to oversee the preparation and publication of the *BP* rather than to do so itself.

The BP Commission held its first meeting in December 1928.[6] Sir Donald MacAlister defined its role and listed the subcommittees it should appoint, including ones for biologicals and medicinal substances of natural origin as well as clinical and pharmacology; there were also committees for pharmacy, and analysis and testing. Dr Charles Hampshire – who was qualified in pharmacy, chemistry, and medicine – was appointed as permanent secretary and remained in that post until 1950.[7] The GMC still had the legal duty to 'cause [the *BP*] to be published' and the BP Commission reported twice yearly to the GMC's Pharmacopoeia Committee, whose secretary attended its meetings. It presented its first report in May 1929, having met weekly for thirteen weeks. Lists of proposed additions and deletions were circulated as before to relevant bodies in Britain and to 'all the Governments and Administrations of the Empire.' The BP Commission received 'a large number of valuable suggestions.'[8]

India and most Dominions established national pharmacopoeia committees to consider revisions; South Africa established a joint committee of pharmacists and doctors. The Canadian Committee on Pharmaceutical Standards had submitted its recommendations earlier.[9] In India the request was received by its Commission on Pharmacopoeial Revision, which forwarded it to the Pharmacopoeia Committee of the Bombay Medical Union.[10] It had no criticisms to make, but suggested the inclusion of anti-plague vaccine, anti-cholera vaccine, and anti-venom serum, along with organic antimonials.[11] It again requested that certain plant medicines be included in the main text of the BP, including Cannabis and its preparations, and Indian ginger. It also requested that standards be set for specific gravities at higher temperatures. By November 1931 the draft of the BP was complete. First proofs were signed off by subcommittees, and in May 1932 the GMC's Pharmacopoeia Committee approved the text; thirty thousand copies were printed and it became official on 8 October 1932.[12]

Acknowledgement of contributions received from colonies reflected changes in the empire; Trans-Jordan and the Irish Free State submitted suggestions.[13] There was no response from most smaller colonies or from Basutoland, the Gambia, Sierra Leone, or Swaziland. The Dominions were now the principal partners in pharmacopoeia development; the voices of smaller colonies – mainly in tropical areas – were gradually marginalized. The BP 1932 represented a further step away from inclusivity and comprehensiveness towards science and standardization. Whilst it included 127 new monographs, 357 listed in the 1914 BP were deleted. The new ones included those devoted to chemical medicines, gases (nitrous oxide and oxygen), and biological medicines (toxins, antitoxins, vaccines, and insulin, first isolated in 1922). Its twenty-one appendices listed reagents and test methods, biological assays for antitoxins, and three methods for sterilizing solutions.

Hampshire later reflected that the trend was 'towards definitive curative treatment by means of specific agents of animal origin, or produced by the resources of synthetic organic chemistry, and away from the use –

often empirical – of vegetable or mineral drugs for the relief of symptoms.' The greatest change was 'the reduction in the number of vegetable products used as drugs.' Although some continued to be used in large quantities, 'the range becomes more and more restricted, largely as the result of pharmacological investigation.'[14] Whilst some items listed in the *Indian and Colonial Addendum* had been included in the 1914 BP, almost all were omitted from that of 1932, the exceptions being Indian podophyllum, arachis oil, and sesame oil.[15] Sixty crude drugs listed in 1914 were excluded, twenty-four of which were 'of interest principally in India or the Dominions and Colonies.' The BP Commission agreed not to include substances or preparations having mainly a local use, as 'Addenda dealing with the drugs especially applicable to India and the various parts of the Empire would be produced by the authorities of the states concerned,' who were authorized to 'issue such supplementary lists of substances or preparations as may seem necessary or expedient for local needs.'[16] Official plant medicines needed to be powdered and standardized. Five were included: digitalis, belladonna, ergot, ipecacuanha, and nux vomica. Biological assays were provided for digitalis and strophanthin.

Hampshire made it clear that plant medicines would play little part in future pharmacopoeias, but biologicals would increase. The Therapeutic Substances Act 1925 applied to Great Britain and Northern Ireland, but most of the substances listed in its regulations were included in the BP, 'in order to provide standards in other parts of the British Empire in which the Pharmacopoeia is the legal authority.'[17] The implications for pharmacy education were clear; 'Xrayser,' writing in *Chemist and Druggist*, concluded that 'if we [pharmacists] are to maintain our position as the trusted guardians of the purity of medicines and the skilled providers of the requirements of the doctor, our training must henceforth be less that of a botanist and more of a biologist.'[18]

CONTINUING CALLS
FOR AN INDIAN PHARMACOPOEIA

In India the continued refusal to allow an Indian pharmacopoeia was viewed mainly as a trade issue. Bhattacharya notes that 'the British medical establishment used Indian drugs widely but denied the necessity for an official Indian pharmacopeia to facilitate the import of British and American drugs within the large and lucrative Indian market.'[19] The British authorities clearly had a strong incentive to discourage colonies and Dominions from producing their own. Doctors in India were left in no doubt that the BP Commission would not be including any of the plant drugs it had requested in the BP itself. In August 1930 the Government of India appointed its own committee of inquiry to make recommendations about the import, manufacture, and sale of drugs, and the regulation of pharmacy. Its remit included the role of pharmacopoeias. Drug regulation remained largely ineffective, although a 1930 Dangerous Drugs Act extended the Opium Act to a wider range of substances.[20]

The Drugs Enquiry Committee was chaired by Ram Nath Chopra, professor of pharmacology at Calcutta, and reported in 1932.[21] It sought the opinion of doctors on whether to compile an Indian pharmacopoeia or adopt that of Britain, the United States, or some other jurisdiction. Of 235 responses, 202 favoured an Indian pharmacopoeia, 4 were against it, and 29 thought that an Indian addendum to the BP would serve the purpose. Singh noted that 'the one great desire of the medical profession in India – to have a pharmacopoeia of their own – became apparent from the very first stage in the inquiry.'[22] The committee supported the majority view and looked forward 'to a day when India will have its own pharmacopoeia, based largely on minerals and plants obtainable in this country, with standardized preparations and assay laboratories.' There was 'no reason why India should not in future have a large export trade in medicinal plants, rather than be dependent almost entirely on imported chemicals.' The medicinal future of India would be based on plant rather than chemical medicines.

Doubts were expressed about the wisdom of the proposal at the time. An editorial in the *Indian and Eastern Druggist* noted that 'whether the Committee's recommendation that an Indian Pharmacopoeia shall be compiled is a wise one, and likely to receive endorsement from authoritative quarters, is rather open to doubt.' It suggested that 'the medical profession in India preferred to adopt the BP – in which the special requirements of India were not overlooked – as their standard and guide.'[23]

When the proposal was put to the Government of India it was rejected.[24] The doctors' views had to be balanced against those of others. David Hooper, the government's former economic botanist, strongly opposed an Indian pharmacopoeia. 'In representing Ayervedic [*sic*] and Unani medical systems' it would effectively 'return conditions to the sixteenth century.' The wisest course for India was to follow the BP, which had 'just been edited by the highest authorities in medicine and pharmacy.'[25] But his views were not shared by Indian colleagues; N.B. Dutta, economic botanist to the Patiala Government, reported that 158 drugs listed in the *BP* 1914 were of vegetable origin and that 103 of those readily grew in India. He thought that a national Indian pharmacopoeia 'should be impartial and comprehensive in the choice of drugs'.[26] The government was in no hurry to implement the recommendations of the Drugs Enquiry Committee, but having rejected an Indian pharmacopoeia it had to consider an alternative. It recommended that India compile a local supplement to the *BP*; its preparation would have to wait until after the Second World War.

UPDATING THE *BP*

The Macmillan Report had recommended that the *BP* 'be revised and re-issued at stated intervals of ten years, supplements being issued between successive editions as required.' It should 'contain only standard drugs in general use throughout the Empire'.[27] Whilst Dominions and colonies could publish their own addenda, the *BP* Commission itself could also do so, which would mainly reflect advances in medicine, pharmacy, and chemistry. Work began on the first one before the end of 1932, with a focus on standards for vitamin products and biological standards. By May 1935 monographs had been prepared for vitamins A, B_1, C, and D_2, and their preparations, along with ones for gas gangrene antitoxin, staphylococcus antitoxin, and anti-pneumococcus serum.[28] Its cooperation with the Committee of Revision for the *United States Pharmacopoeia* (*USP*) increased as that with the empire diminished; selective consultation with the empire was undertaken only after the draft addendum was complete in May 1936; the *BP* Commission received comments 'from committees in India and certain of the Dominions'.[29] The GMC Pharmacopoeia Committee approved the final text and it was published in July.

In November 1936 the GMC Pharmacopoeia Committee agreed that it 'would be desirable to alternate at five-year intervals with the *USP*'. The next *BP* would be published in 1941. New committees were appointed, and experts employed in the industry were recruited. When Boots sought to gain a foothold in New Zealand the company emphasized not only its high ethical standards but the fact that some of its employees served on *BP* committees and on legal and educational bodies.[30] The *BP* Commission compiled lists of drugs of decreasing use or doubtful therapeutic value, and the list of proposed additions and deletions was sent to government departments and medical bodies, to the Governments of India and the Dominions, and to officers of the Colonial Medical Service.[31] Consultation with the empire remained important and a large number of comments were received. The BP Commission concluded that the BP 'should include a larger number of preparations that were frequently prescribed in general practice' as it needed to better reflect medical practice in the metropole.[32] By May 1938, 522 monographs had been completed. The BP Commission reported in May 1939, on the eve of another war.

The separation of pharmacopoeias from drug regulation was cemented in a Pharmacy and Poisons Act in 1933. This provided for the appointment of inspectors, making it clear that it was 'the duty of the Pharmaceutical Society alone to inspect the premises of chemists'. But it was the duty of local authorities independently to ensure that 'persons other than chemists' were complying with the act 'by means of inspection and otherwise'.[33] The act made no reference to the BP.

In 1935 the PSGB sought to establish the extent to which both the BP and the *British Pharmaceutical Codex* (BPC) had statutory status in Dominions and colonies.[34] Most confirmed that the situation was as described in the Macmillan Report. The governor of Newfoundland reported that 'both are legal standards in this country and are so referred to in the various Acts dealing with professional matters'.[35] In Britain use of the BP by hospital doctors was declining. P. Hamill of St Bartholomew's Hospital, London, noted that 'the BP ... has tended to become at each revision more and more a book of standards for substances to be used in medicine and less and less a formulary'.[36] E. Lewis Lilley – chairman of the National Formulary Committee – complained that 'the BP at each successive revision has ceased to take in new medicaments unless they have reached a stage of reasonably satisfactory standardization, and hence the range of its contents is always considerably narrower than the contemporary practice of the profession'.[37] The formulary was largely the work of general medical practitioners.

THE *BP* AND PATENT MEDICINES

The issue of whether pharmacists should focus on dispensing official medicines rather than selling patent medicines received considerable attention in many parts of the empire. Supplying official medicines was usually more profitable for the chemist, cheaper for the patient, and often more effective than a proprietary medicine. By the 1930s the need for chemists to make up official remedies was reducing rapidly. In South Africa a review of major changes in pharmacy since 1910 noted that the chemists' business had altered dramatically.[38] The increased use and sale of patent medicines had resulted in a reduction in both the number of prescriptions dispensed and the demand for chemists' own remedies. Large wholesale businesses increasingly used mass-production methods to manufacture a wide range of pills, tablets, mixtures, and extracts; retail chemists bought BP products ready-made from wholesalers rather than make them themselves. At the same time a growing proportion of patent medicines were sold by general merchants and storekeepers.[39]

A reader of the *South African Pharmaceutical Journal* pleaded to pharmacists not to neglect 'the rich mine of therapeutic remedies to be found in the BP and BPC.' These should not, he advised, 'be replaced too readily with expensive patent medicines.'[40] He offered the case of a medical practitioner who claimed to have prescribed every patent preparation available for a patient with coronary insufficiency without effect, but when he prescribed 'Compound Digitalis Pills' of the BPC the patient experienced relief.[41] Pharmacists faced further difficulties as the popularity of Western medicines with the Indigenous population decreased. As Pratik Chakrabarti has shown, the commercialization of African 'native medicine' was encouraged and competed with Western biomedicine from the 1920s for the rapidly growing African population, particularly in cities.[42]

Markku Hakkanen has demonstrated how British occupation of South-Central Africa (Southern and Northern Rhodesia and Nyasaland) in the late nineteenth century tied the region to new trade networks, global markets, the British Empire, and to mission-based Christianity.[43] It was a highly pluralistic region where Europeans brought medical therapies, ideas, and practices into an area with a rich Indigenous medical culture.[44] Yet the attitude of the British authorities to drug regulation was driven by the interests of the metropole rather than the colonies. Abena Dove Oseo-Asare has shown how Europeans appropriated African knowledge and technology to satisfy the needs of the emerging global medical market.[45] The seeds of strophanthin – a substance used in African arrow poisons – became a valuable export item in West and Central Africa in the late nineteenth century and were included in the BP. Yet the response of the British authorities was to outlaw the use of poison arrows in the Gold Coast rather than to attempt to introduce any form of control over the seeds.

226 Pharmacopoeias, Drug Regulation, and Empires

PATENTING MODERN MEDICINES

In Britain the authorities became more concerned with the 'new' patent medicines than with the old. These were chemical and biological substances subject to patents or trademarks. In May 1934 the BP Commission raised with the GMC Pharmacopoeia Committee the matter of including them in the BP. The medical profession was generally opposed to the patenting of medicines, although many of the drugs they prescribed emanated from the pharmaceutical industry and were subject to patent protection. The issue received considerable attention in the medical press.[46] Manufacturers were often keen to have their products 'made official'. In 1932 Burroughs Wellcome relinquished its patent rights to Ernutin (ergotoxine) in order to facilitate its inclusion in the BP. The company was anxious to separate research from commercial activities in order 'to attract dedicated research workers who otherwise would not have joined a commercial organization'.[47] But the GMC Pharmacopoeia Committee decided that such substances should still be excluded, except where multiple licences to manufacture had been granted, or where the patent would expire shortly after publication of a new edition or addendum.[48]

The rules on patent compliance were soon relaxed. In 1937 the GMC Pharmacopoeia Committee overturned the rule excluding substances 'for which the only practical method of preparation was protected by patent'. A year later it proposed the inclusion of more synthetic drugs such as sulphanilamide and theophylline with ethylene diamine.[49] The issue arose again during the war in the light of a decision by US authorities that products covered by patents or trademarks could be included in the United States Pharmacopoeia (USP), 'the question of therapeutic value only being considered'.[50] In May 1943 the GMC Pharmacopoeia Committee recommended that, in selecting items for inclusion, the BP Commission 'need not consider its choice limited by actual or potential rights in manufacture'. The recommendation was accepted by the full GMC Council and duly implemented, but the impact of patents on the content of the BP continued. Mann observed that 'the shape of the contemporary pharmacopoeia is to no small extent fashioned by the Patent Act'.[51]

A key aim of the imperial pharmacopoeia had been to discourage publication of separate pharmacopoeias in the colonies and Dominions rather than supplements to the BP. The Pharmaceutical Society of Ireland, originally founded in 1875, informed the GMC Pharmacopoeia Committee that 'the Pharmacopoeia Act of 1931 makes provision for a Pharmacopoeia for the Irish Free State. Section 2 adopts the BP for the time being in force in GB subject to any modifications which may be made by the Medical Registration Council.[52] The GMC was well aware of calls in India and Canada for separate pharmacopoeias. In March 1936, the chairman of the BP Commission, Arthur Beddard, wrote to Sir Henry Dale at the National Institute for Medical Research insisting that 'Special steps should be taken to try to make the next BP – in all important points such as standards, assays, and nomenclature – an agreed pharmacopoeia throughout the Empire ... It seems to me that unless the process is checked it won't be long before Canada at least has a pharmacopoeia of its own. Further, unless the Empire can and does speak with one voice, the difficulties of an International Agreement will be greatly increased.'[53]

OUTBREAK OF WAR

The work of the BP Commission was interrupted by the outbreak of the Second World War in September 1939. The whole empire was drawn into it, often without consultation. In India 'the Viceroy ... closely followed the 1914 precedent and declared war without consulting any Indian political representatives.'[54] Supplies of medicines were again disrupted. As in the First World War, the Dominions and colonies needed to find their own solutions to any shortages. The BP Commission's November report included proposals for dealing with such problems. Addenda followed in quick succession. In June 1940 cod liver oil emulsion and several vitamin preparations were added. Substitutions were again authorized: arachis, cottonseed, or sesame oil could be used in place of olive oil in ointments and liniments; fatty bases could be replaced by simple ointment. In November adaptations to official formulas were approved to meet wartime shortages of glycerine, sugar, and other items.[55] By January 1941 monographs were added for previously imported drugs now made by British manufacturers, including carbachol, mepacrine, nikethamide, and stibophen.

The Ministry of Health produced a *National War Formulary* in 1941 following the classification of medicines by the Medical Research Council's Therapeutic Requirements Committee into essential drugs, drugs essential for certain purposes, and non-essential drugs. The BP Commission developed standards for its preparations.[56] An addendum in October 1941 introduced changes to methods of sterilization and added digoxin, ephedrine, and the first sulphonamide – sulphanilamide. Penicillin and its preparations made their official appearances only after the

228   Pharmacopoeias, Drug Regulation, and Empires

war; they were added directly to the *BP* through announcements in the *London, Edinburgh, Belfast,* and *Dublin Gazettes* in June 1946.[57]

In May 1942, eighteen formulas for concentrated preparations were added, making substantial savings in alcohol use. In August new additions included nicotinamide, riboflavin, and stilboestrol. The addendum of February 1945 was the largest since the first. Five new sulphonamides were added along with amphetamine, cyclopropane, and steroids including oestrone and progesterone. Thirty-four monographs for tablets were added; these included standards for uniformity of weight, limits of tolerance, assays, and disintegration tests. The wartime addenda were adopted by most Dominions and colonies, although some produced their own. The Canadian Committee on Pharmaceutical Standards was replaced by a new Committee on Pharmacopoeial Standards, which published several Canadian supplements to the *BP*. It also recommended Canadian standards for *BP* medicines, which were subsequently published by the Canadian government.[58]

Despite the surge in synthetic pharmaceuticals, medicinal plants saw a revival during the war. Many chemical medicines were sourced from plants, and a national medicinal plant collection scheme using volunteers was established to augment supplies available to manufacturers.[59] But only a fraction of the vegetable drugs required could be sourced from native wild and cultivated plants; Britain continued to rely on its empire to supply drugs not available domestically. Exotic medicinal plants – along with supplementary quantities of those available locally – were shipped to Britain.[60] Tanzania supplied camphor, and Ceylon produced quinine from cinchona after the Dutch East Indies were lost to Japan. Kenya, Zanzibar, Malaya, and India grew chamomile, ipecacuanha, cascara, and other warm-climate plants; Australia provided *Dubosia* from which hyoscine was sourced; stramonium and *Hyoscyamus* (for atropine) were imported from Egypt and the Sudan; and supplies of plants including digitalis, belladonna, and stramonium were augmented from New Zealand.[61] But for most of the empire's population the new synthetic remedies were largely irrelevant unless they had access to mission or other Western clinics, where the emphasis was usually on transmissible diseases.

THE INDIAN RESPONSE

In India a Drugs Technical Advisory Board was set up in 1944, and the government asked it 'to prepare the material for a list of drugs in India

GOVERNMENT OF INDIA
DEPARTMENT OF HEALTH

THE INDIAN PHARMACOPŒIAL LIST 1946

CALCUTTA : PRINTED BY THE MANAGER
GOVERNMENT OF INDIA PRESS   1946

Figure 10.1 The *Indian Pharmacopoeial List* 1946.

[that] – although not included in the BP – are of sufficient medicinal value to justify their inclusion in an official pharmacopoeia, and recommend what standards should be prescribed to secure uniformity, and what tests should be used to establish identity and purity'.[62] The list would be issued by the government and known as the *Indian Pharmacopoeial List* (IPL); it would constitute 'the official Indian Supple-

ment to the BP.'[63] An eleven-man committee was appointed, of whom seven were medically qualified, two were chemists, and two had pharmaceutical affiliations, although were not pharmacists themselves.[64] Sir Ram Nath Chopra was appointed its chair.[65] The initiative was widely welcomed in India and a large number of items were suggested for inclusion.[66]

The *IPL* was approved by the government and published in 1946, shortly before Indian gained independence (figure 10.1).[67] It was a substantial volume containing around 180 monographs and several appendices on similar lines to those of the *BP*.[68] Nearly 100 monographs were for vegetable drugs indigenous to India, along with preparations made from them. The *IPL* Committee 'exercised special care in sifting the pharmacological and clinical evidence and in conducting original work to establish sound scientific grounds for selection.'[69] The *Pharmaceutical Journal* commended the cautious approach taken but considered that the inclusion of 'list' in the title was misleading since the book not only enumerated the drugs concerned but also laid down standards for them.[70]

The medicinal plants included those suggested by the Indian Commission on Pharmacopoeial Revision for inclusion in the *BP* 1932 but not accepted by the *BP* Commission. Forty-eight monographs were for locally available substitutes for drugs listed in the *BP*. They included acacia, aloes, lobelia, and rhubarb, along with oils such as chaulmoogra and pudina. But the *IPL* also included some chemical medicines not listed in the *BP* and local amendments to *BP* preparations. The use of the synthetic dye amaranth was authorized for use as a colouring agent, and appendices gave details of methods of determination referred to in the monographs, particularly those relating to vitamin and biological preparations.[71] It was more a colonial pharmacopoeia than a supplement to the *BP*.

Work began on compiling a *Pharmacopoeia of India* (*PI*) soon after independence in 1947. The Ministry of Health appointed an Indian Pharmacopoeia Committee in November 1948 with the director general of health services as its chairman.[72] The Indian Pharmacopoeia Committee's composition was severely criticized as members were selected on the basis of the position they held rather than on their expertise.[73] By 1950 a draft list of drugs had been drawn up and circulated for comment.[74] Part A included Western biomedical drugs; part B listed Indian traditional drugs judged to be of proven efficacy. However, it was noted that 'procedures followed with respect to the British and United States pharmacopoeias had been ignored.'[75] Furthermore, the clash of medical and pharmaceutical interests that had been a feature of the British experience was in danger of being repeated in India; the government planned to place publication of the pharmacopoeia under the control of the Indian Medical Council. The Indian Pharmaceutical Association objected, and it was made a joint responsibility of the Indian Medical Council and the Pharmacy Council of India.[76]

The *IPL* provided the nucleus of the *PI*, with additional material freely drawn from the *BP*, the *USP*, and the *International Pharmacopoeia* published in 1950.[77] It contained 1,001 pages, the first 751 covering monographs for drugs, chemicals, and pharmaceutical preparations. In many ways it followed the pattern of the *BP*, but a special feature was the inclusion of indigenous drugs and their preparations, including many that had been suggested for inclusion in the *BP* in the 1890s – such as *Aristolochia*, datura, and ispaghula. The *PI* was finally published in 1955 under the title *Pharmacopoeia of India*. It was made statutory from 20 August 1956 under the 1944 Drugs Act. Singh noted that, in containing both Western and traditional drugs, it was effectively an update of the 1868 edition, which included all the drugs official in the 1867 *BP* but also incorporated indigenous products.[78]

When a supplement was published in 1960, virtually all the monographs added were for chemical medicines.[79] Many more were added for a new edition published in 1966, and a large number of monographs included in the 1955 pharmacopoeia and its supplement were deleted, most of which were for traditional medicines and galenicals – although three new ones were added.[80] As Bhattacharya notes, 'when finally published, the official Indian Pharmacopoeia sabotaged its raison d'être – dreamed of initially by its colonial advocates – and instead of utilizing Indian drugs, relegated these to a marginal status.'[81] In practice, the post-independence *PI* differed little from the *BP*.

A PHARMACOPOEIA FOR
THE BRITISH COMMONWEALTH OF NATIONS

With the end of the war the *BP* Commission in London planned a new edition of the *BP*. But the goal of an imperial pharmacopoeia had not entirely died. As before, the *BP* Commission consulted throughout the empire. It received 'a large number of valuable suggestions from medical and pharmaceutical authorities', including twenty-four responses from the American, West Indian, Mediterranean, Indian, African, and

Australasian Divisions. Others came from the national pharmacopoeia commissions in Canada, Australia, South Africa, and India.[82] The BP Commission drew up a list of proposed additions and deletions, approved 580 monographs, and in May 1946 sent proofs to the Dominions as well as the United States Pharmacopoeia Committee of Revisions and the British Pharmaceutical Codex Revision Committee.[83]

When the seventh edition of the BP was published in 1948 it consisted of monographs and twenty-four appendices mainly concerned with chemical and biological assay methods. It included some drugs still under patent. 'In so far as such substances are protected by Letters Patent', it noted that 'their inclusion in this Pharmacopoeia neither conveys, nor implies licences to manufacture.'[84] The BP Commission declared that its aim had been to produce a pharmacopoeia 'suitable for the whole British Commonwealth of Nations'. Drugs in general use throughout the empire were included, but 'substances and preparations having mainly a local use in particular parts of the Empire are omitted'. Such drugs would be considered by governments across the empire.[85]

The BP Commission and the PSGB's British Pharmaceutical Codex Revision Committee liaised closely. The latter committee provided the BP Commission with BPC monographs showing how it planned to use official pharmacopoeial materials.[86] A number of drugs of Indian origin that first appeared in the BP 1867 continued to appear in the BPC until the 1949 edition, although their official descriptions often differed from their common names. Further editions appeared at five-year intervals after 1949.[87] They were normally published around eighteen months after publication of the BP. The 1948 BP continued the practice of including a list of 'alternative preparations sanctioned for use in tropical, sub-tropical, and other parts of the British Empire'.[88] It also included a 'precautionary legal notice' stating that 'in some parts of the British Empire the BP is of statutory force, and in some parts ... there are local laws dealing with certain of the substances which are the subject of the monographs which follow'. Wherever this situation arose 'a caution has been affixed to the monograph, but it must not be assumed that where no caution appears, the subject of the monograph is free from legal restrictions.'[89] Such cautions mainly related to antitoxins and vaccines; thus 'in any part of the British Empire in which Diphtheria Antitoxin is controlled by law, care must be taken that provisions of such law are duly complied with.'[90]

Local law trumped the authority of the *BP*: 'Where the preparation or use of any substance is governed by local law, the directions of the Pharmacopoeia as far as possible are followed as well as those of the local law, provided that any direction of the Pharmacopoeia which is contradictory or inconsistent with the local law is deemed thereby to be superseded.'[91] The *BP* might be official, but it did not necessarily have statutory force.

THE LAST DAYS OF EMPIRE

Indian independence in 1947 marked the beginning of the end of the British Empire. Decolonization was to be carefully orchestrated; the official line was that 'withdrawal from India need not appear to be forced upon us by our weakness nor to be the first step in the dissolution of the Empire.'[92] As Wm Roger Louis noted, 'to the world at large, the British would be seen as remaining in control of events. History would record a commitment to self-government that had been planned and fulfilled.'[93] In the event Britain 'had to reshape the old imperial structure into a new framework of more or less equal partners'. Nationalism would be channelled into 'constructing nations in harmony with British interests. British imperialism would be sustained by means other than domination'. What emerged, Louis suggested, was 'mutual accommodation based on self-interest.'[94]

As colonies gained independence from Britain – many in the 1950s and '60s (table 10.1) – the relevance of an imperial pharmacopoeia was increasingly questioned, although the *BP* continued to be official in many colonies long after independence. In Nigeria a 1948 revision of the Pharmacy Ordinance declared that the 'names of substances and preparations in the *BP* or *BPC*, or names closely resembling them, should not be applied to substances of a different composition.'[95] In Canada British texts including the *BP* and *BPC* continued to be used throughout pharmacy apprenticeships and in everyday practice.[96] *BP* addenda continued to be published, with advice having been received from across the empire: that of 1951 noted that the *BP* Commission had received valuable input from authorities in Australia, Canada, South Africa, and New Zealand. This had been of great assistance 'in the endeavour to adjust the Addendum to the needs of the Commonwealth.'[97]

Proofs of the next edition of the *BP* were circulated to medical and pharmaceutical bodies in the four Dominions.[98] India and Pakistan

Table 10.1
Year of independence of selected British Dominions and colonies

Division of empire	Colony or Dominion	Year granted independence	Division of empire	Colony or Dominion	Year granted independence
India	India (Dominion)	1947	Australasia	Australia (Dominion)	1986
Africa	Bechuanaland Protectorate	1966		Fiji	1970
	Gambia (The Gambia)	1965		New Zealand (Dominion)	1986
	Gold Coast (Ghana)	1957	Mediterranean	Cyprus	1960
	Kenya	1963		Gibraltar	2002 (BOT)
	Nigeria	1960		Malta	1964
	Nyasaland (Malawi)	1964	North America	Canada (Dominion)	1982
	Sierra Leone	1961		Newfoundland (Dominion)	1982
	South Africa (Dominion)	1961	West Indies	Barbados	1966
	Southern Rhodesia (Zimbabwe)	1965 (UDI) 1980		British Guiana (Guyana)	1966
Eastern	Ceylon (Dominion)	1972		British Honduras (Belize)	1981
	Hong Kong	1997 (to China)		Grenada	1974
	Mauritius	1968		Jamaica	1962
	Seychelles	1976		St Lucia	1979
	Singapore	1963		Trinidad and Tobago	1962

Source: Wikipedia, s.v. "List of Countries That Have Gained Independence from the United Kingdom," last modified 4 December 2023, 17:28, https://en.wikipedia.org/wiki/List_of_countries_that_have_gained_independence_from_the_United_Kingdom.
Note: BOT: British Overseas Territory. UDI: Unilateral declaration of independence.

continued to be involved in its preparation as members of the Commonwealth until 1963, as did Malaya and Singapore. Few suggestions were received from smaller colonies. Whilst most West Indian colonies had suggested additions to the 1900 *Indian and Colonial Addendum*, by 1932 only the Bahamas, Jamaica, and Trinidad commented, and by 1953 no suggestions at all were received from the West Indian colonies.

In Britain the 1950 Medical Act, which replaced that of 1858, enlarged the scope of the *BP* to include 'medicines, preparations, materials, and articles used in the practice of medicine, surgery, and midwifery'.[99] This brought blood products and surgical catgut into its remit. It would now be much more than a compendium of standards for drugs. But whilst its content expanded, its imperial ambitions remained unchanged: 'In deciding on the scope of the new edition ... regard was made to the practice of medicine and pharmaceutics both in the United Kingdom and in the British Commonwealth and the Colonies'. Selection remained firmly in the hands of the doctors; advice on additions, deletions, and retentions was provided by 'the Clinical Medicine and Doses Committee and the Pharmacology Committee'.[100] Professional and other bodies in Britain and the empire were again consulted, and broader networks became more prominent. The 'helpful cooperation' of the industry was acknowledged, including 'the Association of the British Pharmaceutical Industry, the Association of British Chemical Manufacturers, and the British Disinfectant Manufacturers' Association'.[101] The *BP* Commission also reported that it had derived much assistance in its work from the 'cordial and active cooperation' of the United States Pharmacopoeia Committee of Revision: substantial harmony in titles and standards in the two pharmacopoeias had been achieved.[102] Cooperation continued for the 1951 addendum and the *BP* 1953.[103] American willingness to assist may have been partly motivated by the large number of American pharmaceutical companies establishing subsidiaries in Britain in the post-war period.[104]

The eighth edition of the *BP* became official on 1 September 1953. Membership of the *BP* Commission was increased from nine to eleven and twenty-one committees were appointed. Only one was entirely medical – the Clinical Medicines and Doses Committee chaired by Professor Derek Dunlop. There was a Nomenclature Committee and three concerned with biologicals, but the remaining sixteen were concerned solely with pharmaceutical and chemical standards for drugs and preparations.[105] They were chaired by pharmacists or chemists. A 1955 addendum added yet more new chemical medicines, including cortisone and insulin, along with new tablet monographs. One commentator noted that 'the official British attitude towards new miracle drugs seems in the past to have been rather more sceptical than, for instance, the North Amer-

236   Pharmacopoeias, Drug Regulation, and Empires

ican attitude. In this edition, however, some of the most modern drugs have received official recognition.[106] Phenylbutazone was added to the BP 1953 but had to be dropped from the 1958 edition because of concerns about its safety.[107] It was a stark reminder that the safety of new chemical medicines was often little understood and frequently neglected.

By the 1950s the statutory position of the BP in the empire was becoming increasingly complex as new colonial, British, and international legislation appeared. The 1953 BP included a revised precautionary legal notice clarifying its status in the Commonwealth: 'Substances described in monographs of the BP may be subject to legal control in the UK or in parts of the British Commonwealth in which the BP may have statutory force. Legal control may be concerned with the preparation and labelling of, and the standards for, substances described in the Pharmacopoeia.'[108]

In 1957 all former and current British territories were asked to agree a treaty protocol that would end the 1930 Agreement on the Unification of Pharmacopoeial Formulae for Potent Drugs.[109] It would be superseded by ratification of the *International Pharmacopoeia* (*IP*), which had been produced under the auspices of the World Health Organization, and whose two-volume first edition had been published in 1955.[110] Nearly all colonial governments accepted the protocol, but ratification of the *IP* created difficulties for some; in practice, the legal status of both the BP and the *IP* needed to be recognized, so the BP Commission asked colonial governments to confirm whether there was any local statutory provision regarding the BP. The situation varied greatly: whilst most accepted BP standards, few had made statutory provision to enforce them. British Guiana had statutory provision under a 1956 Pharmacy and Poisons Ordinance, which made the BP the 'standard of quality or composition and preparation of all drugs'. In Dominica there was no statutory provision, but the BP was accepted.[111] Mediterranean colonies all had legislation; in Malta, for example, the Medical and Kindred Professions Ordinance required that 'every apothecary shall in the preparation of medicinal substances be guided by the British Pharmacopoeia'.[112] In Hong Kong a new Pharmacopoeia Ordinance was passed in 1958.[113] The BP could then 'be admitted in evidence in the Courts'. It would 'remove uncertainty as to what are the proper ingredients and proportions of drugs bought and sold'.[114]

THE LAST DAYS OF THE BP COMMISSION

The new edition of the *BP* was signed off by the GMC Pharmacopoeia Committee and published in 1958. The *BP* Commission had met forty-two times and its twenty-two committees nearly two hundred times.[115] Under a new Medical Act in 1956 the GMC retained responsibility for producing it. The PSGB Council agreed that publication of the *BPC* should coincide with that of the *BP* 'so that new versions of the two books could come into effect on the same dates'. The aim was to ensure continuity of standards 'for those drugs and preparations that cease to be the subjects of monographs in the *BP* and become the subjects of monographs in the Codex, and vice versa'.[116] New editions of the *BP* were published at five-year intervals with addenda in between; a 1960 addendum contained fifty-seven new monographs. The tenth edition of the *BP* was published in 1963; an addendum containing sixty new monographs appeared a year later, and a second addendum contained seventy-two more was published in 1966. The *BP* Commission recommended that medicine containers – until then labelled 'the tablets' or 'the mixture' – should give the name of the contents to aid identification, whilst the director of revision of the USP noted that 'the topic given the greatest attention ... is the full achievement of the change-over from the Imperial system to the Metric system of weights and measures'.[117]

The 1963 *BP* consolidated the relationship between the *BP* and the *BPC*. Once the *BP* Commission had decided what to include and exclude there remained many substances that were included in the previous edition that 'still enjoy the confidence of medical practice' or 'are new and becoming increasingly important'. The number of such substances was large, and they were considered 'suitable for inclusion in the *BPC*', whose publication had previously followed eighteen months after that of the *BP*. Of more than one hundred deletions from the *BP* 1958, ninety remained official by inclusion in the new edition of the *BPC*.[118] Of the 211 new monographs included in the *BP* 1963 at least sixty-two substances and preparations had already appeared in the 1959 *BPC*.

The *BP* Commission again noted that 'cordial relations' had been maintained with overseas bodies including the Dominions, India, the United States, the Nordic Pharmacopoeia Council, and the World Health Organization's Pharmaceuticals Unit.[119] Staff of British drug

238 Pharmacopoeias, Drug Regulation, and Empires

companies played increasing roles through membership of subcommittees. The size and pharmacist representation on the BP Commission grew with each new edition. In 1948 it had 10 members, 3 of whom were pharmacists, as was the secretary; there were 4 doctors. The final BP Commission in 1968 had 13 members, 6 of whom – including the secretary and scientific director – were pharmacists. Two other members were chemists. At its end doctors were a minority; the BP was finally a collaborative work by a wide range of experts operating in concert.

THE ASCENDANCY OF DRUG SAFETY

As large numbers of new chemical medicines were marketed during the therapeutic revolution of the 1950s and '60s the BP Commission remained firmly focused on standards and quality. Medicine safety was not explicitly included in the remit of the GMC under the Medical Act. Yet few safeguards were in place to ensure that medicines were safe in all regards, and drug-related tragedies involving multiple deaths or serious harm were increasingly reported. In 1961 large numbers of babies were born deformed after their mothers took the drug thalidomide for the treatment of morning sickness. The thalidomide disaster was a catastrophic demonstration of the failure of drug regulation.[120]

In 1963 the British minister of health, Kenneth Robinson, noted that 'The House [of Commons] and the public suddenly woke up to the fact that any drug manufacturer could market any product – however inadequately tested, however dangerous – without having to satisfy any independent body as to its efficacy or safety.'[121] Thalidomide had not been added to the BP, but the disaster drew attention to the fact that quality and standards were emphasized at the expense of efficacy and safety. In its aftermath the Ministry of Health made wide-ranging recommendations for change. They included a proposal to transfer responsibility for producing the BP – along with other functions – to a new organization. The BP would no longer be published under the authority of the GMC, and its Pharmacopoeia Committee would no longer appoint and approve the work of the BP Commission. The work would be carried out by a new Medicines Commission, which would be responsible directly to the minister of health.[122]

A PHARMACOPOEIA
SUITABLE FOR THE WHOLE OF EUROPE

The new arrangements applied only to Great Britain – not to the empire, Dominions, or colonies. It gave the new body explicit responsibility for drug safety. The shift from Pharmacopoeia Commission to Medicines Commission coincided with Britain's increasing cooperation with its European neighbours. In 1963 the Ministry of Health was contacted about the possibility of establishing a common pharmacopoeia to serve the needs of several European countries. In one of its last acts, the GMC Pharmacopoeia Committee commented on the proposal – part of the preliminary discussions that lead to the creation of the *European Pharmacopoeia* (EP) in 1964.[123] On 17 March 1964 the 'Convention on the Elaboration of a European Pharmacopoeia' was adopted by the Committee of Ministers. In July 1964 Lord Cohen – then chairman of the BP Commission and president of the GMC – reported that a European Pharmacopoeia Commission established under a Council of Europe convention had been signed by Belgium, France, Germany, Italy, Luxembourg, the Netherlands, Switzerland, and the United Kingdom. An EP was to be published, and measures taken to ensure that the monographs included would 'become the official standards applicable within their respective countries as from such dates as should be agreed in respect of each monograph.'[124]

In September 1964 Herbert Grainger was nominated as the first head of the Technical Secretariat. Grainger was a British pharmacist who had previously been chief pharmacist at the Westminster Hospital in London.[125] Former European colonial powers came together to agree a pharmacopoeia suitable for the whole of Europe, and the first edition of the EP was published in 1964. For most countries the EP replaced their national pharmacopoeias, but for Britain it supplemented rather than replaced the BP. Sir Frank Hartley – the last chairman of the BP Commission in 1968 – led the British delegation to meetings of the European Pharmacopoeia Commission in Strasbourg. Grainger recalled that Hartley's 'first and firmest principle was to ensure that nothing got into the *European Pharmacopoeia* that was not of the nature or quality suitable for the BP.'[126] Hartley made it clear, 'spoken or implied, that the *European Pharmacopoeia* could never rise to the quality of the BP.'[127] Only a pharmacopoeia based on British standards would be acceptable: British imperialism had been reaffirmed in Europe.

Conclusion

In this final chapter I draw together insights from this examination of the use of the term 'pharmacopoeia' across the four perspectives considered in this book: the 'cross-disciplinary perspective', in which the different ways in which scholars from a variety of disciplines used the term were examined; the 'cross-imperial power perspective', in which the various approaches to official pharmacopoeias taken by other European colonial powers were considered as a means of identifying ways in which the British approach differed from them; the 'cross-colony perspective', in which ways in which the responses to metropolitan and colonial pharmacopoeias differed between British colonies were identified; and the 'temporal perspective', where ways in which the meanings and functions, legal status, content, and use of the term 'pharmacopoeia' changed over time as well as space were explored.

This book has illustrated how use of the term in scholarly writing has become problematic as a result of its meaning becoming so broad as to be a serious obstacle to further scholarly insight. It has become a ubiquitous umbrella term encompassing everything from the materia medica of Indigenous communities to a diverse range of pharmaceutical texts that may or may not have been issued by a recognized authority and that may or may not have been embedded in statute. The consequences of leaving things unchanged are considerable. A new generation of scholars now use the term without questioning its possible ambiguity. Yet in doing so opportunities for collaboration, for learning from other disciplines, and new avenues of research, are missed. These exist as much in ethnopharmacological research as in the history of medicine, and embrace medical practice, international trade, and drug regulation.

Conclusion   241

Terms are used to convey information and to aid understanding. But their meaning and use change over time; their boundaries expand, subdivisions are created, and new terms invented. This has long been the pattern in scholarly writing, not least in the history of science, technology, and medicine, where the value of terms including 'medical marketplace' and 'colonial science' have already been questioned. This book has shown that the term 'pharmacopoeia' is now overdue for such scrutiny.

PHARMACOPOEIAS FROM
A CROSS-DISCIPLINARY PERSPECTIVE

Following Crawford and Gabriel's observation that the term is now most commonly found in anthropological and ethnobotanical scholarship, chapter 1 illustrated how pharmacopoeias have become the subject of much scholarly activity in recent years, across many different disciplines, and that the term has come to have a great variety of meanings.[1] Whilst most are concerned with materials used for medical purposes (the materia medica) in Indigenous communities, many are not.

Yet if the term 'pharmacopoeia' is used without explanation the meaning is often unclear and misleading. Whether the pharmacopoeia is unwritten – those passed on by word of mouth – or a written text, it may relate only to items of plant origin, to ones of animal, vegetable, and mineral origin, include items used for medical but not medicinal purposes, or items used for other purposes such as food. If referring to a text, use of 'pharmacopoeia' does not signify whether it is a list of items used for medicinal purposes, or a list of those items plus recipes for the forms in which it is used. Nor does it indicate whether it is issued under some official authority or whether that authority is underpinned by law. Chapter 1 illustrated some of the ways in which ambiguity has crept into scholarly discourse about pharmacopoeias and how this can lead to confusion, uncertainty, and error.

Avoiding such uncertainty is important for many reasons, not least because scholarly volumes play vital roles in shaping doctoral studies and research agendas. Terms used by leading scholars are replicated by early career researchers. For example, in one of her books Londa Schiebinger states that 'by the sixteenth century "wonder drugs" such as quinine, jalap, and ipecacuanha had been found, and were soon to be introduced into the pharmacopoeia of major European commercial centres.[2] This suggests that quinine was recognized as a drug in the sixteenth century (it was only extracted from cinchona bark by Pelletier and Caventou in 1820), and that it appeared in the official pharmacopoeias of cities that had introduced them by 1700, such as Amsterdam and London. Or does she just mean that they were used as medicinal items in some European cities?

'Pharmacopoeia' has come to describe such a broad range of ideas, practices, and publications that further elucidation and understanding of their place in the history of medicine may be hampered without greater clarification of the intended meaning of that term, not least in exploring the role they played in the transition of Indigenous remedy to Western medicine, and in the international drug trade. As this book has shown, much of the current literature makes little distinction between official and other types of pharmacopoeias, and the examples given also illustrate how loose use of the term can lead to misunderstandings in the interpretation of the relationship between official pharmacopoeias and drug regulation. Jenner and Wallis suggest that two themes have largely dominated discussion of pharmacopoeias in medical history: the relationship between medicines, trade, and pharmacopoeias, and the relationship between official pharmacopoeias, the regulation of medicines, and praxis.[3]

Hal Cook and Roy Porter identified the rise of specific drugs as an important factor in the growth of the medical marketplace; commodities including tea, coffee, and tobacco moved from the medical marketplace to the wider world of goods.[4] Bhattacharya's assertion that pharmacopoeias can only be understood in the context of markets – 'of the product of the drugs and therapeutics market in India'[5] – may be true for India in the nineteenth and early twentieth centuries, but it works less well over a longer time scale and across a wide range of imperial contexts. The history of pharmacopoeias cannot easily be segregated from the history of drug regulation; a better understanding of the complex interaction between the two is essential for more informed historical analysis of drugs and empires.

The historical value of pharmacopoeias has nevertheless proved enduring. They serve as records of authority and as depositories of knowledge. They help us to track the advance of science as applied to drugs, and they illuminate the interconnectedness of metropole with periphery through the movement of people, goods, and ideas. The search for 'buried treasure' in old pharmacopoeias has extended to all communities across all time frames. Ancient and modern texts continue to be a promising source of discovery of items with therapeutic potential. In Britain several Anglo-Saxon manuscripts reporting medicinal formulations used in England from the tenth century survive, and studies of medicinal plants listed in sixteenth- and seventeenth-century texts have suggested that some were effective and have led to the identification and isolation of new natural compounds.[6] Further insights may emerge through multidisciplinary projects exploring the content of early manuscripts leading to the discovery of metabolites with potential pharmacological applications.

Crawford and Gabriel suggest that analysing 'a diverse array of actors enriches our understanding of the historical genealogy of pharmacopoeias as tools of communication, standardisation, and control.' An additional factor that made them valuable as historical sources was that 'in many cases they emerged out of the intersection of knowledge and the aspirations of state power.'[7] Pablo Gomez noted that the purpose of pharmacopoeias in the early modern period 'was to create an idea of order and structure. A framework of codified knowledge that both practitioners and regulators knew was aspirational.'[8] Pharmacopoeias were a mirage, but nevertheless powerful. They were 'the physical representation of a regime sustained in what could not be said, aspirational attempts at bringing to light what functioned as the basis of obscurity.'

Studies of traditional and official pharmacopoeias also have important contributions to make to contemporary debates, such as those around the historical origins of processes of medicalization, pharmaceuticalization, and biomedicalization.[9] Traditional pharmacopoeias contained only items of natural origin – plant, animal, or mineral; official pharmacopoeias also contained preparations and single chemical entities. Pharmacopoeias illustrate processes of biomedicalization and pharmaceuticalization, yet these literatures are rarely cross-referenced. Further insights must surely result from closer collaboration between scholars from a range of disciplines working on these issues.

PHARMACOPOEIAS FROM
A CROSS-COLONIAL POWER PERSPECTIVE

Chapter 3 explored the development of official pharmacopoeias in other European countries and their place in their respective empires, as a means of identifying factors that might distinguish the British

244 Pharmacopoeias, Drug Regulation, and Empires

approach to pharmacopoeial development and the use of such texts in its colonies from that of its European rivals. Important differences were found in a wide range of issues, including under whose authority they were issued (table 3.1). This changed over time, with early pharmacopoeias issued under the authority of city states rather than national bodies. They ranged from church authorities (Portugal and Italy), monarchs (Spain and Denmark), colleges of physicians (Edinburgh), colleges of apothecaries (Valencia), to medical officers (Naples). Few pharmacopoeias had statutory authority – being embedded in legislation passed by a parliament – before the late eighteenth century.

European pharmacopoeias varied in who was involved in compiling them. Sometimes it was doctors, sometimes it was apothecaries or pharmacists, and sometimes it was both groups working together. Yet this factor had a dramatic impact on the outcome; ones compiled solely by apothecaries tended to be extremely large volumes listing every drug and preparation stocked by apothecaries (Italy); those left entirely in the hands of doctors sometimes failed to deliver an agreed volume (Portugal). At least some level of advice from apothecaries appears to have been essential. Yet the degree of collaboration between the groups varied greatly and has been a key factor in the content and comprehensiveness of pharmacopoeias, as illustrated in the British experience; relations between doctors and pharmacists were at the heart of pharmacy professionalization.[10] In most European countries pharmacy and medicine existed as separate professions from at least the seventeenth century,[11] a fact that had an important impact on the practice of pharmacy in France's overseas colonies, such as Vietnam.[12] This was equally true of most other European colonial powers. The transition of apothecaries into general medical practitioners rather than pharmacists set the progress of British pharmacy back by 150 years compared with the rest of Europe, and this had an important impact on the approach taken in its colonies.[13]

An examination of the ways in which European colonial powers dealt with issues of drug regulation and pharmacopoeias in their colonies demonstrates a considerable degree of uniformity. Despite very different institutional, political, and social circumstances in their metropoles – and very different colonial contexts – most countries simply imposed their national pharmacopoeias across their empires. In most no attempt was made to imperialize the pharmacopoeia by including items primarily used by practitioners working in the colonies – items that could be substituted for ones not available locally – or by adapting formulas to take account of tropical climates or religious sensibilities. Britain alone undertook the imperialization of its pharmacopoeia in the late nineteenth century. At least one European colonial power planned to produce a colonial addendum to its national pharmacopoeia (the Netherlands), but the attempt was unsuccessful.

Little evidence has been found that colonial practitioners played any substantial role in determining the content of national pharmacopoeias. Even where account was taken of colonial conditions (France) no provision was made for local consultation. Pressure to create a standardized national pharmacopoeia updated with the latest knowledge came from metropolitan rather than colonial doctors, although some of those would doubtless have had extensive practical experience in the colonies. Typically, no attempts were made to accommodate the needs of empire; most metropolitan pharmacopoeias were imposed unaltered.

The question as to whether official pharmacopoeias were comprehensive and exclusive, or selective and permissive, also varied considerably. The promise that such volumes should contain all the medicines used in daily practice was always very ambitious, and one on which it would be very difficult to deliver. The result was almost always massive, unwieldy volumes, such as those produced by the Italian apothecaries. The final publication was usually a compromise list of medicines commonly prescribed by doctors and stocked by apothecaries, subject to varying degrees of personal preference and scientific evidence. The history of pharmacopoeias is littered with complaints about omissions – whether of favoured remedies or local substitutes for pharmacopoeial items. There were far fewer complaints about included items that needed to be deleted, whether because they were no longer used, there was a lack of evidence about their efficacy, or concerns about their safety. Most European pharmacopoeias focused on the drugs to be used rather than the methods by which their preparations might be made; they were more medical than pharmaceutical volumes.

These themes informed the subsequent discussion about the evolving nature of pharmacopoeias in Britain and their use in the empire, which was transformed during the course of the nineteenth century. A number of features have been shown to define the British way of dealing with pharmacopoeias in the imperial context by the end of that century. The British authorities chose to develop an imperial pharmacopoeia rather than to impose a metropolitan one; they chose to consult and engage with colonial practitioners rather than leaving it in the hands of metropolitan physicians; and doctors alone would be responsible for its compilation, although they would seek the advice of pharmacists and chemists. The volume would aim to include all medicines regularly prescribed by doctors and dispensed by pharmacists throughout the empire, provided that there was enough evidence to do so; and the final publication would be more a medical than a pharmaceutical work. The British way of dealing with pharmacopoeias in the colonial context therefore stands out as an exception to the norm.

PHARMACOPOEIAS FROM A CROSS-COLONY PERSPECTIVE

A cross-colony perspective has highlighted the fact that the relationship between metropole and empire with regard to pharmacopoeias was by no means homogenous: many differences existed between Britain and its colonies, Dominions, and India, largely based on the origins of their British connections. In some colonies ordinances mandated the use of particular pharmacopoeias – the *London Pharmacopoeia* (LP) in South Africa for example – although with passage of the 1868 Pharmacy and Poisons Act most colonies passed ordinances requiring that, if a drug listed in the *British Pharmacopoeia* (BP) was required, it must only be supplied in the form of a preparation described within it. By the early twentieth century Canada and Australia had compiled local formularies listing preparations authorized for use locally. Such developments highlighted the movement of news and information across the empire and between its various constituent parts, movement that was facilitated by the wide distribution of journals such as the *Pharmaceutical Journal* and *Chemist and Druggist*. They also highlighted the important role of networks in pharmacy, medicine, and science.

The role of networks in the development of empires has received considerable attention from historians.[14] Roy MacLeod described the web of connections between scientists across and between empires as a tangle of 'multiple engagements'.[15] Mark Harrison suggests that 'the more we examine the intricacies of colonial science, the more it seems to be characterized by "multiple engagements" both within and with-

Conclusion 247

out individual colonies.[16] These relationships are clearly demonstrated in discussions about the role of British pharmacopoeias in the empire. The approach in the early 1890s to medical and pharmaceutical authorities in all seventy colonies of the British Empire exemplified the representation of colonial scientific relationships as a wheel, with metropolitan bodies at the hub, and colonial practitioners as the spokes. Yet as the goal of a single imperial pharmacopoeia faded after the First World War the channels of communication began to resemble more the 'polycentric communications network' described by David Wade Chambers and Richard Gillespie, with multiple layers of authority and interaction, as colonial governments established specialist committees to share information between themselves and to channel information and advice to the centre, and those interactions increasingly included ones with agencies beyond the empire, notably the US Pharmacopoeia Commission.[17]

The experience with pharmacopoeias in India was different to that in much of the rest of the empire. Both the *Bengal Pharmacopoeia* and the *Pharmacopoeia of India* were official in being prepared on the orders of the Government of India, compiled under the authority of a committee appointed by it, and published on its orders; but neither was statutory since neither was incorporated in legislation. The reasons why a government would make a pharmacopoeia official without giving it the backing of law are complex. As this book has shown, no relevant legislation existed in Britain before the 1868 Pharmacy and Poisons Act, and even that gave very limited backing to the *BP*. No such act was passed in India. Making any aspect of either the *Bengal Pharmacopoeia* or the *Pharmacopoeia of India* statutory would have been impossible; metropolitan Medical Acts, Pharmacy and Poisons Acts, and Food and Drugs Acts did not apply in India, and no such legislation had been enacted locally. India was a vast country with a very large native-born population where a variety of medical belief systems held sway. The volume of drugs used in Western medicine was tiny in comparison with the total volume of drugs supplied through bazaars. Any attempt to impose a system of inspection, testing, and prosecution would have attracted fierce opposition from local practitioners and people.

If making a pharmacopoeia statutory was likely to be practically or politically impossible, it might seem strange to make it official in the first place. Many factors were involved, but it was undoubtedly at least in part a reflection of the influence of senior medical officers and trade interests in India promoting the use of local products not only in India but also in Britain, with the aim of having these added to the *BP*. Medical officers were a powerful group in a strong position to influence the Government of India and authorities in London. They sought official approval to substitute local plant medicines for equivalent items listed in metropolitan pharmacopoeias and were keen to see those of proven value added to them. But a colonial pharmacopoeia was not the only solution. The government could have adhered to the line taken by most other colonial powers and insisted that the metropolitan pharmacopoeia be fully complied with, banning local variation such as substitution. Potentially useful items from the colonies could be referred to the Pharmacopoeia Committee in London for consideration.

Previous texts on Indian materia medica had failed to have much impact on the content of the *BP*. Making them official in India was a means of drawing the attention of the authorities to worthy Indian plant medicines that might enter everyday use in the metropole, open up new trade opportunities, and find a place in the metropolitan pharmacopoeia. In India allowing an official pharmacopoeia produced by British doctors with experience of India enabled the government to allow the use of some local substitutes in place of equivalent items listed in the *BP*. Had the *Bengal Pharmacopoeia* and the *Pharmacopoeia of India* not been official, with the selection of items decided by an individual and publication through a commercial publisher, their status would have been no different to any other compilation of materia medica. In making them official the government sanctioned the use of items that would not otherwise have been available; they could be obtained by the medical stores and distributed to hospitals and clinics around the country. This book has demonstrated that whilst pharmacopoeias had many meanings, they also had many functions.

PHARMACOPOEIAS FROM
A TEMPORAL PERSPECTIVE

Those many functions are clearly highlighted when viewed from a temporal perspective. Over three and a half centuries both the functions and intended audiences of pharmacopoeias changed. They invariably had multiple aims. Initially they were a useful way of controlling the activities of the apothecaries whilst ostensibly protecting the public. They might be used to control the range of remedies available, or to exclude certain substances from legitimate use. They played important parts in regulating pharmacy practice and medicines; and they reflected relations between doctors and pharmacists, scientific progress, and political ambition in diverse climatic, political, and cultural spaces. Their principal users also changed; these have variously been physicians and apothecaries, chemist and druggist apprentices preparing for examinations, and laboratory staff in pharmaceutical companies testing standards of manufactured products.

Purpose was reinforced by content and structure. By the exclusion of information about the medical indications for prescribed medicines in the *LP* 1618 the physicians hoped to maintain their monopoly over the practice of medicine and the subservience of the apothecaries.[18] Its use of Latin was designed to make it accessible to physicians and apothecaries, but not the wider public. The 1746 *LP* marked the transition of their primary function from instrument of control to vehicle for standardization. But it also had implicit aims, including demonstrating the authority of the Royal College of Physicians, emphasizing one medical philosophy over another, and exhibiting national identity.

For emerging empires official pharmacopoeias served as incentives for bioprospectors to plunder traditional pharmacopoeias, promote their use in the metropole, and establish an international trade in medicinal items. In settler communities their roles were little different to those in the metropole. But pharmacopoeias had non-statutory as well as statutory functions where laws had been passed; they provided guidance and advice and were tools of encouragement and persuasion. The functions of enabling, controlling, standardizing, and regulating were often incorporated into a single pharmacopoeia, with non-statutory functions being dominant in India and other large colonies with diverse populations. Official pharmacopoeias served as instruments of soft colonial power – a connection that has to date received little attention from medical and imperial historians.

Pharmacopoeias became essential badges of national identity during the sixteenth century.[19] Although the authority of most was initially limited to a city state their application to larger territories soon followed. When the 1618 *LP* was published it was addressed to apothecaries 'within the realme of England or the dominions thereof.'[20] The later publication of the *Edinburgh* and *Dublin Pharmacopoeias* provided clear statements of national identity and distinctiveness from the London physicians.[21] Functions changed as the geographical reach expanded; content varied according to whether the intended usage was in the colonies, the Dominions, or the Commonwealth, and ultimately across Europe and throughout the world. By the nineteenth century their value as instruments of imperialism had been recognized.[22] They were a means of assuring uniformity in strength and purity across national boundaries, and of joining disparate colonies and dependencies into a united empire with a common identity.

In the early twentieth century attention focused on efficacy and purity; safety was largely a peripheral concern. What changed was the dominance of one function over others, whether political or economic. Their economic roles have received some attention from historians over the years; in 1951 George Urdang observed that among these were meeting the 'economic needs of the area concerned by including products of its own soil and industry, and excluding – as far as possible – products of foreign origin.'[23] But as well as their role in trade they sometimes had unanticipated functions, such as controlling costs of drugs to the state (New Zealand), or as negotiating tools in the taxing of medicines (South Africa).

Imperializing the pharmacopoeia was never going to be easy; in the end it proved impossible. It demanded the resolution of too many conflicting aims. Compiling a volume that would not only be a comprehensive guide to all the drugs and preparations needed in any part of the empire, but would also bind together disparate communities, was a massive task that was eventually overtaken by political events and scientific developments. But by the mid-nineteenth century the most contested and fundamental issue was whether new medicinal plants requested by colonies should be included in the pharmacopoeia, or whether it should be confined to new chemical medicines, about which there was rarely any dispute. Scientification had been gradual; Western pharmacopoeias included chemical tests for assessing the quality of drugs from the late eighteenth century as a result of advances in chemistry. Few plant medicines had been subjected to rigorous testing – the very feature now emphasized in pharmacopoeias – and most were rejected.

STATUTORY AND NON-STATUTORY
OFFICIAL PHARMACOPOEIAS

The distinction between official pharmacopoeias and those that were also statutory was intimately bound up with drug regulation. As this book has shown official pharmacopoeias that were not statutory were

Conclusion 251

often ineffective as a result of a lack of legally enforceable arrangements for inspection, prosecution, and sanction. Some form of rudimentary drug regulation sometimes existed prior to the publication of pharmacopoeias, such as the fourteenth-century employment of garblers to inspect sacks of imported items at the ports, and later the inspection of premises by physicians. But those who acted as inspectors needed guidance as to what counted as good quality and what as bad, and pharmacopoeias provided a means of doing so. But pharmacopoeias were not a prerequisite for drug regulation; they were independent of it.

Drug regulation is today embedded in legislation, but historically this was not always the case. As this book has shown there were several forms of regulation, from the very weak to the very strong. Over the course of several centuries ways of regulating medicines progressed from the individual to the state via professional regulation and legislation. Official pharmacopoeias were one of the means available to the authorities for standardizing medicines and controlling those who made and supplied them. But there was nothing inevitable about their development. Markets provided a crude but uncertain means of ensuring quality; dissatisfied customers did not return. But it was unrealistic to expect members of the public to be able to judge the quality of medicines themselves; state intervention was necessary. What form that intervention took was a matter of debate, and the nature of that debate varied from place to place.

The professional responsibility of the apothecary transformed into the personal liability of the pharmacist; and the authority of separate colleges of physicians was replaced first by a General Medical Council and later a Medicines Commission reporting directly to government. Holloway's principal models of drug regulation – consumer sovereignty, occupational control, and bureaucratic regulation – all played a part in the development of pharmacopoeias, with early ones intended to ensure that the medicines received by patients were of the standard expected. Occupational control – where responsibility for the inspection of apothecaries' premises and the destruction of medicines was placed in the hands of physicians – was the dominant model applied across the empire; doctors regulated both the practice of pharmacy and the control of poisons. It was only with passage of the 1868 Pharmacy and Poisons Act that a bureaucratic system of drug regulation was assumed by the state.

252 Pharmacopoeias, Drug Regulation, and Empires

Linking poisons control with pharmacy regulation had been necessary to secure legislative backing in the second half of the nineteenth century. Yet history has judged that link to be a disaster for the pharmacy profession. Sir Hugh Linstead concluded that 'this unfortunate legislative association of pharmacy with poisons' led to Parliament placing increasing reliance on 'mechanical safeguards such as the poison label and the poison bottle, in preference to reliance upon the knowledge and sense of professional responsibility of the seller.'[24] One consequence was that corporate bodies were enabled to run pharmacies, and medicines continued to be regulated under poisons legislation until the 1968 Medicines Act. Consideration of intrinsic drug safety came late to both drug regulation and pharmacopoeias. But there was a difficult balance to be reached; in 1980 Sir Derek Dunlop reflected that whilst inadequate legislation could compromise public safety, excessive legislation could also be prejudicial. 'It would be a pity if in our desire to improve the health of the public an excessive regulation of medicines is allowed to develop.'[25]

Arrangements resulting from legislative compromise and largely considered unsatisfactory at the time were nevertheless introduced across much of the empire; most colonies passed legislation based on the 1868 Pharmacy Act, which required that drugs listed in the pharmacopoeia be supplied only in the form of preparations prescribed therein. But some territories did not; in India repeated attempts to introduce legislation failed. In colonies with large and diverse populations the imposition of bureaucratic arrangements for regulating drugs was unrealistic. Even in European enclaves a great deal of determination and commitment was required. In the absence of incentives and sanctions compliance with BP requirements was unlikely; any attempt to impose such standards at the bazaars would be strongly resisted. Inevitable price pressures forced many manufacturers to cut corners and engage in substitution and adulteration. But pharmacopoeias often had ripple effects beyond the items listed; Stebbings suggests that – in Britain – the recognition that medicine stamp duty gave to the BP contributed to regulating the quality of patent medicines.[26]

The challenges of drug regulation were not limited to official pharmacopoeias; the same is now true of the content of traditional pharmacopoeias. Those in colonies seeking to have plant medicines included in pharmacopoeias struggled to come up with evidence in support of their claims. The importance of empirical evidence where

Conclusion

scientific evidence is limited or absent continues to be a challenge for regulating traditional plant medicines. In 1998 the World Health Organization carried out a worldwide review of the herbal medicine regulatory situation; it indicated that traditional plant medicines are now strictly regulated in many countries.[27] Tools have since been developed to systematically collate and evaluate bibliographic data for traditional health claims, which provide additional pathways to operationalize such data in an evidence-based policy framework.[28] Yet historical questions about drug regulation in Indigenous pharmacopoeias – what constraints existed regarding excessive or inappropriate use, what safeguards existed to prevent the ingestion of harmful substances – remain largely unexplored. Understanding the roles of village elders and healers in these issues offer new insights into processes of appropriation and bioprospecting.

PHARMACOPOEIAS
IN SCHOLARLY WRITING

How then can our use of the term 'pharmacopoeia' be made less problematic in scholarly writing? In many cases more appropriate descriptors can be used and indeed sometimes are. Lists of materia medica, with instructions about how to prepare and use them, existed in early civilizations. They were referred to as formularies, *antidotaria*, dispensatories, herbals, codices, and vade mecums, as well as pharmacopoeias.[29] There is no denying that these titles were used rather loosely in the past, but with the vast expansion of scholarly writing in recent years their more specific use might at least offer a degree of discrimination between diverse texts. Guides to the use of medicines of plant origin are commonly referred to as herbals; lists of medicinal recipes are usually called formularies; non-official guides to the use of medicinal substances and their preparations are more helpfully described as dispensatories. To use these terms interchangeably is to miss important historical distinctions and to fail to recognize the way in which they came to mean different things over time.

Whilst 'ethno-pharmacopoeia' and 'Indigenous pharmacopoeia' at least offer some distinction from Western pharmacopoeias, they also lack definition; they give no hint as to whether they include plant items only or also those of animal and mineral origin, and whether they include preparations and instructions on how to make them. The literature on Indigenous pharmacopoeias has revealed many themes that have received little attention from historians to date. We know a great deal about the influence of neighbours' pharmacopoeias – and those of visitors from abroad – on the pharmacopoeias of Indigenous communities, but much less about their historical origins. The geographer Robert Voeks was not the first to question the idea that the knowledge and practices of Indigenous healers in the Americas 'derived exclusively from some ancient wisdom of tropical rainforests that predated European colonialism'. He argued for a more diffuse origin and coined the phrase 'disturbance pharmacopoeia'. Whilst these were based on Indigenous and traditional remedies used by American folk healers, they were enhanced by new medicinal foods, ornamental plants, and weeds brought by European colonizers.[30] He suggests that viewing Indigenous practices as disturbance pharmacopoeias 'recognizes and recasts folk healing traditions as dynamic and historical enterprises rather than storehouses of timeless knowledge'.[31]

This enhancement of Indigenous pharmacopoeias with medicinal items brought by Europeans continues to receive considerable attention from ethnobotanists and economic botanists, who have shown that Indigenous communities had few qualms about adding to their pharmacopoeias items brought by the colonizers that they thought might be beneficial. As indicated in chapter 1 ethnobotanists have tested the diversification hypothesis, which suggests that exotic plant species are selected to fill therapeutic vacancies due to novel bioactivity, thereby diversifying available treatment options.[32] They found support for the hypothesis, in that exotic and native plants contained significantly different proportions of certain compounds.[33] The diversification hypothesis may also have utility for historians examining how exotic plants came to be included in traditional pharmacopoeias. So, too, might the apparency hypothesis, which predicts that the 'apparent' plants (those most easily found in the vegetation) will be the most commonly collected and used as medicines.[34]

But if 'pharmacopoeia' has come to have a broad range of meanings in its non-official sense, its official sense is no less capacious. Yet terms such as 'official' or 'non-official', 'statutory' or 'non-statutory', and 'formal' and 'informal' with regard to pharmacopoeias are also subject to considerable ambiguity. Nandini Bhattacharya, for example, describes the 'inclusions and exclusions of drugs from the formal and informal formularies', and explores 'the principal themes of circulation, marginalization and formalization of drugs in both text and praxis in colonial India?[35] Are we to suppose that 'formal formularies' are in fact 'official pharmacopoeias' published by a recognized authority such as a government and embedded in statutory law, or could they simply be lists of formulas compiled by someone with acknowledged expertise? This book has argued that an important distinction needs to be made between official and statutory pharmacopoeias, and that official pharmacopoeias can only be understood in the context of drug regulation.

THE PROBLEMATIZATION OF 'PHARMACOPOEIA'

The aim of this book has been to problematize the use of the term 'pharmacopoeia' in scholarly writing. For historians of medicine and empire its central message is that better clarification of meaning – particularly in distinguishing between traditional and official pharmacopoeias, between those that are statutory and those that are not, and in recognizing their relationship to drug regulation – will not only more accurately inform issues surrounding drugs and medicines in the colonial context but will also open up new avenues of research and inquiry. But anthropologists, ethnobotanists, and pharmacologists also need to better explain how they are using the word, for not to distinguish Indigenous pharmacopoeias from official ones is to miss important distinctions between them based on the origin, authenticity, and acceptance of particular medicines in specific contexts. The contents of official pharmacopoeias changed in response to changing medical philosophies and practices, to scientific developments (chemistry, physiology, pharmacology, and botany), and to technological developments (microscopes, balances, and dosage forms). As John Pickstone has shown the 'history of STM [science, technology, and medicine] is not a matter of successions, or the replacement of one kind of knowledge by another; rather it is a matter of complex cumulation and of simultaneous variety, contested over time, not least when new forms of knowledge partially displace old forms'[36]

This book has drawn evidence from a broad range of both primary and secondary sources. Many of these have received little attention to date in wider studies of the history of pharmacy. Jonathan Simon has called for 'an all-inclusive history of pharmacy that integrates social, institutional, practical, experimental, and theoretical analyses'. He has also drawn attention to the lack of comparative studies between different national contexts, suggesting that such studies 'promise to reveal much about the development of pharmacy'.[37] In Britain the position of the pharmacist was much less formalized than in France, and no serious attempt was made to reform pharmacy there in the late eighteenth century as there had been in France. 'The schism in nineteenth century British pharmacy was between those who remained apothecaries and those who became physicians', Simon argues. 'There is much to learn from the difference in the trajectory of French pharmacy when compared to other countries'.[38]

This book has made explicit the relationship between pharmacopoeias, drug regulation, and empire, and illuminated how states exercised power, either directly through legislation or indirectly by delegation to professional organizations. The BP continues to be used in over one hundred countries, about a quarter of which were once part of the British Empire.[39] It is still referred to in the legislation of many of them. It is mentioned in Hong Kong's Pharmacy and Poisons Regulations, alongside the pharmacopoeia of the People's Republic of China, the *European Pharmacopoeia*, the *International Pharmacopoeia*, the *Pharmacopoeia of Japan*, and the *United States Pharmacopoeia*.[40] Reflecting on its future in 2014, Samantha Atkinson – the then scientific director of the British Pharmacopoeia Commission – considered that one of its ongoing roles should be to 'build on international relationships, to increase collaborative use of pharmacopoeial texts, and to encourage harmonization by default'.[41]

In 1999 the United Kingdom's Department of Heath asked a senior civil servant, Roy Cunningham, to conduct a consultation on the future of the two volumes of the BP and its companion volumes. In his report Cunningham declared that, in addition to its other roles, 'the BP was an instrument of economic development and assistance to developing countries and Eastern Europe, for example by helping their regulatory authorities police markets in counterfeit drugs'.[42]

Today 'pharmacopoeia' has many meanings and serves a multitude of functions beyond merely setting standards for drugs. The language has changed, but the call for an 'imperial British pharmacopoeia' – first made in 1813 – echoed down the centuries.

Notes

INTRODUCTION

1 Emily Beck, 'The *Ricettario Fiorentino* and Manuscript Recipe Culture in Sixteenth-Century Florence,' in *Drugs on the Page: Pharmacopoeias and Healing Knowledge in the Early Modern Atlantic World*, ed. Matthew James Crawford and Joseph Gabriel (Pittsburgh, PA: University of Pittsburgh Press, 2019), 45–62.

2 Vivian Nutton, *Ancient Medicine* (Abingdon, UK: Routledge, 2013), 175.

3 Ibid., 176.

4 *The Old English Illustrated Pharmacopoeia*, MS Facsimile 494/27, 1998, British Library.

5 Maria Amalia D'Aronco, 'The Old English Pharmacopoeia,' *Avista Forum Journal* 13, no. 2 (2003): 11.

6 G.E. Trease, *Pharmacy in History* (London: Bailliere, Tindall & Cox, 1964), 45.

7 The process of garbling commenced in 1393. See Trease, *Pharmacy in History*, 65.

8 J. Worth Estes, 'The European Reception of the First Drugs from the New World,' *Pharmacy in History* 37, no. 1 (1995): 3–23.

9 Ibid., 3.

10 Ibid., 18–19.

11 Andrew Chevalier, *The Encyclopedia of Medicinal Plants* (London: Dorling Kindersley, 1996).

12 Londa Schiebinger, *Plants and Empire: Colonial Bioprospecting in the Atlantic World* (Cambridge, MA: Harvard University Press, 2007), 193.

13 Francisco Guerra, 'Medical Colonization of the New World,' *Medical History* 7, no. 2 (1963): 147–54.

258 Notes to pages 8–10

14 The phrase 'Columbian Exchange' is taken from the title of Alfred W. Crosby's book *The Columbian Exchange: Biological and Cultural Consequences of 1492* (Westport, CT: Greenwood, 1972). It divided exchanges into three groups: diseases, animals, and plants.

15 Nathan Nunn and Nancy Qian, 'The Columbian Exchange: A History of Disease, Food, and Ideas', *Journal of Economic Perspectives* 24, no. 2 (2010): 163–88.

16 Worth Estes, 'European Reception', 19.

17 David L. Cowen, 'The British North American Colonies as a Source of Drugs', *Proceedings of the International Society for the History of Pharmacy* 28 (1966): 47–59.

18 David L. Cowen, 'The History of Pharmacy and the History of the South', *Report of Rho Chi* 38 (1967): 18–25. Reprinted in *Apothecary's Cabinet* 6 (2003): 1–5.

19 Worth Estes, 'European Reception', 3–23.

20 John K. Crellin, *A Social History of Medicines in the Twentieth Century* (New York: Pharmaceutical Products Press, 2004), 32.

21 Patrick Wallis, 'Exotic Drugs and English Medicine: England's Drug Trade c.1550–c.1800', *Social History of Medicine* 25, no. 1 (2011): 26.

22 Louis De Vorsey, 'The Tragedy of the Columbia Exchange', in *North America: The Historical Geography of a Changing Continent*, ed. Thomas F. McIlwraith and Edward K. Muller (Lanham, MD: Rowman and Littlefield, 2001), 27.

23 Zachary Dorner, *Merchants of Medicines: The Commerce and Coercion of Health in Britain's Long Eighteenth Century* (Chicago: University of Chicago Press, 2020), 41–70.

24 Renate Wilson, 'Trading in Drugs through Philadelphia in the Eighteenth Century: A Transatlantic Enterprise', *Social History of Medicine* 26, no. 3 (2013): 352–63; William I. Roberts III, 'Samuel Storke: An Eighteenth-Century London Merchant Trading to the American Colonies', *Business History Review* 39, no. 2 (1965): 147–70; Nicholas L. Wood, 'Private Lives, Quaker Connections, and Overseas Trading: The Family Journal and Account Book of Thomas Mayleigh, 1671–1732', *Pharmaceutical Historian* 51, no. 4 (2019): 106–17; C.H. Spiers, 'Drug Suppliers of George Washington and other Virginians', *Pharmaceutical Historian* 7, no. 1 (1977): 2–3.

25 Mark S.R. Jenner and Patrick Wallis, 'The Medical Marketplace', in *Medicine and the Market in England and Its Colonies, c.1450–c.1850*, ed. Jenner and Wallis (London: Palgrave Macmillan, 2007), 11.

26 Cited in Jenner and Wallis, 'The Medical Marketplace', 15.

Notes to pages 11–12

27 David L. Cowen, 'The Impact of the Materia Medica of the North American Indian on Professional Practice', *Proceedings of the International Society for the History of Pharmacy* 53 (1984): 51–63.

28 Letitia McCune and Alain Cuerrier, 'Traditional Plant Medicines and the Protection of Traditional Harvesting Sites', in *Plants, People and Places: The Roles of Ethnobotany and Ethnoecology in Indigenous Peoples' Land Rights in Canada and Beyond*, ed. Nancy Turner (Montreal and Kingston: McGill-Queen's University Press, 2020), 154.

29 Danielle C.A. Spoor, Louis C. Martineau, Charles Leduc, Ali Benhaddou-Andaloussi, Bouchra Meddah, Cory Harris, Andrew Burt, Marie-Hélène Fraser, Jason Coonishish, Erik Joly, Alain Cuerrier, Steffany A.L. Bennett, Timothy Johns, Marc Prentki, John T. Arnason, and Pierre S. Haddad, 'Selected Plant Species from the Northern Quebec Cree Pharmacopoeia Possess Anti-diabetic Potential', *Canadian Journal of Physiology and Pharmacology* 84, nos 8–9 (2006): 847–58.

30 McCune and Cuerrier, 'Traditional Plant Medicines', 155.

31 Ibid., 163.

32 Audrey M. Martin, *Pharmacy in Canada: Highlights of Its History from Early to Recent Times* (Vancouver: Pharmaceutical Association of British Columbia, 1955), 8.

33 F.W. Howay, ed., *Builders of the West: A Book of Heroes* (Toronto: Ryerson Press, 1929).

34 Martin, *Pharmacy in Canada*, 8.

35 Harold J. Cook and Timothy D. Walker, 'Circulation of Medicine in the Early Modern Atlantic World', *Social History of Medicine* 26, no. 3 (2013): 337–51.

36 Matthew James Crawford, *The Andean Wonder Drug: Cinchona Bark and Imperial Science in the Spanish Atlantic World, 1630–1800* (Pittsburgh, PA: Pittsburgh University Press, 2016).

37 Guy Attewell, 'Interweaving Substance Trajectories: Circulation and Therapeutic Transformation in the Nineteenth Century', in *Crossing Colonial Historiographies: Histories of Colonial and Indigenous Medicines in Transnational Perspective*, ed. Anne Digby, Waltraud Ernst, and Projit B. Mukharji (Newcastle, UK: Cambridge Scholars, 2010), 1–20.

38 Nandini Bhattacharya, 'Between the Bazaar and the Bench: Making of the Drugs Trade in Colonial India, c.1900–1930', *Bulletin of the History of Medicine* 90 (2016): 62.

39 Cowen, 'British North American Colonies', 47–59.

40 Stefanie Gänger, *A Singular Remedy: Cinchona across the Atlantic World, 1751–1820* (Cambridge: Cambridge University Press, 2020).

260 Notes to pages 12–15

41 Sabine Anagnostou, Florike Egmond, and Christoph Friedrich, eds, *A Passion for Plants: Materia Medica and Botany in Scientific Networks from the Sixteenth to Eighteenth Centuries* (Stuttgart: Wissenschaftliche Verlagsgesellschaft, 2011).

42 Londa Schiebinger, *Secret Cures of Slaves: People, Plants and Medicines in the Eighteenth-Century Atlantic World* (Stanford, CA: Stanford University Press, 2017), 149. For knowledge brokers, see Simon Schaffer, Lissa Roberts, Kapil Raj, and James Delbourgo, eds, *The Brokered World: Go-Betweens and Global Intelligence, 1770–1820* (Sagamore Beach, MA: Watson Publishing International, 2009).

43 Lucile H. Brockway, *Science and Colonial Expansion: The Role of British Royal Botanic Gardens* (New Haven, CT: Yale University Press, 2002).

44 Chandra Mukerji, 'Dominion, Demonstration, and Domination', in *Colonial Botany: Science, Commerce, and Politics in the Early Modern World*, ed. Londa Schiebinger and Claudia Swan (Philadelphia: University of Pennsylvania Press, 2005), 25–6.

45 Mukerji, 'Dominion', 27.

46 Pratik Chakrabarti, *Medicine and Empire, 1600–1960* (London: Palgrave Macmillan, 2014): 31. See also Pratik Chakrabarti, *Materials and Medicine: Trade, Conquest, and Therapeutics in the Eighteenth Century* (Manchester: Manchester University Press, 2014).

47 Chakrabarti, *Medicine and Empire*, 27–8.

48 Ibid., 26.

49 Andreas-Holger Maehle, *Drugs on Trial: Experimental Pharmacology and Therapeutic Innovation in the Eighteenth Century* (Amsterdam: Rodopi, 1999), 223–310.

50 Pratik Chakrabarti, 'Medical Marketplaces beyond the West: Bazaar Medicines, Trade, and the English Establishment in Eighteenth-century India', in Jenner and Wallis, *Medicine and the Market*, 209–10.

51 Chakrabarti, 'Medical Marketplaces', 210.

52 Jonathan Simon, *Chemistry, Pharmacy and Revolution in France, 1777–1809* (Aldershot, UK: Ashgate, 2005).

53 Andrew Duncan Jr, *Edinburgh New Dispensatory*, 3rd ed. (Edinburgh: Printed for William Creech,1803), vii.

54 Chakrabarti, 'Medical Marketplaces', 210.

55 Andrew Duncan Jr, *Supplement to Edinburgh New Dispensatory* (Edinburgh: Printed for Bell & Bradfute, 1829), 4–5. Cited in Chakrabarti, 'Medical Marketplaces', 210.

56 Worth Estes, 'European Reception', 19.

57 Nandini Bhattacharya, 'From Materia Medica to the Pharmacopoeia:

Notes to pages 15–17

Challenges of Writing the History of Drugs in India', *History Compass* 14, no. 4 (2016): 131.

58 Hal Cook, *Matters of Exchange: Commerce, Medicine, and Science in the Dutch Golden Age* 2007 (New Haven, CT: Yale University Press), 416. Anna Winterbottom, *Hybrid Knowledge in the Early East India Company World* (London: Palgrave Macmillan, 2016), 2.

59 Mark Harrison, 'Science and the British Empire', *Isis* 96, no. 1 (2005): 57.

60 Ibid., 58.

61 Roy MacLeod, 'On Visiting the Moving Metropolis: Reflections on the Architecture of Imperial Science', in *Scientific Colonialism*, ed. Nathan Reingold and Marc Rothenberg (Washington, DC: Smithsonian Institution Press, 1987), 217–49.

62 Michael Worboys, 'The Imperial Institute: The State and the Development of the Natural Resources of the Colonial Empire, 1887–1923', in *Imperialism and the Natural World*, ed. John M. MacKenzie (Manchester: Manchester University Press, 1990), 164–86.

63 Cook, *Matters of Exchange*, 416.

64 See Chakrabarti, *Medicine and Empire*, 14. Nandini Bhattacharya, *Disparate Remedies: Making Medicines in Modern India* (Montreal and Kingston: McGill-Queen's University Press, 2023), 47–54; Dorner, *Merchants of Medicines*, 145–7.

65 Hal Cook, *Matters of Exchange*, 416.

66 Winterbottom, *Hybrid Knowledge*, 2.

67 Steven Shapin, *The Scientific Revolution* (Chicago: University of Chicago Press, 1996), 28.

68 M. Elisabeth Moreau Complexion, 'Temperament and Four Humor Theory in the Renaissance', in *Encyclopedia of Renaissance Philosophy*, ed. Marco Sgarbi (Cham, CH: Springer, 2020).

69 Bhattacharya, 'From Materia Medica to Pharmacopoeia', 131.

70 Ibid.

71 Laurence Monnais, *The Colonial Life of Pharmaceuticals: Medicines and Modernity in Vietnam* (Cambridge: Cambridge University Press, 2019), 2.

72 Schiebinger, *Plants and Empire*, 73–104.

73 Maehle, *Drugs on Trial*, 4.

74 S.F. Gray, *A Supplement to the Pharmacopoeia* (London: Printed for Thomas and George Underwood, 1821).

75 Nicholas Culpeper, *A Physicall Directory, or a Translation of the London Dispensatory* (London: Peter Cole, 1649), 2.

76 Anne Van Arsdall, *Medieval Herbal Remedies: The Old English Herbarium and Anglo-Saxon Medicine* (Abingdon, UK: Routledge, 2012); Sinead

262 Notes to pages 17–19

Spearing, *Old English Medical Remedies* (Barnsley, UK: Pen & Sword, 2018); Lori Ann Garner, *Hybrid Healing: Old English Remedies and Medical Texts* (Manchester: Manchester University Press, 2022).

77 Gabrielle Hatfield, *Memory, Wisdom and Healing: The History of Domestic Plant Medicine* (Stroud, UK: History Press, 1999).

78 Mary Chamberlain, *Old Wives' Tales: The History of Remedies, Charms and Spells* (Stroud, UK: History Press, 2010).

79 For the early history of pharmacy in Britain see George E. Trease, *Pharmacy in History* (London: Bailliere, Tindall & Cox, 1964); Leslie G. Matthews, *History of Pharmacy in Britain* (London: E. & S. Livingstone, 1962); F.N.L. Poynter, ed., *Evolution of Pharmacy in Britain* (London: Pitman Medical, 1965).

80 For the history of the Society of Apothecaries see Penelope Hunting, *A History of the Society of Apothecaries* (London: Society of Apothecaries, 1998); C.R.B. Barrett, *History of the Society of Apothecaries of London* (London: Elliot Stock, 1905).

81 For the history of pharmacy in Britain in the nineteenth century see Jacob Bell and Theophilus Redwood, *Historical Sketch of the Progress of Pharmacy in Great Britain* (London: Pharmaceutical Society of Great Britain, 1880); S.W.F. Holloway, *Royal Pharmaceutical Society of Great Britain, 1841–1991: A Political and Social History* (London: Pharmaceutical Press, 1991).

82 Jenner and Wallis, 'The Medical Marketplace', 9.

83 Patrick Wallis, 'Competition and Cooperation in the Early Modern Medical Economy', in Jenner and Wallis, *Medicine and the Market*, 53. For accounts of the relationship between physicians and apothecaries in the early modern period see Hunting, *Society of Apothecaries*; Juanita G.L. Burnby, 'A Study of the English Apothecary from 1660 to 1760', in *Medical History* (London: Wellcome Institute for the History of Medicine, 1983), 24–61.

84 Wallis, 'Competition and Cooperation', in Jenner and Wallis, *Medicine and the Market*, 59–60.

85 Ibid., 60n67.

86 Ibid., 62.

87 Ibid., 63.

88 Ronald L. Numbers, 'Introduction', in *Medicine in the New World: New Spain, New France and New England*, ed. Ronald L. Numbers (Knoxville: University of Tennessee Press, 1987), 1–11.

89 Ronald L. Numbers, 'Conclusion', in Numbers, *Medicine in the New World*, 154–7.

Notes to pages 19–25   263

90 Ibid., 156.
91 Thomas Packenham, *The Scramble for Africa* (London: Abacus History, 1992).
92 Matthew James Crawford, 'An Imperial Pharmacopoeia? The *Pharmacopoeia Matritensis* and Materia Medica in the Eighteenth-century Spanish Atlantic World', in Crawford and Gabriel, *Drugs on the Page*, 78.
93 Matthew James Crawford and Joseph M. Gabriel, 'Introduction: Thinking with Pharmacopoeias', in Crawford and Gabriel, *Drugs on the Page*, 4.
94 Ibid., 8.
95 Ibid.
96 Ibid., 9.
97 C.J.S. Thompson, *The Mystery and Art of the Apothecary* (London: John Lane and Bodley Head, 1929), 136.
98 Bhattacharya, *Disparate Remedies*, 73–96.
99 Ibid., 4–5.
100 Ibid.

CHAPTER ONE

1 George Urdang, 'The Development of Pharmacopoeias: A Review with Special Reference to the Pharmacopoeia Internationalis', *Bulletin of the World Health Organisation* 4 (1951): 578.
2 Antoine Lentacker, 'The Codex Nationalized: Naming People and Things in the Wake of a Revolution', in *Drugs on the Page: Pharmacopoeias and Healing Knowledge in the Early Modern Atlantic World*, ed. Matthew James Crawford and Joseph M. Gabriel (Pittsburgh, PA: University of Pittsburgh Press, 2019), 225.
3 Paula de Vos, 'Pharmacopoeias and the Textual Tradition in Galenic Pharmacy', in Crawford and Gabriel, *Drugs on the Page*, 43.
4 James Grier, *A History of Pharmacy* (London: Pharmaceutical Press, 1937), 45.
5 Emily Beck, 'Authority, Authorship, and Copying: The *Ricettario Fiorentino* and Manuscript Recipe Culture in Sixteenth-Century Florence', in Crawford and Gabriel, *Drugs on the Page*, 52.
6 *The Pharmacopoeia of the Royal College of Physicians of London, 1809*, trans. Richard Powell, 3rd ed. (London: Royal College of Physicians, 1815), ii.
7 Grier, *History of Pharmacy*, 46.
8 Powell, *Pharmacopoeia of Royal College of Physicians*, ii.

264   Notes to pages 25–8

9 For a review of early pharmaceutical texts see de Vos, 'Pharmacopoeias and the Textual Tradition', 19–44.

10 Garcia D'Orta, *Coloquios dos Simples e Drogas he Cousas Medicinai da India* [Dialogues on simples and drugs] (Lisbon, 1563).

11 Jose Pardo-Tomas, 'Natural Knowledge and Medical Remedies in the Book of Secrets', in *A Passion for Plants: Materia Medica and Botany in Scientific Networks from the Sixteenth to Eighteenth Centuries*, ed. Sabine Anagnostou, Florike Egmond, and Christoph Friedrich (Stuttgart: Wissenschaftliche Verlagsgesellschaft, 2011), 93–108.

12 Christopher J. Duffin, 'Some Notes on the Gart der Gesundheit, 1485', *Pharmaceutical Historian* 50, no. 3 (2020): 91–6.

13 Urdang, 'Development of Pharmacopoeias', 581.

14 Ibid.

15 "Notes", in Crawford and Gabriel, *Drugs on the Page*, 270n13.

16 Crawford and Gabriel, 'Introduction: Thinking with Pharmacopoeias', in *Drugs on the Page*, 8.

17 Franz Boas, 'The History of Anthropology', *Science* 20, no. 512 (1904): 512–24.

18 Ibid., 522.

19 Alfred C. Haddon, *History of Anthropology* (Cambridge: Cambridge University Press, 1934).

20 Thomas Hylland Eriksen and Finn Sivert Nielsen, *History of Anthropology* (London: Pluto Press, 2013).

21 Efram Sera-Shriar, *The Making of British Anthropology, 1813–1871* (London: Pickering and Chatto, 2013).

22 See Francis J. Clune, 'Witchcraft, the Shaman, and Active Pharmacopoeia', 5–10, and Janet Belcove, 'The Traditional Folk Medicine of Taos, New Mexico', 103–4, both in *Medical Anthropology*, ed. Francis X. Grollig and Harold B. Haley (Berlin: De Gruyter Mouton, 1976).

23 Pablo Gomez, *The Experiential Caribbean: Creating Knowledge and Healing in the Early Modern Atlantic* (Chapel Hill, NC: University of North Carolina Press, 2017).

24 Peter Conrad, 'Parallel Play in Medical Anthropology and Medical Sociology', *American Sociologist* 28, no. 4 (1997): 90–100.

25 Norman A. Scotch, 'Medical Anthropology', in *Biennial Review of Anthropology*, no. 3, ed. Bernard J. Siegel (Redwood City, CA: Stanford University Press, 1963), 30–68.

26 Conrad, 'Parallel Play in Medical Anthropology', 96.

27 Sjaak Geest and Susan Reynolds White, eds, *Context of Medicines in*

Developing Countries: Studies in Pharmaceutical Anthropology (London: Palgrave Macmillan, 1988).

28 Linda K. Sussman, 'Use of Herbal and Biomedical Pharmaceuticals in Mauritius', in Geest and Reynolds White, *Studies in Pharmaceutical Anthropology*, 199. Sussman lists a large number of publications dating from 1971. None include any references to pharmacopoeias.

29 Nina L. Etkins, 'Cultural Constructions of Efficacy', in Geest and Reynolds White, *Studies in Pharmaceutical Anthropology*, 302.

30 Siva Krishnan, 'Traditional Herbal Medicines: A Review', *International Journal of Research and Analytical Reviews* 5, no. 4 (2018): 611–14.

31 Ibid., 611.

32 Londa Scheibinger, *Plants and Empire: Colonial Bioprospecting in the Atlantic World* (Cambridge, MA: Harvard University Press, 2007), 16.

33 Nina L. Etkin and Elaine Elisabetsky, 'Seeking a Transdisciplinary and Culturally Germane Science: The Future of Ethnopharmacology', *Journal of Ethnopharmacology* 100, nos 1–2 (2005): 23–6.

34 Nina L. Etkin, 'A Hausa Herbal Pharmacopoeia: Biomedical Evaluation of Commonly used Plant Medicines', *Journal of Ethnopharmacology* 4, no. 1 (1981): 75–98.

35 Peter Delaveau, 'Evaluation of Traditional Pharmacopoeias', in *Natural Products as Medicinal Agents*, ed. J.L. Beal and E. Reinhard (Stuttgart: Hippokrates Verlag, 1981), 395–404.

36 Joseph W. Bastien, 'Pharmacopeia of Qollahuaya Andeans', *Journal of Ethnopharmacology* 8, no. 1 (1983): 97–111. Kevin D. Janni and Joseph W. Bastien, 'Establishing Ethnobotanical Conservation Priorities: A Case Study of the Kallawaya Pharmacopoeia', *Sida Contributions to Botany* 19, no. 2 (2000): 387–98.

37 See, for example, W. McClatchey, 'The Ethnopharmacopoeia of Rotuma', *Journal of Ethnopharmacology* 50, no. 3 (1996): 147–56.

38 Kevin D. Janni and Joseph W. Bastien, 'Exotic Botanicals in the Kallawaya Pharmacopoeia', *Economic Botany* 58 (2004): S274–9; Bradley C. Bennett and Ghilean T. Prance, 'Introduced Plants in the Indigenous Pharmacopoeia of Northern South America', *Economic Botany* 54, no. 1 (2000): 90–120.

39 María Eugenia Suárez, 'Medicines in the Forest: Ethnobotany of Wild Medicinal Plants in the Pharmacopeia of the Wichí People of Salta Province (Argentina)', *Journal of Ethnopharmacology* 231, no. 11 (2019): 525–44.

40 Orou G. Gaoue, Michael A. Coe, Matthew Bond, Georgia Hart, Barnabas C. Seyler, and Heather McMillen, 'Theories and Major Hypotheses in Ethnobotany', *Economic Botany* 71 (2017): 269–87.

Notes to pages 31–3

41 Nélson Leal Alencar, Thiago Antonio de Sousa Araújo, Elba Lúcia Cavalcanti de Amorim, and Ulysses Paulino de Albuquerque, 'The Inclusion and Selection of Medicinal Plants in Traditional Pharmacopoeias: Evidence in Support of the Diversification Hypothesis', *Economic Botany* 64, no. 1 (2010): 68–79.

42 Łukasz Łuczaj, Marija Jug-Dujaković, Katija Dolina, Mirjana Jeričević, and Ivana Vitasović-Kosić, 'Insular Pharmacopoeias: Ethnobotanical Characteristics of Medicinal Plants Used on the Adriatic Islands', *Frontiers in Pharmacology* 12 (2021): 1–21.

43 Ibid., 12.

44 Laurent Pordié, 'Pharmacopoeia as an Expression of Society: A Himalayan Study', in *From the Sources of Knowledge to the Medicines of the Future*, ed. Jacques Fleurentin, Jean-Marie Pelt, and Guy Mazars (Paris: IRD Éditions, 2002), 195–204.

45 Ibid., 195.

46 Alexander N. Shikov, Olga N. Pozharitskaya, Valery G. Makarov, Hildebert Wagner, Rob Verpoorte, and Michael Heinrich, 'Medicinal Plants of the Russian Pharmacopoeia: Their History and Applications', *Journal of Ethnopharmacology* 154, no. 3 (2014): 481–536.

47 Reinaldo Farias Paiva de Lucena, Patricia Muniz de Medeiros, Elcida de Lima Araújo, Angelo Giuseppe Chaves Alves, and Ulysses Paulino de Albuquerque, 'The Ecological Apparency Hypothesis and the Importance of Useful Plants in Rural Communities from North-eastern Brazil', *Journal of Environmental Management* 96, no. 1 (2012): 106–15.

48 Alejandro Lozano, Elcida Lima Araújo, Maria Franco Trindade Medeiros, and Ulysses Paulino Albuquerque, 'The Apparency Hypothesis Applied to a Local Pharmacopoeia in the Brazilian Northeast', *Journal of Ethnobiology and Ethnomedicine* 10, no. 2 (2014): 111–12.

49 Bradley C. Bennett and Ghillean T. Prance, 'Introduced Plants in the Indigenous Pharmacopoeia of Northern South America', *Economic Botany* 54, no. 1 (2000): 90–102.

50 Ibid., 90.

51 Marc-Alexandre Tareau, Alexander Greene, Marianne Palisse, and Guillaume Odonne, 'Migrant Pharmacopoeias: An Ethnobotanical Survey of Four Caribbean Communities in Amazonia (French Guiana)', *Economic Botany* 76, no. 2 (2022): 176–88.

52 Ibid., 185.

53 A. Waldstein, 'Mexican Migrant Ethnopharmacology: Pharmacopoeia, Classification of Medicines, and Explanations of Efficacy', *Journal of Ethnopharmacology* 108, no. 2 (2006): 299–310.

54 Melissa Ceuterick, Ina Vandebroek, Bren Torry, and Andrea Pieroni, 'Cross-Cultural Adaptation in Urban Ethnobotany: The Colombian Folk Pharmacopoeia in London', *Journal of Ethnopharmacology* 120, no.3 (2008): 342–59.

55 Andrea Pieroni and Cassandra L. Quave, 'Traditional Pharmacopoeias and Medicines among Albanians and Italians in Southern Italy: A Comparison', *Journal of Ethnopharmacology* 101, nos 1–3 (2005): 258–70.

56 C.L. Quave, A. Pieroni, and B.C. Bennett, 'Dermatological Remedies in the Traditional Pharmacopoeia of Vulture-Alto Bradano, Inland Southern Italy', *Journal of Ethnobiology and Ethnomedicine* 4, no. 5 (2008): 5.

57 Taline Cristina da Silva, Patrícia Muniz Medeiros, Alejandro Lozano Balcazár, Thiago Antônio de Sousa Araújo, Ana-lia Pirondo, and Maria Franco Trindade Medeiros, 'Historical Ethnobotany: An Overview of Selected Studies', *Ethnobiology and Conservation* 3, no. 4 (2014): 1–12.

58 See Maria G.L. Brandão, Gustavo P. Cosenza, Cristiane F.F. Grael, Nilton L. Netto Junior, and Roberto L.M. Monte-Mór, 'Traditional Uses of American Plant Species from the First Edition of the Brazilian Official Pharmacopoeia', *Revista Brasileira de Farmacognosia* 19 (2009): 478–87; Maria G.L. Brandão, Naiara N'S. Zanetti, Patricia Oliveira, Cristiane F.F. Grail, Aparecida C.P. Santos, and Roberto L.M. Monte-Mór, 'Brazilian Medicinal Plants Described by Nineteenth Century European Naturalists and in the Official Pharmacopoeia', *Journal of Ethnopharmacology* 120, no. 2 (2008): 141–8; Łukasz Jakub Łuczaj, 'A Relic of Medieval Folklore: Corpus Christi Octave Herbal Wreaths in Poland and Their Relationship with the Local Pharmacopoeia', *Journal of Ethnopharmacology* 142, no.1 (2012): 228–40.

59 Diego Rivera, Alonso Verde, Concepción Obón, Francisco Alcaraz, Candelaria Moreno, Teresa Egea, José Fajardo, José Antonio Palazón, Arturo Valdés, Maria Adele Signorini, and Piero Bruschi, 'Is There Nothing New Under the Sun? The Influence of Herbals and Pharmacopoeias on Ethnobotanical Traditions in Albacete (Spain)', *Journal of Ethnopharmacology* 195, no.1 (2017): 96–117.

60 Rivera et al., 'Is There Nothing New Under the Sun?', 115.

61 C. Simon and M. Lamla, 'Merging Pharmacopoeia: Understanding the Historical Origins of Incorporative Pharmacopoeial Processes among Xhosa Healers in Southern Africa', *Journal of Ethnopharmacology* 33, no. 3 (1991): 237–42.

62 Maria Franco Trindade Medeiros and Ulysses Paulino de Albuquerque, 'The Pharmacy of the Benedictine Monks: The Use of Medicinal Plants in Northeast Brazil during the Nineteenth Century (1823–1829)', *Journal of Ethnopharmacology* 139, no.1 (2012): 280–6.

268 Notes to pages 35–8

63 V. Davidov, 'Amazonia as Pharmacopoeia', *Critique of Anthropology* 33, no. 3 (2013): 243–62.

64 Kerri Brown, 'Pharmaceutical Territories: Contested Pharmacopoeias and Environmental Debates in Brazil" (PhD diss., Southern Methodist University, 2018).

65 M.F.T. Medeiros, R.H.P. Andreata, and L. Senna-Valle, 'Identification of Nineteenth-Century Terms Relating to Medicinal Plants Used in the Monastery of Saint Benedict of Rio de Janeiro, Brazil', *Acta Botanica Brasilica* 24, no. 3 (2010): 780–9.

66 See Melina Giorgetti, Giuseppina Negri, and Eliana Rodrigues, Brazilian Plants with Possible Action on the Central Nervous System: A Study of Historical Sources from the Sixteenth to Nineteenth Centuries', *Journal of Ethnopharmacology* 109, no. 2 (2007): 338–47; M.G.L. Brandão et al., 'Brazilian Medicinal Plants', 141–8. N. Scalco, M. Giorgetti, L. Rossi, J.F.L. Santos, R.D. Otsuka, and E. Rodrigues, 'Ancient Literature (Eighteenth and Nineteenth Centuries) with Reports of Native Medicinal Plants Found in Institutions of Four Brazilian Cities', in *Historical Aspects of Ethnobiological Research*, ed. M.F.T. Medeiros (Recife, BR: NUPEEA, 2010), 73–102.

67 M.F.T. Medeiros et al., 'Identification of Nineteenth-Century Terms', 780–9.

68 Domingos Tabajara de Oliveira Martins, Eliana Rodrigues, Laura Casu, Guillermo Benítez, and Marco Leonti, 'The Historical Development of Pharmacopoeias and the Inclusion of Exotic Herbal Drugs, with a Focus on Europe and Brazil', *Journal of Ethnopharmacology* 240, no. 2 (2019): 2.

69 Crawford and Gabriel, 'Introduction: Thinking with Pharmacopoeias', in *Drugs on the Page*, 4.

70 Chandra Mukerji, 'Dominion, Demonstration, and Domination', in *Colonial Botany: Science, Commerce and Politics in the Early Modern World*, ed. Londa Schiebinger and Claudia Swan (Philadelphia: University of Pennsylvania Press, 2005), 25.

71 Londa Schiebinger, 'Prospecting for Drugs', in Schiebinger and Swan, *Colonial Botany*, 120–1.

72 Ibid., 132.

73 Ibid., 122.

74 W.F. Bynum, 'Treating the Wages of Sin', in *Medical Fringe and Medical Orthodoxy, 1750–1850*, ed. W.F. Bynum and Roy Porter (London: Croom Helm, 1987), 17.

75 Crawford and Gabriel, 'Introduction: Thinking with Pharmacopoeias', *Drugs on the Page*, 5.

76 Paula de Vos, 'Pharmacopoeias and the Textual Tradition in Galenic Pharmacy', in Crawford and Gabriel, *Drugs on the Page*, 42–3.

77 Mark S.R. Jenner and Patrick Wallis, 'The Medical Marketplace', in *Medicine and the Market in England and Its Colonies, c.1450–c.1850*, ed. Mark S.R. Jenner and Patrick Wallis (London: Palgrave Macmillan, 2007), 15.

78 Ibid.

79 Mark Harrison, 'Medicine and Orientalism', in *Health, Medicine and Empire: Perspectives on Colonial India*, ed. Biswamoy Pati and Mark Harrison (Hyderabad, IN: Orient Longman, 2001), 77.

80 Poonam Bala, *Imperialism and Medicine in Bengal* (New Delhi: Sage, 1991).

81 Nandini Bhattacharya, 'From Materia Medica to the Pharmacopoeia: Challenges of Writing the History of Drugs in India', *History Compass* 14, no. 4 (2016): 131.

82 Nandini Bhattacharya, *Disparate Remedies: Making Medicines in Modern India* (Montreal and Kingston: McGill-Queen's University Press, 2023), 131.

83 Ibid., 132.

84 Bhattacharya, 'Materia Medica to Pharmacopoeia', 133.

85 Sara Press, 'Ayahuasca on Trial: Bio-colonialism, Biopiracy, and the Commodification of the Sacred', *History of Pharmacy and Pharmaceuticals* 63, no. 2 (2021): 347.

86 Ibid., 333.

87 Ashley Buchanan, 'An Empire of Materia Medica at the Late Medici Court', *History of Pharmacy and Pharmaceuticals* 63, no. 2 (2021): 157.

88 Ibid., 159.

89 Ellen Amster, 'Head of a Serpent, a Pinch of Rue: Women, Indigenous Pharmacology, and the Patriarchy of French Colonizing Science in Morocco', *History of Pharmacy and Pharmaceuticals* 63, no. 2 (2021): 198.

90 Ibid., 195.

91 Rachael A. Hill, 'Making Scientific Sense of Traditional Medicine: Efficacy, Bioprospecting, and the Enduring Hope of Drug Discovery in Ethiopia', *History of Pharmacy and Pharmaceuticals* 63, no. 2 (2021): 277.

92 John Mason Good, *The History of Medicine, So Far as It Relates to the Profession of the Apothecary, from the Earliest Accounts to the Present Period* (London: C. Dilly, 1795), 115.

93 Good, *The History of Medicine*, vi.

94 Jacob Bell and Theophilus Redwood, *Historical Sketch of the Progress of Pharmacy in Great Britain* (London: Pharmaceutical Society of Great Britain, 1880).

270   Notes to pages 41–2

95 A.C. Wootton, *Chronicles of Pharmacy*, vol. 2 (London: Macmillan, 1910), 59–69; C.J.S. Thompson, *The Mystery and Art of the Apothecary* (London: John Lane and Bodley Head, 1929), 136–50.

96 Thompson, *Mystery and Art*, 136.

97 James Grier, *A History of Pharmacy* (London: The Pharmaceutical Press, 1937), 39–47.

98 Ibid., 45–6.

99 George Urdang, *Pharmacopoeia Londinensis of 1618, Reproduced in Facsimile, with a Historical Introduction by George Urdang* (Madison: State Historical Society of Wisconsin, 1944). See also George Urdang, *Bulletin of the History of Medicine* 12, no. 2 (1942): 304–13. For a list of Urdang's publications in English and German, see *Pharmacy in History* 24, no. 3 (1982): 106–14.

100 William Munk, *The Roll of the Royal College of Physicians of London* (London: Royal College of Physicians, 1878), 1.

101 George Urdang, 'Pharmacopoeias as Witnesses of World History', *Journal of the History of Medicine and Allied Sciences* 1, no. 1 (1946): 46–70.

102 Urdang, 'Development of Pharmacopoeias', 581.

103 Ibid.

104 David L. Cowen, *Pharmacopoeias and Related Literature in Britain and America, 1618–1847* (Aldershot, UK: Ashgate Variorum, 2001), 55–66; David L. Cowen, 'The Edinburgh Pharmacopoeia', *Medical History* 1, no. 2 (1957): 123–39 and 340–53. For a full list of Cowen's publications, see *Pharmacy in History* 48, no. 1 (2006): 30–4.

105 David L. Cowen, 'The Edinburgh Pharmacopoeia', in *The Early Years of the Edinburgh Medical School*, ed. R.G.W. Anderson and A.D.C. Simpson (Edinburgh: Royal Scottish Museum, 1976), 1–20.

106 Cowen, *Pharmacopoeias and Related Literature*, 31.

107 David Cowen, 'The Influence of the Edinburgh Pharmacopoeia and the Edinburgh Dispensatories', *Pharmaceutical Historian* 12, no. 1 (1982): 1–7.

108 David L. Cowen, 'The Spread and Influence of British Pharmacopoeial and Related Literature', in *Pharmacopoeias and Related Literature*, 79–184.

109 Leslie G. Matthews, *History of Pharmacy in Britain* (London: E. & S. Livingstone, 1962), 89.

110 Robert Multhauf, 'Medical Chemistry and the Paracelsians', *Bulletin of the History of Medicine* 28, no. 2 (1954): 106.

111 George E. Trease, *Pharmacy in History* (London: Bailliere, Tindall & Cox, 1964), 241.

Notes to pages 43–8

112 Betty Jackson, 'From Papyri to Pharmacopoeia: The Development of Standards for Crude Drugs', in *Evolution of Pharmacy in Britain*, ed. F.N.L. Poynter (London: Pitman Medical, 1965), 151–64.

CHAPTER TWO

1 C.J.S. Thompson, *The Mystery and Art of the Apothecary* (London: John Lane and Bodley Head, 1929), 136.

2 David L. Cowen, 'The Edinburgh Pharmacopoeia', in *The Early Years of the Edinburgh Medical School*, ed. R.G.W. Anderson and A.D.C. Simpson (Edinburgh: Royal Scottish Museum, 1976), 1.

3 *Cambridge English Dictionary*, 4th ed. (2022), s.v. 'statutory'.

4 *Report of the Sub-committee on the British Pharmacopoeia of the Committee of Civil Research*, Cmd 3101 (London: His Majesty's Stationery Office, 1928), 9, para. 22 (hereafter cited as Macmillan Report).

5 Macmillan Report, 24, para. 56.

6 Stuart Anderson, *Pharmacy and Professionalization in the British Empire, 1780–1970* (London: Palgrave Macmillan, 2021), 36–67.

7 Lembit Rägo and Budiono Santoso, 'Drug Regulation: History, Present and Future', *WHO Policy Perspectives on Medicines*, no. 7 (Geneva: WHO, 2003), 67.

8 "Principal Medicines Regulatory Functions', in *WHO Policy Perspectives on Medicines*, no. 7 (Geneva: WHO, 2003).

9 Pliny, *Natural History*, 11:14, trans. John Bostock and H.T. Riley (London, 1856), 3:13.

10 Ernst W. Stieb, *Drug Adulteration: Detection and Control in Nineteenth Century Britain* (Madison: University of Wisconsin Press, 1966), 3–4.

11 Nandini Bhattacharya, *Disparate Remedies: Making Medicines in Modern India* (Montreal and Kingston: McGill-Queen's University Press, 2023), 125.

12 Ibid., 126.

13 Gregory Haines, *Pharmacy in Australia: The National Experience* (Deakin: Pharmaceutical Society of Australia, 1988), 63.

14 Cited in Haines, *Pharmacy in Australia*, 72.

15 Nandini Bhattacharya, 'From Materia Medica to the Pharmacopoeia: Challenges of Writing the History of Drugs in India', *History Compass* 14, no. 4 (2016): 136. See also Nandini Bhattacharya, 'Between the Bazaar and the Bench: Making of the Drugs Trade in Colonial India, c.1900–1930', *Bulletin of the History of Medicine* 90, no. 1 (2016): 61–91.

Notes to pages 48–51

16 Haines, *Pharmacy in Australia*, 115. See also Arnold V. Raison, *A Brief History of Pharmacy in Canada* (Ottawa: Canadian Pharmaceutical Association, 1967), and Mike Ryan, *History of Organized Pharmacy in South Africa, 1885–1950* (Cape Town: Society for the History of Pharmacy in South Africa, 1986).

17 See, for example, Joseph Brown, *Antidotaria; or, a Collection of Antidotes against the Plague, and Other Malignant Diseases* (London: printed for J. Wilcox, 1721), https://wellcomecollection.org/works/jxb2z3u7.

18 See Myles D.B. Stephens, *The Dawn of Drug Safety* (Winchester, UK: George Mann Publications, 2010).

19 Barbara Griggs, *Green Pharmacy: A History of Herbal Medicine* (London: Jill Norman and Hobhouse, 1981), 109.

20 For discussion of this point see Ole Peter Grell, Andrew Cunningham, and Jon Arrizabalaga, eds, *It All Depends on the Dose: Poisons and Medicines in European History* (Abingdon, UK: Routledge, 2018).

21 George Urdang, *Pharmacopoeia Londinensis of 1618, Reproduced in Facsimile, with a Historical Introduction by George Urdang* (Madison: State Historical Society of Wisconsin, 1944), 89–96.

22 William Withering, *An Account of the Foxglove and Some of Its Medical Uses* (London: C.G.J. and J. Robinson, 1785). See also Kees van Grootheest, 'The Dawn of Pharmacovigilance: An Historical Perspective,' *International Journal of Pharmaceutical Medicine* 17, nos 5–6 (2003): 196; Michael D. Rawlins, 'Pharmacovigilance: Paradise Lost, Regained, or Postponed?,' *Journal of the Royal College of Physicians of London* 29, no. 1 (1995): 41–8.

23 Philip Routledge, '150 Years of Pharmacovigilance,' *The Lancet* 351, no. 9110 (1998): 1200–1.

24 R.D. Mann, 'From Mithradatium to Modern Medicine: The Management of Drug Safety,' *Journal of the Royal Society of Medicine* 81, no. 12 (1988): 725–8.

25 Zachary Dorner, *Merchants of Medicines: The Commerce and Coercion of Health in Britain's Long Eighteenth Century* (Chicago: University of Chicago Press, 2020), 55.

26 Letter Thomas Corbyn to Robert James, 1744, Ms. 5442, Corbyn & Co. papers, Wellcome Library.

27 S.W.F. Holloway, 'The Regulation of the Supply of Drugs in Britain before 1868,' in *Drugs and Narcotics in History*, ed. Roy Porter and Mikulas Teich (Cambridge: Cambridge University Press, 1997), 77. See also V. Krzyzyk, 'The History of Drug Regulation,' *Bulletin of the Parenteral Drug Association* 31, no. 3 (1977): 156–60.

Notes to pages 52–3 273

28 Holloway, 'Regulation of Supply of Drugs', 77.
29 Christoph Gradmann and Jonathan Simon, *Evaluating and Standardizing Therapeutic Agents, 1890–1950* (London: Palgrave Macmillan, 2010), 1.
30 Ibid.
31 Stuart Anderson, 'From Bespoke to Off-the-Peg: Community Pharmacists and the Retailing of Medicines in Great Britain, 1900 to 1970', in *From Physick to Pharmacology: Five Hundred Years of British Drug Retailing*, ed. Louise Hill Curth (Aldershot, UK: Ashgate, 2006), 105–42.
32 T.A.B. Corley, 'UK Government Regulation of Medicinal Drugs, 1890–2000', *Business History* 47, no. 3 (2005): 338.
33 *The Garbling Act, with Short Remarks Relating to the East India Company* (1708), Ms. CUP 645.b.11(1), Petitions, General Reference Section, British Library.
34 P. Weedle, F. Crean, and L. Clarke, 'Historical Development of Medicines and Pharmacy Law', in *Pharmacy and Medicines Law in Ireland*, ed. Peter Weedle and Leonne Clarke (London: Pharmaceutical Press, 2011), 12.
35 G.E. Trease, *Pharmacy in History* (London: Bailliere, Tindall & Cox, 1964), 65.
36 Ibid., 65–6.
37 "London's Drug Market and the Romance of Mincing Lane', *Chemist & Druggist* 108, no. 2525 (1928): 855.
38 See P.H. Ditchfield, *The City Companies of London and Their Good Works: A Record of Their History, Charity and Treasure* (London: J.M. Dent, 1904).
39 Robin E. Ferner and Jeffrey K. Aronson, 'Medicines Legislation and Regulation in the United Kingdom, 1500–2020', *British Journal of Clinical Pharmacology* 89, no. 1 (2023): 80–92.
40 John P. Griffin, 'Venetian Treacle and the Foundation of Medicines Regulation', *British Journal of Clinical Pharmacology* 58, no. 3 (2004): 317–25. See also John P. Griffin, 'A History of Drug Regulation in the UK', in *The Textbook of Pharmaceutical Medicine*, ed. John P. Griffin, John Posner, and Geoffrey R. Barker, 7th ed. (London: John Wiley & Sons, 2013), 317–46.
41 *Kremers and Urdang's History of Pharmacy*, ed. Glenn Sonnedecker, 4th ed. (Madison, WI: American Institute of the History of Pharmacy, 1976), 111.
42 George Clark, *History of the Royal College of Physicians*, vol. 2 (London: Clarendon Press, 1970), 1704–35.
43 Weedle, Crean, and Clarke, 'Historical Development', 11–23.
44 C.R.B. Barrett, *The Society of Apothecaries of London* (London: Society of Apothecaries, 1905), xxxiv.

274 Notes to pages 53–8

45 Act of Parliament, 10 George I, c. 22. See Jacob Bell and Theophilus Redwood, *Historical Sketch of the Progress of Pharmacy in Great Britain* (London: Pharmaceutical Press, 1880), 21.

46 Bell and Redwood, *Historical Sketch*, 21; Barrett, *Society of Apothecaries*, 132; *Chemist & Druggist* 105 (1926): 198.

47 Stuart Anderson, 'James Goodwin's Bonfire of Medicines', *Pharmaceutical Journal* 283, no. 7401 (2005): 705–6.

48 Thomas Ferguson, 'History of Pharmacy in Scotland', *Chemist & Druggist* 116, no. 2733 (1932): 695.

49 Colin Dollery, 'Medicine and the Pharmacological Revolution', *Journal of the Royal College of Physicians of London* 28, no. 1 (1994): 59–69.

50 Ibid.

51 Ibid., 84.

52 Stieb, *Drug Adulteration*, 232.

53 For more on this point see Anderson, *Pharmacy and Professionalization*, 49–51.

54 Weedle, Crean, and Clarke, 'Historical Development', 23.

55 S.W.F. Holloway, *Royal Pharmaceutical Society of Great Britain, 1841–1991: A Political and Social History* (London: Pharmaceutical Press, 1991), 42.

56 Gradmann and Simon, *Evaluating and Standardizing Therapeutic Agents*, 2.

57 Ibid., 3.

58 Haines, *Pharmacy in Australia*, 81.

59 Ibid.

60 See Harold J. Cook, 'The Rose Case Reconsidered: Physicians, Apothecaries, and the Law in Augustan England', *Journal of the History of Medicine and Allied Sciences* 45 (1990): 527–55.

61 For the history of the Pharmaceutical Society of Great Britain see Holloway, *Royal Pharmaceutical Society of Great Britain* (London: Pharmaceutical Press, 1991).

62 Ibid., 244.

63 Peter Bartrip, 'A Pennurth of Arsenic for Rat Poison: The Arsenic Act 1851 and the Prevention of Secret Poisoning', *Medical History* 36 (1992): 53–69. See also James A. Whorton, *The Arsenic Century: How Victorian Britain Was Poisoned at Home, Work, and Play* (Oxford: Oxford University Press, 2010).

64 Holloway, 'The Regulation of the Supply of Drugs', 95.

65 For more on this point see Anderson, *Pharmacy and Professionalization*, 51.

66 Michael Brown, 'Medicine, Quackery, and the Free Market: The 'War' against Morison's Pills and the Construction of the Medical Profession,

Notes to pages 58–61

c.1830–c.1850; in *Medicine and the Market in England and Its Colonies, c.1450–c.1850*, ed. Mark S.R. Jenner and Patrick Wallis (Basingstoke, UK: Palgrave Macmillan, 2007), 238.

67 *The Lancet* 31 (1838): 63. Cited in Brown, 'Medicine, Quackery, and the Free Market', 258.

68 Brown, 'Medicine, Quackery, and the Free Market', 251.

69 Ibid., 254.

70 "The Report of the Committee on the Sale of Poisons Bill', *Pharmaceutical Journal* 17, no. 9 (1858): 446.

71 Cited in Holloway, 'The Regulation of the Supply of Drugs', 94.

72 Ibid., 86.

73 R.G. Penn, 'The State Control of Medicines: The First 3,000 Years', *British Journal of Clinical Pharmacology* 8 (1979): 293–305.

74 Derrick Dunlop, 'The Growth of Drug Regulation in the United Kingdom', *Journal of the Royal Society of Medicine* 73 (1980): 405–7.

75 Ronald D. Mann, *Modern Drug Use: An Enquiry on Historical Principles* (Lancaster, UK: MTP Press, 1984), 552.

76 Marion Hodges, 'Control of the Safety of Drugs, 1868–1968 (Part 1)', *Pharmaceutical Journal* 239, no. 6444 (1987): 119–22; Marion Hodges, 'Control of the Safety of Drugs, 1868–1968 (Part 2)', *Pharmaceutical Journal* 239, no. 6445 (1987): 150–3. See also A. Goldberg, 'Development of Drug Regulating Authorities', *British Journal of Clinical Pharmacology* 22, suppl. 1 (1986): 67S–70S.

77 Dorner, *Merchants of Medicines*, 55.

78 Bhattacharya, 'From Materia Medica to the Pharmacopoeia', 126.

79 Stieb, *Drug Adulteration*, 3.

80 Ibid., 24.

81 Gradmann and Simon, *Evaluating and Standardizing Therapeutic Agents*, 1.

82 Ibid., 2.

83 John V. Pickstone, *Ways of Knowing: A New History of Science, Technology, and Medicine* (Manchester: Manchester University Press, 2000), 14.

84 James H. Mills and Patricia Barton, *Drugs and Empires: Essays on Modern Imperialism and Intoxication, c.1500 to c.1930* (Basingstoke, UK: Palgrave Macmillan, 2007).

85 Described by David T. Courtwright in his review of *Drugs and Empires* in *Social History of Medicine* 21, no. 2 (2008): 404.

86 William O. Walker III, 'A Grave Danger to the Peace of the East: Opium and Imperial Rivalry in China, 1895–1920', in Mills and Barton, *Drugs and Empires*.

276   Notes to pages 61–6

87 William McAllister, 'The Trade-Off: Chinese Opium Traders and Antebellum Reform in the United States, 1815–1860, in Mills and Barton, *Drugs and Empires.*

88 Stuart Anderson and Virginia Berridge, 'Opium in Twentieth Century Britain: Pharmacists, Regulation and the People', *Addiction* 95, no. 1 (2000): 23–36.

89 See "Severe Penalties" in Dorothy W. Goyns, *Pharmacy in the Transvaal, 1894–1994* (Braamfontein: Pharmaceutical Society of South Africa, 1995), 30.

CHAPTER THREE

1 James Matthew Crawford, 'An Imperial Pharmacopoeia?', in *Drugs on the Page: Pharmacopoeias and Healing Knowledge in the Early Modern Atlantic World*, ed. Matthew James Crawford and Joseph Gabriel (Pittsburgh: University of Pittsburgh Press, 2019), 63.

2 "Decreto del Tribunal del Real Proto-Medicato', in *Pharmacopoeia Matritensis* (Madrid: Typis Antonii Perez de Soto, 1739).

3 Crawford, 'An Imperial Pharmacopoeia?', 64.

4 For histories of European colonialism see, for example, H.L. Wesseling, *The European Colonial Empires: 1815–1919* (Abingdon, UK: Routledge, 2004). For postcolonial comparisons see Miguel Bandeira Jerónimo and António Costa Pinto, *The Ends of European Colonial Empires: Cases and Comparisons* (London: Palgrave Macmillan, 2016); V.G. Kiernan, *European Empires from Conquest to Collapse 1815–1960* (Leicester: Leicester University Press, 1982); Matthew G. Stanard, *European Overseas Empire, 1879–1999: A Short History* (London: Wiley Blackwell, 2018).

5 Antonio González Bueno, 'An Account on the History of the Spanish Pharmacopoeias', International Society for the History of Pharmacy, 2022, https://www.histpharm.org/ISHPWG%20Spain.pdf.

6 González Bueno, 'An Account on the History of the Spanish Pharmacopoeias."

7 Paula de Vos, 'Pharmacopoeias and the Textual Tradition in Galenic Pharmacy', in Crawford and Gabriel, *Drugs on the Page*, 43.

8 For the introduction of the pharmacopoeia across the Spanish Empire, see *Estatutes del Real Colegio de Professores Boticarios de Madrid, aprobados y confirmados por su Megestad, que Dios guarde* [Statutes of the Royal College of Apothecary Professors of Madrid, approved and confirmed by His Highness, may God preserve] (Madrid: Imprenta Real, 1737), cited

Notes to pages 66–8

by Paula de Vos, 'Pharmacopoeias and the Textual Tradition in Galenic Medicine', in Crawford and Gabriel, *Drugs on the Page*, 277n78.

9   Crawford, 'An Imperial Pharmacopoeia?', 72.

10 Matthew James Crawford, personal communication, 7 July 2021.

11 Linda A. Newson, *Making Medicines in Early Colonial Lima, Peru: Apothecaries, Science and Society* (Leiden: Brill, 2017). See also Linda A. Newson, 'Alchemy and Chemical Medicines in Early Colonial Lima, Peru', *Ambix* 67, no. 2 (2020): 107–34.

12 Liliana Schifter and Patricia Aceves, 'The Role of Mexican Pharmacopoeias in the Construction of a National Identity', International Society for the History of Pharmacy, 2022, https://www.histpharm.org/ISHPWG %20Mexico.pdf.

13 Paula S. De Vos, *Compound Remedies: Galenic Pharmacy from the Ancient Mediterranean to New Spain* (Pittsburgh: University of Pittsburgh Press, 2020).

14 Schifter and Aceves, *Mexican Pharmacopeias*, 3.

15 Ibid., 2.

16 For the history of the Portuguese Empire see Charles Ralph Boxer, *The Portuguese Seaborne Empire 1415–1825* (London: Hutchinson, 1969); Liam Matthew Brockey, *Portuguese Colonial Cities in the Early Modern World* (Farnham, UK: Ashgate, 2008); A.R. Disney, *History of Portugal and the Portuguese Empire*, vols 1 and 2 (Cambridge: Cambridge University Press, 2009).

17 See, for example, J.R. Pita and A.L. Pereira, 'The Beautiful Age of the First Portuguese Pharmacopoeia: 300 Years of Medicine in Beira Interior from Prehistory to the Twentieth Century', *Culture Notebooks* 19 (2005): 74–82.

18 João Rui Pita, 'Brief History of Portuguese Pharmacopoeias (18th–20th Century)', International Society for the History of Pharmacy, 2022, https://www.histpharm.org/ISHPWG%20Portugal.pdf.

19 João Rui Pita, 'A Publicação da Primeira Farmacopeia Oficial: Pharmacopeia Geral (1794)', *Revista de História das Ideias* 20 (1999): 47–100.

20 Ana Leonor Pereira and João Rui Pita, 'Liturgia Higienista no Século XIX. Pistas para um Estudo', *Revista de História das Ideias* 15 (1993): 462.

21 *Pharmacopêa Portugueza* (Lisboa: Imprensa Nacional, 1876), xi.

22 João Rui Pita, 'Sanitary Normalization in Portugal: Pharmacies, Pharmacopoeias, Medicines, and Pharmaceutical Practices', in *European Health and Social Welfare Policies*, ed. Laurinda Abreu (Brno, CZ: Brno University of Technology/VUTIUM Press, 2004), 438.

278   Notes to pages 68–70

23 Ibid., 439.
24 Ibid.
25 Madhusudan Joshi, 'Pharmacy Profession in Goa during the Portuguese Period, 1842–1961', *Proceedings of World Congress of Pharmacy and Pharmaceutical Sciences* (Lisbon: International Pharmaceutical Federation, 2010), H4-03.
26 Jorge Varanda, 'Crossing Colonies and Empires: The Health Services of the Diamond Company of Angola', in *Crossing Colonial Historiographies: Histories of Colonial and Indigenous Medicines in Transnational Perspective*, ed. Anne Digby, Waltraud Ernst, and Projit B. Mukharji (Newcastle: Cambridge Scholars Publishing, 2010), 169.
27 Ibid., 170.
28 Ibid., 174.
29 For the history of the Dutch colonial empire see C.R. Boxer, *The Dutch Seaborne Empire 1600–1800* (London: Hutchinson, 1965).
30 Kerry Ward, *Networks of Empire: Forced Migration in the Dutch East India Company* (Cambridge: Cambridge University Press, 2009), 322–42.
31 Toine Pieters, 'The Battle between David and Goliath: Drug Making and the Dutch Pharmacist versus the International Pharmaceutical Industry, 1865–2020', *History of Pharmacy and Pharmaceuticals* 63, no. 1 (2021): 47.
32 A.M.G. Rutten, *Dutch Transatlantic Medicine Trade in the Eighteenth Century under the Cover of the West India Company* (Rotterdam: Erasmus, 2000), 23.
33 Ibid.
34 Ibid., 22.
35 Ibid., 24.
36 A.M.G. Rutten, *Blue Ships: Dutch Ocean Crossing with Multifunctional Drugs and Spices in the Eighteenth Century* (Rotterdam: Erasmus, 2008), 107.
37 Pieter van der Wielen, 'De eerste Nederlandsche Pharmacopee', *Pharmaceutisch Weekblad* 73 (1936): 545–64; Pieter Hendrik Vree, "De Vermeerdering Onzer Kennis': Bereiding en Onderzoek van Geneesmiddelen in Nederlandse Farmacopees (1851–1966)" (PhD diss., Leiden University, 2020), 20.
38 P.H. Brans, 'Zur Geschichte der in Niederländisch-Indien Gebrauchten Pharmakopöen', in *Festschrift zum 65 Geburtstag von Georg Edmund Dann*, ed. Wolfgang-Hagen Hein and Herbert Hugel (Stuttgart: Wissenschaftliche Verlagsgesellschaft, 1963), 9–20. https://publikationsserver .tu-braunschweig.de/servlets/MCRFileNodeServlet/dbbs_derivate _00048183/Ea-837-21.pdf.

Notes to pages 70–3

39 Loepold van Itallie, *Overzicht van de uit Oost-Indië door de Pharmacopee-commissie Ontvangen Rapporten Omtrent in de Pharmacopee Gewenschte Wijzigingen* (Dieren, NL, 1900), cited in Brans, 'Zur Geschichte.'

40 P.H. Brans, 'Zur Geschichte', 18.

41 Ibid.

42 Ibid.

43 Ibid.

44 Pieters, 'David and Goliath', 40–60.

45 For the history of drug safety from a Dutch perspective see Kees van Grootheest, 'The Dawn of Pharmacovigilance: An Historical Perspective', *International Journal of Pharmaceutical Medicine* 17, nos 5–6 (2003): 195–200.

46 For the history of the French colonial empire see, for example, Raymond Betts, *Tricouleur: The French Overseas Empire* (London: Gordon and Cremonesi, 1978); Robert Aldrich, *Greater France: A History of French Overseas Expansion* (London: Springer, 1996); Martin A. Klein, *Slavery and Colonial Rule in French West Africa* (Cambridge: Cambridge University Press, 1998).

47 Londa Scheibinger, *Secret Cures of Slaves* (Stanford, CA: Stanford University Press, 2017), 150.

48 James McClellan and Francois Regourd, *The Colonial Machine: French Science and Overseas Expansion in the Old Regime* (Turnhout, BE: Brepols, 2011).

49 Olivier Lafont, 'A Stroll through the Collections of Pharmacopoeias of the Order of Pharmacists in Paris', International Society for the History of Pharmacy, 2022, https://www.histpharm.org/ISHPWG%20France.pdf. See also Jacques Saller, *La Pharmacopee Francaise, dans l'evolution, Scientifique et Professionelle* (Metz, FR: Maisonneuve, 1969), cited by Crawford and Gabriel, 'Introduction: Thinking with Pharmacopoeias', in *Drugs on the Page*, 270n17.

50 Lafont, *Collections of Pharmacopoeias*, 2.

51 David A. Guba, *Taming Cannabis: Drugs and Empire in Nineteenth Century France* (Montreal and Kingston: McGill-Queen's University Press, 2020), 113.

52 Jonathan Simon, *Chemistry, Pharmacy and Revolution in France, 1777–1809* (Aldershot, UK: Ashgate, 2005), 170.

53 Ibid., 49–92.

54 Ibid., 108.

55 For the history of pharmacy in France see, for example, Glenn Sonnedecker, 'The Development in France', in *Kremers and Urdang's His-*

280   Notes to pages 73–7

tory of Pharmacy, ed. Glenn Sonnedecker (Madison, wɪ: American Institute of the History of Pharmacy, 1976), 67–84.

56 Bruno Bonnemain, 'Pharmacopoeias in France after the French Revolution', International Society for the History of Pharmacy, 2022, https://www.histpharm.org/ɪsHPWG%20France2.pdf.

57 Ibid.

58 Simon, *Chemistry, Pharmacy and Revolution*, 2005.

59 Bruno Bonnemain, 'Colonisation et pharmacie, 1830–1962: Une présence diversifiée de 130 ans des pharmaciens français', *Revue d'histoire de la pharmacie* 56, no. 359 (2008): 311–34. See also Bruno Bonnemain, 'Contribution à l'histoire de la pharmacie française en Indochine 1861–1954', *Revue d'histoire de la pharmacie* 57, no. 362 (2009): 125–44.

60 Antoine Lentacker, 'The Codex Nationalized: Naming People and Things in the Wake of a Revolution', in Crawford and Gabriel, *Drugs on the Page*, 222.

61 Bruno Bonnemain, 'Le Formulaire des Hôpitaux Militaires de Coste, Publié à Newport, pour l'armée de Rochambeau en 1780', *Revue d'histoire de la pharmacie* 68, no. 407 (2020): 303–14.

62 Christopher Parsons, 'Consuming Canada: *Capillaire du Canada* in the French Atlantic World', in Crawford and Gabriel, *Drugs on the Page*, 162.

63 Ibid., 169.

64 Laurence Monnais, *The Colonial Life of Pharmaceuticals: Medicines and Modernity in Vietnam* (Cambridge: Cambridge University Press, 2019), 149.

65 Ibid., 112.

66 Ibid., 113.

67 Maria del Carmen France Causape, Maria Cristian de Frutos Quitanilla, and Joe Ivan Pando Marcos, *Aportacion a la Farmacia Vietnamita en y tras la Epoca Colonial Francesa en el Signo XX* (Madrid: Catedratica de Universidad, 2021), 12.

68 For the history of pharmacy in Germany see, for example, Glenn Sonnedecker, 'The Development in Germany', in *Kremers and Urdang*, 85–98.

69 Christoph Friedrich, 'German Pharmacopoeias', International Society for the History of Pharmacy, 2022, https://www.histpharm.org/ɪsHPWG %20Germany.pdf.

70 Friedrich, 'German Pharmacopoeias.'

71 Christoph Friedrich and Wolf-Dieter Müller-Jahncke, 'Von der Frühen Neuzeit bis zur Gegenwart', *Geschichte der Pharmazie* 16 (2005): 573–6, 579–81.

Notes to pages 77–8

72 Michael Heinrich and Sabine Anagnostou, 'From Pharmacognosia to DNA-Based Medicinal Plant Authentication: Pharmacognosy through the Centuries', *Planta Medica* 83, nos 14–15 (2017): 1110–16.

73 Domingos Tabajara de Oliveira Martins, Eliana Rodrigues, Laura Casu, Guillermo Benítez, and Marco Leonti, 'The Historical Development of Pharmacopoeias and the Inclusion of Exotic Herbal Drugs with a Focus on Europe and Brazil', *Journal of Ethnopharmacology* 240, no. 2 (2019): 1–11.

74 Josef Bernhard Theodor Ketteler, 'Arzneimittelverkehr und Apothekenwesen in den Deutschen Kolonien" [Drug trade and pharmacy in the German colonies] (Dr math.-nat. diss., Friedrich-Schiller-Universität, Jena, Germany, 1941), 75. For a summary see Josef Ketteler, 'Arzneimittelverkehr und Apothekenwesen in den Deutschen Kolonien', *Süddeutsche Apothekerzeitung* 81 (1941): 52, 57, 67, 71, available at https://leopard.tu-braunschweig.de/rsc/viewer/dbbs_derivate_00041697/max/00000062.jpg?logicalDiv=log_b511fed4-9384-42f4-800c-e6fd46c1a58d.

75 Günter Klatt, 'Geschichte und Entwicklung des Apotheken- und Arzneimittelwesens in Tansania unter besonderer Berücksichtigung der Deutschen Kolonialpharmazie" [History and development of the pharmacy and pharmaceutical industry in Tanzania with special consideration of German colonial pharmacy] (Dr rer. nat. diss., Philipps Universität, Marburg, Germany, 1969), 284.

76 André Schön, Untersuchungen von Arzneidrogen und Giften aus den ehemaligen deutschen Kolonien West-und Sudwestafrikas, vornehmlich an Beliner Instituten, 1884–1918" [Investigation of medicinal drugs and poisons of the former German colonies in West and South West Africa, especially at Berlin Institutes] (Sr res. nat. diss., Philipps Universität, Marburg, Germany, 2017), 87–154.

77 André Schön, personal communication, 4 July 2021.

78 Sabine Anagnostou, 'Forming, Transfer, and Globalization of Medical-Pharmaceutical Knowledge in Southeast Asian Missions', *Journal of Ethnopharmacology* 167, no. 1 (2015): 78–85.

79 Schön, 'Drugs and Poisons of the Former German Colonies."

80 For the history of the Danish Empire see Michael Bregnsbo and Kurt Villads Jensen, *The Rise and Fall of the Danish Empire* (London: Palgrave Macmillan, 2022).

81 Jens Soelberg, 'Dansk Vestindien og Guldkystens Glemte Lægeplanter', *Theriaca* 45 (2019): 44–73.

82 For background on the history of Greenland see Wikipedia, s.v. "Grønlands historie', last modified 14 July 2023, 18:44, https://da.wikipedia.org/wiki/Grønlands_historie.

282 Notes to pages 79–83

83 Paul Kruse, personal communication, 21 July 2021.
84 E. Dam and A. Schæffer, *De Danske Apotekers Historie* (Copenhagen: E. Munksgaards Forlag, 1947), 687, 692–7; P.H.J. Hansen, *Apotheker-Lovene i Den danske Stat ... fra 1660 til 1859* (Copenhagen: P.H.J. Hansen, 1859), 131.
85 Niklas Thode Jensen, *For the Health of the Enslaved: Slaves, Medicine and Power in the Danish West Indies, 1803–1848* (Copenhagen: Museum Tuscuanum Press, 2012), 206.
86 L. Brimer and G. Hauberg, 'Pamiut/Frederikshåb', *Farmaceutisk Tidende* 89 (1979): 934–41; A. Schæffer, *De Danske Apotekers Historie* (Copenhagen: Nyt Nordisk Forlag, 1947); L.R. Thomsen, 'Medicinleverancen til Grønland', *Archiv for Pharmaci og Chemi* 55 (1948): 434–5.
87 For the history of pharmacy in Italy see Glenn Sonnedecker, 'The Development in Italy', in *Kremers and Urdang*, 56–66.
88 For the history of Italian pharmacopoeias see Giovanni Cipriani, 'Italian Pharmacopoeias: A General Survey', International Society for the History of Pharmacy, 2022, https://www.histpharm.org/ISHPWG%20Italy2 .pdf; Raimondo Villano, 'Pharmacopoeias from the Ducky [*sic*] of Naples to Kingdom of the Two Sicilies', International Society for the History of Pharmacy, 2022, https://www.histpharm.org/ISHPWG%20Italy.pdf; Ernesto Riva, 'Pharmacopoeias in Veneto from the Fall of the Republic until Italian Unification', International Society for the History of Pharmacy, 2022, https://www.histpharm.org/ISHPWG%20Italy3.pdf.
89 Antonio Corvi, 'The Last Pharmacopoeias of the Italian States Prior to Unification, 1853–1858', International Society for the History of Pharmacy, 2022, https://www.histpharm.org/ISHPWG%20Italy4.pdf.
90 Ibid.
91 Giovanni Cipriani, personal communication, 8 July 2021.
92 Cipriani, personal communication.
93 Thomas Pakenham, *The Scramble for Africa: The White Man's Conquest of the Dark Continent from 1876 to 1912* (London: Abacus, 1992).
94 George Urdang, 'Pharmacopoeias as Witnesses of World History', *Journal of the History of Medicine* 1, no. 1 (1946): 46–70.
95 Charles Rice, 'The Study of Pharmacy', *Pharmaceutical Era* 13, no. 2 (1895): 68.
96 Urdang, 'Pharmacopoeias as Witnesses of World History', 64–6.
97 Juan Esteva, 'Las Farmacopeas Hispanas', in *Historia de la Farmacia de Barcelona*, ed. Jose Luis Gomez Caamaño (Barcelona: Facultad de Farmacia, 1980), 103–38.

Notes to pages 84–6

CHAPTER FOUR

1 For the history of the British Empire see *The Oxford History of the British Empire*, 5 vols (Oxford: Oxford University Press, 1998–99); Lawrence James, *The Rise and Fall of the British Empire* (London: Abacus, 1998); Trevor Lloyd, *Empire: A History of the British Empire* (London: Bloomsbury, 2000).

2 For the history of pharmacy in Britain see G.E. Trease, *Pharmacy in History* (London: Bailliere, Tindall & Cox, 1964); Leslie G. Matthews, *History of Pharmacy in Britain* (London: E. & S. Livingstone, 1962); N.L. Poynter, ed., *The Evolution of Pharmacy in Britain* (London: Pitman Medical, 1965); S.W.F. Holloway, *Royal Pharmaceutical Society of Great Britain, 1841–1991: A Political and Social History* (London: Pharmaceutical Press, 1991); Stuart Anderson, ed., *Making Medicines: A Brief History of Pharmacy and Pharmaceuticals* (London: Pharmaceutical Press, 2005).

3 For the history of the British Parliament see J.R. Maddicott, *The Origins of the English Parliament* (Oxford: Oxford University Press, 2010), 924–1327; Ann Lyon, *Constitutional History of the UK*, 2nd ed. (Abingdon, UK: Routledge, 2016): Clive Jones, ed., *A Short History of Parliament: England, Great Britain, the United Kingdom, Ireland and Scotland* (Martlesham, UK: Boydell Press, 2009).

4 For the seventeenth-century rivalry between physicians and apothecaries see Penelope Hunting, *A History of the Society of Apothecaries* (London: Society of Apothecaries, 1998), 29–55; George Clark, *A History of the Royal College of Physicians of London*, vol. 1 (Oxford: Clarendon Press, 1964); Juanita G.L. Burnby, 'A Study of the English Apothecary from 1660 to 1760', in *Medical History* (London: Wellcome Institute for the History of Medicine, 1983), 24–61.

5 Clark, *History of the Royal College of Physicians*, 1:58.

6 William Munk, *Roll of the College of Physicians*, vol. 1 (London: Royal College of Physicians, 1855), 2.

7 Clark, *History of the Royal College of Physicians*, 1:158.

8 George Urdang, *Pharmacopoeia Londinensis of 1618, Reproduced in Facsimile with a Historical Introduction* (Madison: State Historical Society of Wisconsin, 1944), 82.

9 Clark, *History of the Royal College of Physicians*, 1:159.

10 D. Jacques, *Essential to the Practick Part of Physic: The London Apothecaries, 1540–1617* (London: Society of Apothecaries, 1992), 47.

11 Hunting, *History of Society of Apothecaries*, 24.

284 Notes to pages 87–9

12 A.C. Wootton, *Chronicles of Pharmacy*, vol. 2 (London: Macmillan & Co., 1910), 60.

13 The full list is printed in William Munk, *Roll of the College of Physicians*, vol. 3 (London: Royal College of Physicians, 1856), 373, cited in Clark, *History of the Royal College of Physicians*, 1:161.

14 Clark, 1:161.

15 Ibid., 1:165.

16 Ibid., 1:199.

17 Ibid., 1:218.

18 Ibid., 1:219.

19 Hunting, *History of Society of Apothecaries*, 32.

20 Clark, *History of the Royal College of Physicians*, 1:159.

21 Hunting, *History of Society of Apothecaries*, 34.

22 Clark, *History of the Royal College of Physicians*, 1:158.

23 Ibid., 1:220.

24 A.C. Wootton, *Chronicles of Pharmacy*, vol. 1 (London: Macmillan & Co., 1910), 256.

25 Ibid., 2:64. See also James Grier, *A History of Pharmacy* (London: Pharmaceutical Press, 1937), 141.

26 Hunting, *History of Society of Apothecaries*, 48.

27 Clark, *History of the Royal College of Physicians*, 1:228.

28 *Pharmacopoea Londinensis, in Qva Medicamenta Antiqva et Nova, Londinensis, Opera Medicorum Collegij*, 1618. First issue of first edition of *London Pharmacopoeia*.

29 Urdang, *Pharmacopoeia Londinensis of 1618*, 77–81; *The Pharmacopoeia Londinensis of 7 May 1618 from the London College of Physicians in Facsimile*, ed. Henry Oakeley (London: Royal College of Physicians, 2018), i–xvi; Claire J. Fowler, *Pharmacopoeia Londinensis 1618 and Its Descendants* (London: Royal College of Physicians, 2018).

30 Clark, *History of the Royal College of Physicians*, 1:228. See also Hunting, *History of Society of Apothecaries*, 268n43.

31 Munk, *Roll of the College of Physicians*, 1:170.

32 Clark, *History of the Royal College of Physicians*, 1:228.

33 *Kremers and Urdang's History of Pharmacy*, ed. Glenn Sonnedecker, 4th ed. (Madison, wi: American Institute of the History of Pharmacy, 1976), 430.

34 W. Brockbank, 'Sovereign Remedies: A Critical Depreciation of the Seventeenth Century London Pharmacopoeia,' *Medical History* 8, no. 1 (1964): 1–14.

35 Urdang, *Pharmacopoeia Londinensis of 1618*, 77–81.

Notes to pages 89–93

36 Ibid., 81.
37 M.P. Earles, 'Pharmacopoeia Londinensis 1618: A New Look at an Old Problem', *Pharmaceutical Historian* 12, no. 2 (1982): 4–5.
38 Ibid., 5.
39 Fowler, *Pharmacopoeia Londinensis 1618*, 79.
40 Ibid., 69.
41 Urdang, *Pharmacopoeia Londinensis of 1618*, 68–70; Paula de Vos, 'Pharmacopoeias and the Textual Tradition in Galenic Pharmacy', in *Drugs on the Page: Pharmacopoeias and Healing Knowledge in the Early Modern Atlantic World*, ed. Matthew James Crawford and Joseph Gabriel (Pittsburgh: University of Pittsburgh Press, 2019), 19–44.
42 Urdang, *Pharmacopoeia Londinensis of 1618*, 68–70.
43 Ibid., 72. For analysis of the content of the 1618 LP see also Brockbank, 'Sovereign Remedies', 1–14.
44 Anna Simmons, 'Medicines, Monopolies, and Mortars: The Chemical Laboratory and Pharmaceutical Trade at the Society of Apothecaries in the Eighteenth Century', *Ambix* 53, no. 3 (2006): 225.
45 Nicholas Culpeper, *A Physicall Directory, or Translation of the London Dispensatory* (London: Peter Cole, 1649), 2.
46 Patrick Wallis, 'Exotic Drugs and English Medicine: England's Drug Trade, c.1550–c.1800', *Social History of Medicine* 25, no. 1 (2011): 26–30.
47 Ibid., 31.
48 Oakeley, *Pharmacopoeia Londinensis*, xiii.
49 Trease, *Pharmacy in History*, 119.
50 Clark, *History of the Royal College of Physicians*, 1:345.
51 R.G. Todd, 'The London Pharmacopoeias 1618, 1650, and 1677', *Pharmaceutical Historian* 10, no. 2 (1980): 10–12.
52 Kenneth Holland, 'Medicine from Animals: From Mysticism to Science', *Pharmaceutical Historian* 24, no. 3 (1994): 9–12.
53 Todd, 'London Pharmacopoeias 1618, 1650, and 1677', 11.
54 Trease, *Pharmacy in History*, 119.
55 Oakeley, *Pharmacopoeia Londinensis*, xiii.
56 Anthony C. Cartwright, *The British Pharmacopoeia, 1864 to 2014: Medicines, International Standards, and the State* (Farnham, UK: Ashgate, 2015), 1–13.
57 Fowler, *Pharmacopoeia Londinensis 1618*, 93.
58 Ibid., 87.
59 Ibid., 104.
60 Jacob Bell and Theophilus Redwood, *Historical Sketch of the Progress of Pharmacy in Great Britain* (London: Pharmaceutical Press, 1880), 7.

Notes to pages 93–8

61 D.A. Jones, 'Nicholas Culpeper and His Pharmacopoeia', *Pharmaceutical Historian* 10, no. 2 (1980): 9–10.

62 Trease, *Pharmacy in History*, 142.

63 W. Ferguson, *Scotland's Relations with England: A Survey to 1707* (Edinburgh: John Donald, 1977), 201.

64 T.M. Devine, *Scotland's Empire, 1600–1815* (London: Penguin Books, 2004), 1.

65 Ibid., 2.

66 Ibid.

67 Ibid., 36.

68 Ibid., 38.

69 Ibid., 39.

70 Ibid., 40.

71 T. M. Devine, *Independence or Union: Scotland's Past and Scotland's Present* (London: Penguin Random House, 2017), 8.

72 Ibid.

73 For events leading up to the union of Scotland with England see Devine, *Independence*, 18–27.

74 Morrice McCrae, *Physicians and Society: A Social History of the Royal College of Physicians of Edinburgh* (Edinburgh: John Donald, 2007), 15.

75 J.F. McHarg, 'Dr John Maklure and the 1630 Attempt to Establish the College', in *Proceedings of the Royal College of Physicians of Edinburgh Tercentenary Congress, 1981* (Edinburgh: Royal College of Physicians, 1982), 49.

76 Clark, *History of the Royal College of Physicians*, 1:284.

77 McCrae, *Physicians and Society*, 15–18.

78 Ibid., 7.

79 Devine, *Scotland's Empire*, 43.

80 McCrae, *Physicians and Society*, 21.

81 Clark, *History of the Royal College of Physicians*, 1:337.

82 McCrae, *Physicians and Society*, 27.

83 Ibid., 37.

84 David L. Cowen, 'The Edinburgh Pharmacopoeia', in *The Early Years of the Edinburgh Medical School*, ed. R.G.W. Anderson and A.D.C. Simpson (Edinburgh: Royal Scottish Museum, 1976), 3.

85 F.P. Hett, *Memoirs of Sir Robert Sibbald, 1641–1722* (Oxford: Oxford University Press, 1932), 93. See also Andrew Cunningham, 'Sir Robert Sibbald and Medical Education, Edinburgh, 1706', *Clio Medica* 13, no. 2 (1978): 136–61.

86 McCrae, *Physicians and Society*, 51,

Notes to pages 98–101   287

87 Cowen, 'The Edinburgh Pharmacopoeia', 3.

88 McCrae, *Physicians and Society*, 34.

89 Ibid., 35.

90 Ibid., 36.

91 W.B. Howie, 'Sir Archibald Stevenson, His Ancestry and the Riot in the College of Physicians at Edinburgh', *Medical History* 11, no. 3 (1967): 269–84.

92 McCrae, *Physicians and Society*, 38.

93 H.L. Coulter, *Divided Legacy: A History of Modern Western Medicine, J.B. Helmont to Claude Bernard* (Berkeley, CA: North Atlantic Books, 2000), 110.

94 Stuart Anderson, 'National Identities, Medical Politics and Local Traditions', in Crawford and Gabriel, *Drugs on the Page*, 212.

95 *Pharmacopoea Collegii Regii Medicorum Edimburgensium, Edimburgi, MDCXCIX* (Edinburgh: Royal College of Physicians, 1699).

96 David L. Cowen, *Pharmacopoeias and Related Literature in Britain and America, 1618–1847* (Aldershot, UK: Ashgate, 2001), 1–73.

97 Stephen Mullen, *The Glasgow Sugar Aristocracy: Scotland and Caribbean Slavery, 1775–1838* (London: University of London Press, 2023).

98 George Clark, *History of the Royal College of Physicians of London*, vol. 2 (Oxford: Clarendon Press, 1966), 456.

99 Ibid.

100 Ibid., 2:487.

101 *Pharmacopoeia Collegii Regalis Medicorum Londinensis* (London: Royal College of Physicians, 1724), 1.

102 Ibid., 2.

103 Ibid., 3.

104 Matthews, *History of Pharmacy*, 79.

105 Bell and Redwood, *Historical Sketch*, 24–5.

106 Clark, *History of the Royal College of Physicians*, 2:487.

107 *Pharmacopoeia Collegii Regalis Medicorum Londinensis* (London: Royal College of Physicians, 1746), i.

108 William Munk, *Munk's Roll*, vol. 3 (London: Royal College of Physicians, 1856), 382.

109 Henry Pemberton, *Dispensatory of the Royal College of Physicians of London, Translated into English with Remarks* (London: Longman and Shewell, 1746), viii–ix.

110 Matthews, *History of Pharmacy*, 79–80.

111 Pemberton, *Dispensatory*, 36–7.

112 Ibid., ix–x.

288 Notes to pages 101–5

113 Clark, *History of the Royal College of Physicians*, 2:497.

114 C.R.B. Barrett, *History of the Society of Apothecaries of London* (London: Society of Apothecaries, 1905), 157.

115 Clark, *History of the Royal College of Physicians*, 2:581.

116 William Heberden, *Antitheriaka: Essay on Mithradatum and Theriaca* (London, 1745).

117 A.I. Bierman, 'Medical Fiction and Pharmaceutical Facts about Theriac', *Pharmaceutical Historian* 24, no. 3 (1994): 8.

118 Robert James, *Pharmacopoeia Universalis: or a New Universal English Dispensatory* (London, 1747), v.

119 Trease, *Pharmacy in History*, 167.

120 Clark, *History of the Royal College of Physicians*, 2:591.

121 William Withering, *An Account of the Foxglove and Some of Its Medical Uses* (London: G.G.J. and J. Robinson, 1785).

122 S.F. Gray, *Supplement to the London Pharmacopoeia 1809* (London: Longman, 1818), i–ix.

123 J.D.H. Widdess, *A History of the Royal College of Physicians of Ireland, 1665–1963* (London: E. & S. Livingstone, 1963), 7; Anderson, 'National Identities', 212–19.

124 T. Percy C. Kirkpatrick, *The Dublin Pharmacopoeias* (Dublin: Royal College of Physicians, 1921), 4.

125 Kirkpatrick, *Dublin Pharmacopoeias*, 4.

126 N.C. Cooper, 'Development of a Pharmaceutical Profession in Ireland', *Pharmacy in History* 29, no. 4 (1987): 165–76.

127 Kirkpatrick, *Dublin Pharmacopoeias*, 5.

128 Hunting, *History of Society of Apothecaries*, 224.

129 Kirkpatrick, *Dublin Pharmacopoeias*, 7.

130 Ibid., 8.

131 For more on this point, see Anderson, 'National Identities', 212–19.

132 Kirkpatrick, *Dublin Pharmacopoeias*, 9.

133 Ibid.

134 *Pharmacopoeia Collegii Medicorum Regis et Retinae in Hibernia* (Dublin: Royal College of Physicians, 1807).

135 Kirkpatrick, *Dublin Pharmacopoeias*, 12.

136 *Pharmacopoeia Collegii Medicorum Regis et Retinae in Hibernia*, i.

137 Ibid.

138 Anderson, 'National Identities', 212.

139 Trease, *Pharmacy in History*, 167.

140 Anthony C. Cartwright and N. Anthony Armstrong, *A History of the Medicines We Take* (Barnsley, UK: Pen & Sword History, 2020), 90.

Notes to pages 106–9   289

141   Stuart Anderson, *Pharmacy and Professionalization in the British Empire, 1780–1970* (London: Palgrave Macmillan, 2021), 35–67.

142   Clark, *History of the Royal College of Physicians*, 2:624.

143   Kirkpatrick, *Dublin Pharmacopoeias*, 11.

144   Richard Powell, *The Pharmacopoeia of the Royal College of Physicians of London, 1809, Translated into English with Notes &c.*, 3rd ed. (London: Royal College of Physicians, 1815), iii.

145   Ibid.

146   Ibid., v.

147   Ibid.

148   Anna Simmons, 'Stills, Status, Stocks and Science: The Laboratories at Apothecaries' Hall in the Nineteenth Century', *Ambix* 61, no. 2 (2014): 151.

149   Clark, *History of the Royal College of Physicians*, 2:686.

150   Bell and Redwood, *Historical Sketch*, 42.

151   Powell, *Pharmacopoeia of the Royal College of Physicians of London*, v.

152   Clark, *History of the Royal College of Physicians*, 2:660.

153   Ibid., 2:661.

CHAPTER FIVE

1   Thomas K. Ford, *The Apothecary in Eighteenth-Century Williamsburg*, 4th ed. (Williamsburg, VA: Colonial Williamsburg Foundation, 1965), 1.

2   *Kremers and Urdang's History of Pharmacy*, ed. Glenn Sonnedecker, (Madison, WI: American Institute of the History of Pharmacy, 1976), 145–60.

3   Harold B. Gill Jr, *The Apothecary in Colonial Virginia* (Williamsburg, VA: Colonial Williamsburg Foundation, 1972), 12.

4   Norman Gevitz, 'Prey Let the Medicines be Good', in *Apothecaries and the Drug Trade*, ed. Gregory J. Higby and Elaine C. Stroud (Madison, WI: American Institute of the History of Pharmacy, 2001), 8.

5   R.C. Anderson, *The Great Migration Begins* (Boston: New England Historic Genealogic Society, 1995), 1807–9.

6   Virginia DeJohn Anderson, 'New England in the Seventeenth Century', in *The Oxford History of the British Empire*, vol. 1, *The Origins of Empire: British Overseas Enterprise to the Close of the Seventeenth Century*, ed. Nicholas Canny (Oxford: Oxford University Press, 1998), 195.

7   P.J. Marshal, ed., *The Eighteenth Century*, vol. 2 of *The Oxford History of the British Empire* (Oxford: Oxford University Press, 1998), 100.

290   Notes to pages 109–10

8 Penelope Hunting, *A History of the Society of Apothecaries* (London: Society of Apothecaries, 1998), 179.

9 Ibid., 178.

10 K. Scott, 'New York Doctors and London Medicines, 1677', *Medical History* 11, no. 4 (1967): 389–98.

11 George E. Osborne, 'Pharmacy in British Colonial America', in *American Pharmacy in the Colonial and Revolutionary Periods*, ed. George A. Bender and John Parascandola (Madison, WI: American Institute of the History of Pharmacy, 1977), 8.

12 Samuel Lee to Nehemiah Grew, in "Letters of Samuel Lee and Samuel Sewall Relating to New England and the Indians', in *Publications of the Colonial Society of Massachusetts, 1911–13*, vol. 14, ed. George Lyman Kittredge (Boston: Colonial Society of Massachusetts, 1913), 146.

13 George Urdang, 'Pharmacy in Colonial North America', *Merck Report*, April 1947, 3–7.

14 Sylvester Judd, *History of Hadley* (Amherst, MA: Metcalf, 1863), 615.

15 David L. Cowen, 'The Boston Editions of Nicholas Culpeper', *Journal of the History of Medicine and Allied Sciences* 11, no. 2 (1956): 156–8, 165.

16 George B. Griffenhagen and James Harvey Young, 'Old English Patent Medicines in America', *Pharmacy in History* 34, no. 4 (1992): 200–28.

17 Gill, *Apothecary in Colonial Virginia*, 63.

18 Hunting, *History of Society of Apothecaries*, 180.

19 See, for example, Roy Porter and Dorothy Porter, 'The Rise of the English Drugs Industry: The Role of Thomas Corbyn', *Medical History* 33, no. 3 (1989): 277–95; William I. Roberts III, 'Samuel Storke: An Eighteenth-Century London Merchant Trading to the American Colonies', *Business History Review* 39, no. 2 (1965): 147–70.

20 Renate Wilson, 'Trading in Drugs through Philadelphia in the Eighteenth Century: A Transatlantic Enterprise', *Social History of Medicine* 26, no. 3 (2013): 352–63.

21 C.H. Spiers, 'The Drug Suppliers of George Washington and Other Virginians', *Pharmaceutical Historian* 7, no. 1 (1977): 2–3. See also table 1 in C.H. Spiers, 'Sidelights on the Supply of Drugs to Pre-revolutionary Virginia', *Pharmaceutical Historian* 32, no. 2 (2002): 20.

22 Spiers, 'Drug Suppliers of George Washington', 2.

23 Spiers, 'Sidelights on Supply of Drugs', 18–25.

24 For pharmacy in colonial Pennsylvania see Renate Wilson and Woodrow J. Savacool, 'The Theory and Practice of Pharmacy in Pennsylvania: Observations on Two Colonial Country Doctors', *Pennsylvania History* 68, no. 1 (2001): 31–65.

25 Zachary Dorner, *Merchants of Medicines: The Commerce and Coercion of Health in Britain's Long Eighteenth Century* (Chicago: University of Chicago Press, 2020), 39.

26 David Cowen, 'Colonial Drugs Pertaining to Pharmacy', *Pharmacy in History* 48, no. 1 (2006): 24.

27 Ibid., 24–30.

28 Dorner, *Merchants of Medicines*, 158.

29 Cowen, *Colonial Drugs*, 27.

30 For the history of the Royal African Company see Kenneth Gordon Davies, *The Royal African Company* (London: Octagon Books, 1975).

31 Stuart Anderson, 'Pharmacy and Slavery: Apothecaries, Medicines and the Slave Trade, 1650 to 1807', *Pharmaceutical Historian* 39, no. 1 (2009): 11–6.

32 Hunting, *Society of Apothecaries*, 164.

33 George Clark, *History of the Royal College of Physicians of London*, vol. 2 (Oxford: Clarendon Press, 1966), 431.

34 Hunting, *Society of Apothecaries*, 165.

35 Dorner, *Merchants of Medicines*, 73.

36 Ibid.

37 Juanita G.L. Burnby, *A Study of the English Apothecary from 1660 to 1760* (London: Wellcome Institute for the History of Medicine, 1993), 62.

38 Hunting, *Society of Apothecaries*, 166–7.

39 David R. Kennedy, 'One Hundred Years of Pharmacy Legislation', in *One Hundred Years of Pharmacy in Canada*, ed. Ernst W. Stieb (Toronto: Canadian Academy for History of Pharmacy, 1969), 26.

40 Kennedy, 'One Hundred Years of Pharmacy Legislation', 27.

41 Gregory Haines, *Pharmacy in Australia: The National Experience* (Deakin: Pharmaceutical Society of Australia, 1988), 18.

42 Stuart Anderson, *Pharmacy and Professionalization in the British Empire, 1780–1970* (London: Palgrave Macmillan, 2021), 285.

43 John Pearn, Andrew F. Petrie, and Gwynneth M. Petrie, 'An Early Colonial Pharmacopoeia: A Drug List and Its Materia Medica for an Australian Convict Settlement', *Medical Journal of Australia* 149, nos 11–12 (1988): 630–4.

44 Haines, *Pharmacy in Australia*, 18.

45 Juanita G.L. Burnby, 'The Early Days of Pharmacy in Australia', *Pharmaceutical Journal* 241, no. 6493 (1988): 56–60.

46 See Anderson, *Pharmacy and Professionalization*, 286–91.

47 Juanita G.L. Burnby, 'Early Years of British Pharmaceutical Journalism', *Pharmaceutical Historian* 24, no. 1 (1994): 9.

Notes to pages 114–16

48 Paula de Vos, 'Pharmacopoeias and the Textual Tradition in Galenic Pharmacy', in *Drugs on the Page: Pharmacopoeias and Healing Knowledge in the Early Modern Atlantic World*, ed. Matthew James Crawford and Joseph Gabriel (Pittsburgh: University of Pittsburgh Press, 2019), 42.

49 For the history of the East India Company see John Keay, *The Honourable Company: A History of the English East India Company* (London: Harper Collins, 1993).

50 See, for example, Douglas M. Peers and Nandini Gooptu, *India and the British Empire* (Oxford: Oxford University Press, 2016); Roderick Matthews, *Peace, Poverty and Betrayal: A New History of British India* (London: Hurst & Co., 2021). See also James Mill, *History of British India* (Abingdon, UK: Routledge, 1997).

51 For the history of medicine in the British Empire see Pratik Chakrabarti, *Medicine & Empire, 1600–1960* (Basingstoke, UK: Palgrave Macmillan, 2014); Mark Harrison, *Medicine in an Age of Commerce and Empire: Britain and Its Tropical Colonies, 1660–1830* (Oxford: Oxford University Press, 2010); *Medicine and the Market in England and Its Colonies, c.1450–c.1850*, ed. Mark S.R. Jenner and Patrick Wallis (Basingstoke, UK: Palgrave Macmillan, 2007).

52 Dorner, *Merchants of Medicines*, 138.

53 Mark Harrison, 'Medicine and Orientalism', in *Health, Medicine and Empire: Perspectives on Colonial India*, ed. Biswamoy Pati and Mark Harrison (New Delhi: Orient Longman, 2001), 77.

54 Ibid., 142.

55 Bombay Military Department, 30 June 1797, IOR/E/4/1012, ff. 611–12, India Office Records, British Library.

56 Repeat orders for the *LP* were placed by the Medical Department in India between 1807 and 1813. See IOR/Z/E/39/A1183; IOR/Z/E/39/B963; IOR/Z/E/39/M1050, India Office Records, British Library.

57 Harkishan Singh, *Pharmacopoeias and Formularies* (Delhi: Vallabh Prakashan, 1994), 23.

58 Singh, *Pharmacopoeias and Formularies*, 142.

59 Zaheer Baber, 'The Plants of Empire: Botanic Gardens, Colonial Power and Botanical Knowledge', *Journal of Contemporary Asia* 46, no. 4 (2016): 659–79; Donal McCracken, *Gardens of Empire: Botanical Institutions of the Victorian British Empire* (Leicester: Leicester University Press, 1997); "Medical Garden at Darjeeling", Aug. 1849–Apr. 1850, IOR/F/4/2444/134239, India Office Records, British Library.

60 Londa Schiebinger, *Plants and Empire: Colonial Bioprospecting in the Atlantic World* (Cambridge, MA: Harvard University Press, 2007), 73.

Notes to pages 116–21

61 B. Bennett and J. Hodge, *Science and Empire: Knowledge and Networks of Science across the British Empire, 1800–1970* (Basingstoke, UK: Palgrave Macmillan, 2011).

62 Ibid., 139.

63 Dorner, *Merchants of Medicines*, 143.

64 Ibid.

65 Ibid., 146.

66 Whitelaw Ainslie, *Materia Indica of Hindoostan* (Madras: published by special permission of the Government of Madras, 1813).

67 Nandini Bhattacharya, 'From Materia Medica to the Pharmacopoeia: Challenges of Writing the History of Drugs in India', *History Compass* 14, no. 4 (2016): 135.

68 Bhattacharya, 'From Materia Medica to the Pharmacopoeia', 135.

69 Singh, *Pharmacopoeias and Formularies*, 29.

70 Neil MacGillivray, 'Sir William Brooke O'Shaughnessy (1809–1889)', *Journal of Medical Biography* 25, no. 3 (2015): 86–196; Mel Gorman, 'Sir William Brooke O'Shaughnessy (1809–1889)', *Notes and Records of the Royal Society of London* 39 (1984): 151–64; Albert Frederick Pollard, 'O'Shaughnessy, William Brooke', *Dictionary of National Biography* 42 (1885–1900): 310–11.

71 Copies of the LP 1836 continued to be sent to India from 1838 to 1842. See IOR/Z/E/4/45/P313; IOR/Z/E/4/45/P321, India Office Records, British Library.

72 Singh, *Pharmacopoeias and Formularies*, 29–30.

73 W.B. O'Shaughnessy, *The Bengal Dispensatory and Pharmacopoeia*, vol. 1, *Dispensatory* (Calcutta: Bishop's College Press, 1841), iii–xxiii.

74 Singh, *Pharmacopoeias and Formularies*, 30.

75 O'Shaughnessy, *Bengal Dispensatory*.

76 W.B. O'Shaughnessy, *The Bengal Pharmacopoeia and General Conspectus of Medicinal Plants* (Calcutta: Bishop's College Press, 1844).

77 O'Shaughnessy, *Bengal Dispensatory*, i.

78 David L. Cowen, 'The Influence of the Edinburgh Pharmacopoeia and the Edinburgh Dispensatories', *Pharmaceutical Historian* 12, no. 1 (1982): 2–4.

79 O'Shaughnessy, *Bengal Pharmacopoeia*, i.

80 Ibid., iii–vii.

81 Ibid., iv.

82 Jenner and Wallis, *Medicine and the Market*, 15.

83 Bhattacharya, 'From Materia Medica to the Pharmacopoeia', 136.

84 Pratik Chakrabarti, *Materials and Medicine: Trade, Conquest, and Thera-*

294 Notes to pages 121–5

peutics in the Eighteenth Century (Manchester: Manchester University Press, 2010), 42–4.

85 O'Shaughnessy, *Bengal Pharmacopoeia*, v.

86 Singh, *Pharmacopoeias and Formularies*, 23.

87 Hindustani translation of *LP*, Dec. 1841–42, IOR/F/4/2012/89830, India Office Records, British Library.

88 Singh, *Pharmacopoeias and Formularies*, 23.

89 David L. Cowen, *Pharmacopoeias and Related Literature in Britain and America, 1618–1847* (Aldershot, UK: Ashgate Variorum, 2001), 181–2.

90 Singh, *Pharmacopoeias and Formularies*, 23.

91 Ibid., 27.

92 Mike Ryan, *A History of Organised Pharmacy in South Africa, 1885–1950* (Cape Town: Society for History of Pharmacy of South Africa, 1986), 1.

93 G.R. Paterson, 'Canadian Pharmacy in Pre-Confederation Medical Legislation', *Journal of the American Medical Association* 200, no. 10 (1967): 849–52.

94 Richard Powell, *Pharmacopoeia of the Royal College of Physicians of London* (London: Royal College of Physicians, 1815), viii.

95 Powell, *Pharmacopoeia of the Royal College*, ix.

96 Clark, *History of the Royal College of Physicians*, 2:661.

97 G.E. Trease, *Pharmacy in History* (London: Bailliere, Tindall & Cox, 1964), 175.

98 Richard Powell, *Translation of Pharmacopoeia of the Royal College of Physicians of London* (London: Royal College of Physicians, 1836), 61–2.

99 Ernst W. Stieb, *Drug Adulteration: Detection and Control in Nineteenth Century Britain* (Madison: University of Wisconsin Press, 1966), 86.

100 Fredrick Accum, *Treatise on Adulterations of Food and Culinary Poisons* (London: J. Mallett, 1820), 18.

101 J.G.L. Burnby, 'Pharmacy in the Mid-nineteenth Century', *Pharmaceutical Historian* 22, no. 1 (1992): 5.

102 Clark, *History of the Royal College of Physicians*, 2:680.

103 T. Percy C. Kirkpatrick, *The Dublin Pharmacopoeias* (Dublin: Royal College of Physicians, 1921), 15.

104 Jacob Bell and Theophilus Redwood, *Historical Sketch of the Progress of Pharmacy in Great Britain* (London: Pharmaceutical Press, 1880), 75.

105 Clark, *History of the Royal College of Physicians*, 2:679–80.

106 Richard Phillips, *Translation of Pharmacopoeia Londinensis 1836* (London: Royal College of Physicians, 1836), 7.

107 Morrice McCrae, *Physicians and Society: A Social History of the Royal College of Physicians of Edinburgh* (Edinburgh: John Donald, 2007), 210.

Notes to pages 125–9

108 Records of the Royal College of Physicians of Edinburgh, College and Council meeting minutes, RCP/COL/2/1/1, 1 May 1848, Royal College of Physicians of Edinburgh Archive.
109 Clark, *History of the Royal College of Physicians*, 2:680.
110 Phillips, *Translation of Pharmacopoeia Londinensis 1836*, xi–xii.
111 Burnby, 'Pharmacy in Mid-nineteenth Century', 5.
112 Clark, *History of the Royal College of Physicians*, 2:680.
113 Phillips, *Translation of Pharmacopoeia Londinensis 1836*, xi.
114 Trease, *Pharmacy in History*, 184–5.
115 Anthony Morson, *Operative Chemyst* (Amsterdam: Rodopi, 1997), 216–17.
116 Ibid., 101.
117 Ibid.
118 Clark, *History of the Royal College of Physicians*, 2:697.
119 Bell and Redwood, *Historical Sketch*, 205.
120 Clark, *History of the Royal College of Physicians*, 2:697.
121 Ruth A. Guy, 'The History of Cod Liver Oil', *American Journal of Diseases of Childhood* 26, no. 2 (1913): 112–16.
122 Bell and Redwood, *Historical Sketch*, 205.
123 Ibid., 206.
124 See, for example, Jonathan Pereira, 'Review', *Pharmaceutical Journal* 11, no. 3 (1851): 143–4; C.P. Cloughly, J.G.L. Burnby, and M.P. Earles, eds, *My Dear Mr Bell* (Madison, WI: American Institute of the History of Pharmacy, 1976), 84.
125 Jacob Bell, 'The New London Pharmacopoeia', *Pharmaceutical Journal* 10, no. 10 (1851): 481.
126 Ibid.
127 Clark, *History of the Royal College of Physicians*, 2:580.
128 Ibid., 2:697.
129 Bell and Redwood, *Historical Sketch*, 227.
130 Ibid., 171.
131 Ibid., 171–2.
132 S.W.F. Holloway, *Royal Pharmaceutical Society of Great Britain, 1841–1991: A Political and Social History* (London: Pharmaceutical Press, 1991), 215–16.
133 Franklin Bache, 'On the Advantages That Would Accrue to English and American Pharmacy by the Adoption of a Single Uniform Pharmacopoeia for the British Empire', *American Journal of Pharmacy* 27 (1855): 11.

CHAPTER SIX

1 For medical reform in Britain see Roger French and Andrew Wear, eds, *British Medicine in an Age of Reform* (Abingdon, UK: Routledge, 2005); Ian Burney, 'The Politics of Particularism: Medicalization and Medical Reform in Nineteenth-Century Britain', in *Medicine, Madness and Social History*, ed. Roberta Bivins and John V. Pickstone (Basingstoke, UK: Palgrave Macmillan, 2007), 46–57; W.F. Bynum and Roy Porter, eds, *Medical Fringe and Medical Orthodoxy, 1750–1850* (Abingdon, UK: Routledge, 1987).

2 S.W.F. Holloway, *Royal Pharmaceutical Society of Great Britain, 1841–1991: A Political and Social History* (London: Pharmaceutical Press, 1991), 83–91.

3 Jacob Bell, 'Restrictions in the Medical Profession', *Pharmaceutical Journal* 3, no. 11 (1844): 509–10; Holloway, *Royal Pharmaceutical Society of Great Britain*, 183n30.

4 Stuart Anderson, *Pharmacy and Professionalization in the British Empire, 1780–1970* (London: Palgrave Macmillan, 2021), 35–67.

5 Nandini Bhattacharya, *Disparate Remedies: Making Medicines in Modern India* (Montreal and Kingston: McGill-Queen's University Press, 2023), 74.

6 Anderson, *Pharmacy and Professionalization*, 35–67.

7 Stuart Anderson, 'From Bespoke to Off-the-Peg: Community Pharmacists and the Retailing of Medicines in Great Britain, 1900 to 1970', *Pharmacy in History* 50, no. 2 (2008): 43–69.

8 George Clark, *History of Royal College of Physicians of London*, vol. 2 (Oxford: Clarendon Press, 1966), 728–9.

9 Robert Christison, *A Dispensatory, or Commentary on the Pharmacopoeias of Great Britain* (Philadelphia, PA: Lea & Blanchard, 1848).

10 Medical Act, 1862, 25 Vict., c. 3, vi. Emphasis added.

11 *Report of the Sub-committee on the British Pharmacopoeia of the Committee of Civil Research*, Cmd 3101 (London: His Majesty's Stationery Office, 1928), 11 (hereafter cited as Macmillan Report).

12 Macmillan Report, 267.

13 Ibid., 271.

14 Jacob Bell and Theophilus Redwood, *Historical Sketch of the Progress of Pharmacy in Great Britain* (London: Pharmaceutical Press, 1880), 272.

15 Holloway, *Royal Pharmaceutical Society*, 135.

16 Anthony Morson, *Operative Chymist* (Amsterdam: Rodopi, 1997), 182.

17 For the correspondence between the Pharmaceutical Society and the RCPS see Bell and Redwood, *Historical Sketch*, 267–72.

Notes to pages 133–5

18 Bell and Redwood, 268–9.

19 Anthony C. Cartwright, *The British Pharmacopoeia, 1864 to 2014: Medicines, International Standards, and the State* (Farnham, UK: Ashgate, 2015), 30.

20 G.E. Trease, *Pharmacy in History* (London: Bailliere, Tindall & Cox, 1964), 195.

21 GMC Minutes, November 1858, General Medical Council Archive, British Library.

22 Geoffrey Tweedale, *At the Sign of the Plough: 275 Years of Allen & Hanburys and the British Pharmaceutical Industry, 1715–1990* (London: John Murray, 1990), 57.

23 John V. Pickstone, *Ways of Knowing: A New History of Science, Technology and Medicine* (Manchester: Manchester University Press, 2000), 85.

24 *British Pharmacopoeia 1867* (London: General Medical Council, 1867), viii.

25 *British Pharmacopoeia 1864* (London: General Medical Council, 1864), xv–xvi.

26 *British Pharmacopoeia 1867*, viii.

27 E.J. Waring, *Remarks on the Uses of Some of the Bazaar Medicines and Common Medical Plants of India* (London: Churchill, 1859).

28 Theophilus Redwood, 'Note on the Tests of Purity of Balsam of Copaiba', *Pharmaceutical Journal* 6 (1846–47): 18.

29 Ernst W. Stieb, *Drug Adulteration: Detection and Control in Nineteenth Century Britain* (Madison: University of Wisconsin Press, 1966), 94.

30 Ibid., 51–69.

31 John Abraham, *Science, Policy, and the Pharmaceutical Industry: Controversy and Bias in Drug Regulation* (London: Routledge, 1995), 40.

32 J. Forrester, 'The *Lancet's* Analytical Sanitary Commission', *The Lancet* 2 (1978): 1360–62.

33 Arthur Hill Hassall, *Adulterants Detected, or Plain Instructions for the Discovery of Frauds in Food and Medicine* (London: Longman, Brown, Green, Longmans, and Roberts, 1857), 57–61.

34 Abraham, *Science, Policy, and the Pharmaceutical Industry*, 40.

35 *Report from the Select Committee on Adulterations of Foods, Drinks, and Drugs, Together with the Proceedings of the Committee, Minutes of Evidence, Appendix, and Index* (London: His Majesty's Stationery Office, 1856), 56–7.

36 *Report from the Select Committee*, 253.

37 M. Hodges, 'Control of the Safety of Drugs, 1868–1968 (Part 1)', *Pharmaceutical Journal* 240, no. 6444 (1987): 119.

38 A.B. Garrod, 'Lectures on the British Pharmacopoeia,' *British Medical Journal* 1, no. 163 (1864): 178–81. Garrod reported that, in smaller doses, cannabis "exalted the mental faculties and for this purpose is used in Eastern countries in the form of haaschisch."

39 Alexander MacDougall Cooke, *History of the Royal College of Physicians of London*, vol. 3 (Oxford: Oxford University Press, 1972), 810.

40 *British Pharmacopoeia 1867*, xv.

41 Macmillan Report, 12.

42 Cartwright, *The British Pharmacopoeia*, 31.

43 *British Pharmacopoeia 1867*, xv.

44 Ibid., viii.

45 Ibid., ix.

46 Ibid., viii. Emphasis added.

47 D.M. Dunlop and T.C. Denston, 'The History and Development of the BP,' *British Medical Journal* 2, no. 5107 (1958): 1251–2.

48 Anderson, *Pharmacy and Professionalization*, 281–309.

49 Ibid., 69–98.

50 Ibid., 113–14.

51 See, for example, Pratik Chakrabarti, *Medicine & Empire, 1600–1960* (Basingstoke, UK: Palgrave Macmillan, 2014), 20–39; Bhattacharya, *Disparate Remedies*; Mark Harrison, *Medicine in an Age of Commerce and Empire: Britain and Its Tropical Colonies, 1660–1830* (Oxford: Oxford University Press, 2010).

52 J.F. Royle, *An Essay on the Antiquity of Hindoo Medicine* (Philadelphia, PA: Lea and Blanchard, 1847); J.F. Royle, *Manual of Materia Medica and Therapeutics* (London: Churchill, 1847).

53 Nandini Bhattacharya, 'From Materia Medica to the Pharmacopoeia: Challenges of Writing the History of Drugs in India,' *History Compass* 14, no. 4 (2016): 135.

54 Bhattacharya, *Disparate Remedies*, 151–61.

55 Harkishan Singh, *Pharmacopoeias and Formularies* (Delhi: Vallabh Prakashan, 1994), 46.

56 Harkishan Singh, 'Edward John Waring (1819–1891) in India,' *Pharmaceutical Historian* 46, no. 4 (2016): 75–8.

57 Singh, *Pharmacopoeias and Formularies*, 47.

58 Government of Madras, G.O. No. 958 (88–90), 22 August 1864, Tamil Nadu Archives, Madras.

59 Government of Madras, 22 August 1864.

60 Home Department, Public Branch, Government of India, No. 14–17, 10 November 1864, National Archives of India, New Delhi.

Notes to pages 139–44

61 Financial Department, Government of India, No. 434, 25 May 1865, National Archives of India, New Delhi.

62 Bhattacharya, *Disparate Remedies*, 74.

63 'Pharmacopoeia of India', *Indian Medical Gazette* 1, no. 1 (1866): 15–19.

64 Ibid., 15.

65 Singh, *Pharmacopoeias and Formularies*, 49.

66 Zachary Dorner, *Merchants of Medicines: The Commerce and Coercion of Health in Britain's Long Eighteenth Century* (Chicago: University of Chicago Press, 2020), 142.

67 S.W.F. Holloway, 'The Regulation of the Supply of Drugs in Britain before 1868', in *Drugs and Narcotics in History*, ed. Roy Porter and Mikulas Teich (Cambridge: Cambridge University Press, 1997), 77.

68 E.J. Waring, *Pharmacopoeia of India* (London: W.H. Allen, 1868).

69 Ibid., vi.

70 Rai Bahadur Kanny Lall Dey, 'Indian Pharmacology: A Review', *Indian Medical Gazette* 30, no. 1 (1895): 25–8.

71 Singh, *Pharmacopoeias and Formularies*, 50.

72 Ibid., 62.

73 Ibid., 54.

74 Government Resolution No. 2889, 19 May 1885, cited in Military Department, Government of Madras, G.O. No. 846 Public, 23 April 1886, Tamil Nadu Archives, Madras, cited in Singh, *Pharmacopoeias and Formularies*, 62.

75 David L. Cowen, *Pharmacopoeias and Related Literature in Britain and America, 1618–1847* (Aldershot, UK: Ashgate Variorum, 2001), 114.

76 'Pharmacopoeia of India', *Pharmaceutical Journal* 10, 2nd ser., no. 6 (1868): 373–5.

77 Ibid., 375.

78 Public Department, Government of Madras, G.O. No. 121, 5 February 1867, Tamil Nadu Archives, Madras.

79 Moodeen Sheriff, *Supplement to the Pharmacopoeia of India* (Madras: Government Gazette Press, 1869).

80 Ibid., 331–5.

81 Review, 'Supplement to the Pharmacopoeia of India', *Madras Monthly Journal of Medical Science* 1, no. 6 (1870): 315–18.

82 Singh, *Pharmacopoeias and Formularies*, 56.

83 *Madras Monthly Journal*, 316.

84 Ibid., 315–18.

85 *Additions to the British Pharmacopoeia of 1867* (London: General Medical Council, 1874).

300 Notes to pages 144–6

86 Holloway, *Royal Pharmaceutical Society*, 243.

87 Anderson, *Pharmacy and Professionalization*, 241.

88 Ibid., 228–9.

89 *Chemist and Druggist* 22 (1880): 83–4.

90 *Chemist and Druggist* 45 (1894): 476.

91 Anderson, *Pharmacy and Professionalization*, 241.

92 IOR/L/MIL/7/15141, File 355, 8 June 1875, India Office Records, British Library.

93 H.P. Cholmeley, revised by W.F. Bynum, 'Fayrer, Sir Joseph (1824–1907)', *Oxford Dictionary of National Biography* (Oxford: Oxford University Press, 2022), https://www.oxforddnb.com/display/10.1093/ref:odnb/9780198614128.001.0001/odnb-9780198614128-e-33099.

94 IOR/L/E/51, File 1420, Feb. 1879–Jan. 1881, India Office Records, British Library.

95 IOR/L/E/6/39, File 233, 16 January 1878, Feb. 1880, India Office Records, British Library.

96 Singh, *Pharmacopoeias and Formularies*, 57.

97 IOR/P/1337, 11 December 1879, Nos 27–53, Dec. 1879–Nov. 1880, India Office Records, British Library.

98 IOR/L/E/6/39, File 233, Feb. 1880, India Office Records, British Library.

99 IOR/P/1337, 9 November 1880, Nos 27–53, Dec. 1879–Nov. 1880, India Office Records, British Library.

100 IOR/L/E/51, 20 January 1881, File 1420, Feb. 1879–Jan. 1881, India Office Records, British Library.

101 Cartwright, *The British Pharmacopoeia*, 33.

102 Ibid.

103 "Preparation of the BP', Memo to Clerk of the General Medical Council, 12 January 1884, PC8/304, The National Archives, Kew.

104 George Barber, *The Pharmaceutical or Medico-Botanical Map of the World* (London: G. Philip & Son, 1870).

105 F.A. Flückiger and D. Hanbury, *Pharmacographia: A History of the Principal Drugs of Vegetable Origin Met with in Great Britain and British India*, 2nd ed. (London: Macmillan & Co., 1879).

106 William Martindale and W. Wynn Westcott, *The Extra Pharmacopoeia of Unofficial Drugs and Chemical and Pharmaceutical Preparations* (London: H.K. Lewis, 1883).

107 Neshat Quaiser, 'Politics, Culture, and Colonialism: Unani's Debates with Doctory', in *Health, Medicine and Empire: Perspectives on Colonial India*, ed. Biswamoy Pati and Mark Harrison (New Delhi: Orient Longman, 2001), 341.

Notes to pages 148–51

108 Macmillan Report, 12.
109 *British Pharmacopoeia 1885* (London: General Medical Council, 1885), i.
110 Abena Dove Osseo-Asare, 'Bioprospecting and Resistance: Transforming Poisoned Arrows into Pills in Colonial Gold Coast, 1885–1922', *Social History of Medicine* 21, no. 2 (2008): 271.
111 Osseo-Asare, 'Bioprospecting and Resistance', 271.
112 Cartwright, *The British Pharmacopoeia*, 33.
113 Government Resolution No. 2889, 19 May 1885, cited in Military Department, Government of Madras, G.O. No. 846 Public, 23 April 1886, Tamil Nadu Archives, Madras.
114 Thomas Pakenham, *The Scramble for Africa* (London: Abacus Books, 1991).
115 Letter No. 837/c, 29 March 1886 from Government of India, Military Department, to Secretary to Government of Bombay, Military Department, cited in Military Department, Government of Madras, G.O. No. 846 Public, 23 April 1886, Tamil Nadu Archives, Madras.
116 Bhattacharya, *Disparate Remedies*, 88.
117 Ibid.
118 IOR/P/1337, 12 March 1880, Nos 27–53, Dec. 1879–Nov. 1880, India Office Records, British Library.

CHAPTER SEVEN

1 Letter No. 837/c, 29 March 1886, from Government of India, Military Department, to secretary to Government of Bombay, Military Department, cited in Military Department, Government of Madras, G.O. No. 846 Public, 23 April 1886, Tamil Nadu Archives, Madras.
2 This issue has been discussed by several historians including Zachary Dorner, *Merchants of Medicines: The Commerce and Coercion of Health in Britain's Long Eighteenth Century* (Chicago: University of Chicago Press, 2020), 142; Anil Kumar, 'The Indian Drug Industry under the Raj, 1860–1920', in *Health, Medicine and Empire: Perspectives on Colonial India*, ed. Biswamoy Pati and Mark Harrison (New Delhi: Orient Longman, 2001), 35; Pratik Chakrabarti, *Medicine & Empire, 1600–1960* (Basingstoke, UK: Palgrave Macmillan, 2014), 20–39; Nandini Bhattacharya, *Disparate Remedies: Making Medicines in Modern India* (Montreal and Kingston: McGill-Queen's University Press, 2023).
3 Home Department, Government of India, Medical-B, April 1886, Nos 5–6, National Archives of India (hereafter NAI), New Delhi.

302 Notes to pages 151–6

4 Stuart Anderson, *Pharmacy and Professionalization in the British Empire, 1780–1970* (London: Palgrave Macmillan, 2021), 69–97.

5 Arnold V. Raison, *A Brief History of Pharmacy in Canada* (Ottawa: Canadian Academy for the History of Pharmacy, 1967), 66.

6 Audrey M. Martin, *Pharmacy in Canada: Highlights of Its History from Early to Recent Times* (Vancouver: Pharmaceutical Association of British Columbia, 1955), 14.

7 Ibid.

8 Thomas Pakenham, *The Scramble for Africa: The White Man's Conquest of the Dark Continent from 1876 to 1912* (London: Random House, 1991); Peter J. Cain and Anthony G. Hopkins, 'Gentlemanly Capitalism and British Expansion Overseas II: New Imperialism, 1850–1945,' *Economic History Review* 40, no. 1 (1987): 1–26.

9 "The Medicines We Dispense," *Chemist and Druggist* 28 no. 1404 (1886): 351–5.

10 S.W.F. Holloway, *Royal Pharmaceutical Society of Great Britain, 1841–1991: A Political and Social History* (London: Pharmaceutical Press, 1991), 308–9.

11 Anthony C. Cartwright, *The British Pharmacopoeia, 1864 to 2014: Medicines, International Standards, and the State* (Farnham, UK: Ashgate, 2015), 43–4; Gregory Haines, *Pharmacy in Australia: The National Experience* (Deakin: Pharmaceutical Society of Australia, 1988), 142.

12 Martin, *Pharmacy in Canada*, 14.

13 Letter Farrar to Privy Council, 4 February 1887, 1, PC8/366, The National Archives, Kew.

14 Letter Farrar to Privy Council, 2.

15 *Report of the Sub-committee on the British Pharmacopoeia of the Committee of Civil Research*, Cmd 3101 (London: His Majesty's Stationery Office, 1928), 28 (hereafter cited as Macmillan Report).

16 Macmillan Report, 12.

17 Cartwright, *The British Pharmacopoeia*, 33.

18 Macmillan Report, 12.

19 Ibid.

20 *1890 Addendum to the British Pharmacopoeia 1885* (London: General Medical Council, 1890), i.

21 Ibid.

22 Peter G. Homan, 'Seidlitz: The Morning After Powder,' *Pharmacy History Australia* 5, no. 37 (2009): 28.

23 W. Dymock, C.J.H. Warden, and D. Hooper, *Pharmacographia India: A History of the Principal Drugs of Vegetable Origin, Met within British India* (London: Kegan Paul, Trübner & Co., 1890).

Notes to pages 156–60

24 Harkishan Singh, 'Moodeen Sheriff and the 1869 Supplement to the Pharmacopoeia of India 1868', *Pharmaceutical Historian* 47, no. 2 (2017): 41.

25 Kanny Lall Dey, *Indigenous Drugs of India: Short Descriptive Notices of the Principal Medicinal Products Met with in British India* (Calcutta: Thacker, Spink & Co., 1867).

26 Nandini Bhattacharya, 'From Materia Medica to the Pharmacopoeia: Challenges of Writing the History of Drugs in India', *History Compass* 14, no. 4 (2016): 136.

27 Letter dated 12 November 1891, IOR/P/5644 March 1899, Nos 89–93, India Office Records, British Library.

28 Letter dated 12 November 1891.

29 Macmillan Report, 13.

30 Cartwright, *The British Pharmacopoeia*, 37.

31 Macmillan Report, 14.

32 Ibid.

33 Harkishan Singh, *Pharmacopoeias and Formularies* (Delhi: Vallabh Prakashan, 1994), 66.

34 Singh, *Pharmacopoeias and Formularies*, 68.

35 Ibid., 66.

36 K.L. Dey, *Indian Pharmacology: A Review* (Calcutta: Thacker, Spink & Co, 1894), xxxi.

37 Kumar, 'The Indian Drug Industry', 357.

38 Home Department, Medical-A, 31 October 1895, No. 24, NAI, New Delhi.

39 G. King, *Report of Central Indigenous Drugs Committee 1896* (Calcutta: Government of India Press, 1901), 151, 165.

40 Singh, *Pharmacopoeias and Formularies*, 66.

41 King, *Report of Central Indigenous Drugs Committee*, 165.

42 Kumar, 'The Indian Drug Industry', 358.

43 Home Department, Medical-A, March 1901, Nos 48–62, NAI, New Delhi.

44 King, *Report of Central Indigenous Drugs Committee*, 150.

45 Ibid.

46 Kumar, 'The Indian Drug Industry', 360.

47 Ibid.

48 Home Department, Medical-A, June 1900, Nos 214–20, NAI, New Delhi. This document provides the background to the CIDC and to the second Madras committee.

49 King, *Report of Central Indigenous Drugs Committee*, 151.

50 Home Department, Medical-A, March 1901, Nos 48–62, NAI, New Delhi.

304 Notes to pages 160–4

51 Kumar, 'The Indian Drug Industry', 359.
52 See "Appendix on Methods Adopted in Preparing the *British Pharmacopoeia* of 1898," in *Report of the Pharmacopoeia Committee, 31 May 1898* (London: General Medical Council, 1898), 436–42.
53 Cartwright, *The British Pharmacopoeia*, 34.
54 "Survey of Pharmacopoeia Drugs," *British Medical Journal* 1 (1895): 724.
55 Macmillan Report, 16.
56 Cartwright, *The British Pharmacopoeia*, 35–7.
57 *Brisbane Courier*, 28 November 1898, 7.
58 *British Pharmacopoeia 1898* (London: General Medical Council, 1898), ix.
59 *British Pharmacopoeia 1898*, appendix 11, 443–4.
60 McAlister was a member of the GMC for forty-four years and its president from 1904 to 1931. See Olive Edis, revised by A.J. Crilly, 'MacAlister, Sir Donald, First Baronet (1854–1934)', *Oxford Dictionary of National Biography* (Oxford: Oxford University Press, 2022), https://www.oxforddnb .com/display/10.1093/ref:odnb/9780198614128.001.0001/odnb-9780198614128-e-1000178.
61 *British Pharmacopoeia 1898, Indian and Colonial Addendum*: "Report of Progress," 29 November 1899, appendix 20, Pharmacopoeia Committee, 745, Minutes of the General Medical Council 1863–1970, British Library.
62 Cartwright, *The British Pharmacopoeia*, 38.
63 Singh, *Pharmacopoeias and Formularies*, 68.
64 *Pharmaceutical Journal* 4, no. 7 (1898): 612.
65 Singh, *Pharmacopoeias and Formularies*, 66.
66 'Report of Progress,' November 1899, 747.
67 'Report of Progress,' 747.
68 *British Pharmacopoeia 1898, Indian and Colonial Addendum*: "Report of Progress," 28 May 1900, appendix A, Pharmacopoeia Committee, 506, Minutes of General Medical Council 1863–1970, British Library.
69 IOR/P/5645 Oct. 1899, 2058–67, Letter Curzon to Hamilton, 26 October 1899, India Office Records, British Library.
70 Home Department, Government of India, Medical-A, May 1901, Nos 273–4, NAI, New Delhi.
71 'Report of Progress,' November 1899, 747.
72 'Report of Progress,' May 1900, 505.
73 Ibid., 506.
74 Singh, *Pharmacopoeias and Formularies*, 68.
75 'Report of Progress,' May 1900, 506.

Notes to pages 164–7

76 'Report of Progress', November 1899, 747.
77 Ibid.
78 Dymock, Warden, and Hooper, *Pharmacographia Indica* (1890).
79 D. Hooper, 'A Pharmacopoeia for India', *Indian Lancet* 7 (1896): 23–4.
80 Harkishan Singh, *Pharmacy Practice* (Delhi: Vallabh Prakashan, 2002), 8.
81 'Report of Progress', November 1899, 748.
82 Ibid., 752.
83 Ibid., 752.
84 J.E. Morrison, 'Some Suggestions for a Canadian Addendum to the British Pharmacopoeia', *Canadian Pharmaceutical Journal* 32, no. 8 (1899): 8–11; J.E. Morrison, 'Some Suggestions for a Canadian Addendum to the British Pharmacopoeia', *Pharmaceutical Journal* 63 (September 1899): 230–3.
85 'Report of Progress', November 1899, 752.
86 'Report of Progress', May 1900, 508.
87 Ibid.
88 Ibid.
89 Anderson, *Pharmacy and Professionalization*, 65.
90 'Report of Progress', May 1900, 508.
91 'Report of Progress', November 1899, 753.
92 Ibid.
93 Ibid.
94 'Report of Progress', May 1900, 505.
95 Paul Cassar, 'Pharmacies and Apothecaries One Hundred Years Ago in Malta', *Journal of the Malta Union of Pharmacists* 1 (1967): 35.
96 *Code of Police Laws* (Malta: Government of Malta, 1883), 41.
97 'Report of Progress', November 1899, 752.
98 Ibid.
99 'Report of Progress', May 1900, 505.
100 'Report of Progress', November 1899, 752.
101 H.H. Johnston, 'The Importance of Africa', *Journal of the Royal African Society* 17, no. 67 (1918): 177–98.
102 H.H. Johnston, *British Central Africa* (London: Methuen, 1897), 442–3, cited in Markku Hokkanen, 'Towards a Cultural History of Medicine(s) in Colonial Central Africa', in *Crossing Colonial Historiographies: Histories of Colonial and Indigenous Medicines in Transnational Perspectives*, ed. Anne Digby, Waltraud Ernst, and Projit B. Mukharji (Newcastle upon Tyne: Cambridge Scholars, 2010), 156.
103 Abena Dove Osseo-Asare, *Bitter Roots: The Search for Healing Plants in Africa* (Chicago: University of Chicago Press, 2014), 13–16.

306 Notes to pages 167–73

104 Hokkanen, 'Towards a Cultural History of Medicine(s)', 156.
105 'Report of Progress', November 1899, 748.
106 Ibid.
107 'Report of Progress', May 1900, 506.
108 Dorothy W. Goyns, *Pharmacy in the Transvaal, 1894–1994* (Braamfontein: Pharmaceutical Society of South Africa, 1995), 26.
109 'Report of Progress', November 1899, 751.
110 Van Dort in "Report of Progress', November 1899, 751.
111 Ibid.
112 'Report of Progress', November 1899, 751.
113 Ibid.
114 Ibid., 752.
115 Ibid.
116 Lee Yong Kiat, *The Medical History of Early Singapore* (Singapore: Southeast Asian Medical Information Centre, 1978), 13.
117 'Report of Progress', May 1900, 507.
118 Haines, *Pharmacy in Australia*, 156.
119 'Report of Progress', November 1899, 749–50.
120 Ibid., 750.
121 Ibid.
122 'Indian and Colonial Addendum', *Australasian Journal of Pharmacy* 14 (1899): 326.
123 'Report of Progress', November 1899, 749.
124 Ibid., 750.
125 'BP Addendum', *Chemist and Druggist of Australasia* 15 (1899): 231.
126 'BP Addendum', 231.
127 *Lyttleton Times*, 24 August 1892, cited in Reg Coombes, *Pharmacy in New Zealand: Aspects and Reminiscences* (Wellington: Pharmaceutical Society of New Zealand, 1981), 21.
128 'Report of Progress', November 1899, 749.
129 Ibid.
130 'Report of Progress', May 1900, 507.
131 Ibid., 505.
132 Ibid., 508.
133 *Indian and Colonial Addendum to the British Pharmacopoeia 1898* (London: General Medical Council, 1900).
134 *British Medical Journal* 2 (1900): 1676–8.
135 Singh, *Pharmacopoeias and Formularies*, 65.
136 Rachel Berger, 'Ayurveda and the Making of the Urban Middle Class in North India, 1900–1945', in *Modern and Global Ayurveda: Pluralism and*

Notes to pages 173–8

Paradigms, ed. Dagmar Wujastyk and Frederick M. Smith (New York: University of New York, 2008), 101–15.

137 Nandini Bhattacharya, 'Between the Bazaar and the Bench: The Making of the Drugs Trade in Colonial India, c.1900–1930', *Bulletin of the History of Medicine* 90, no. 1 (2016): 62–4.

138 Harkishan Singh, 'History of Drugs and Pharmacy Statutes', *Eastern Pharmacist* 42, no. 11 (1999): 31–7.

139 Home Department, Government of India, Medical-A, June 1901, Nos 57–9, NAI, New Delhi.

140 *Army Regulations for India* (Calcutta: Government of India, 1900), vol. 6, para. 958.

141 *Indian and Colonial Addendum to British Pharmacopoeia 1898, Government of India Edition* (London: General Medical Council, 1901).

142 Singh, *Pharmacopoeias and Formularies*, 70.

143 Home Department, Government of India, Medical-B, July 1902, Nos 214–18, NAI, New Delhi.

CHAPTER EIGHT

1 *Indian Medical Record* 20 (1901): 40.

2 Nandini Bhattacharya, 'From Materia Medica to the Pharmacopoeia: Challenges of Writing the History of Drugs in India', *History Compass* 14, no. 4 (2016): 136.

3 In 1902 K.C. Bose published his *Official Indigenous Drugs of India* (Calcutta: Bengal Chemical and Pharmaceutical Works, 1902). An enlarged version was published in 1932 under the title *Pharmacopoeia Indica: Being a Collection of Vegetable, Mineral, and Animal Drugs in Common Use in India* (Calcutta: Book Co., 1932).

4 'Indian and Colonial Addendum', *Indian Medical Gazette* 36 (1901): 62–3.

5 Ibid.

6 'Indigenous Drugs of India', *Chemist and Druggist* 54 (1899): 536.

7 P.C. Ray, *Life and Experiences of a Bengali Chemist* (London: Kegan Paul, 1932), 104.

8 Anil Kumar, 'The Indian Drug Industry under the Raj, 1860–1920', in *Health, Medicine and Empire: Perspectives on Colonial India*, ed. Biswamoy Pati and Mark Harrison (New Delhi: Orient Longman, 2001), 361.

9 'Pharmacy in the Indian Army', *Chemist and Druggist* 64 (1904): 691.

10 Ibid.

308 Notes to pages 178–82

11 Mridula Ramanna, *Health Care in Bombay Presidency, 1896–1930* (Delhi: Primus Books, 2012), 158.

12 Alistair Lloyd, 'Pharmacy in the Australian Colonies: The British Influence', *Pharmaceutical Historian* 19, no. 1 (1989): 6.

13 *Australian Pharmaceutical Formulary* (Melbourne: Victoria Pharmaceutical Association, 1902), i.

14 Gregory Haines, *Pharmacy in Australia: The National Experience* (Deakin: Pharmaceutical Society of Australia, 1988), 142.

15 Ibid., 167.

16 Ibid., 111–12.

17 Ibid., 143.

18 Reg Coombes, *Pharmacy in New Zealand: Aspects and Reminiscences* (Wellington: Pharmaceutical Society of New Zealand, 1981), 102.

19 Ibid., 75–6.

20 Stuart Anderson, *Pharmacy and Professionalization in the British Empire, 1780–1970* (London: Palgrave Macmillan, 2021), 89–90.

21 Arnold V. Raison, *A Brief History of Pharmacy in Canada* (Ottawa: Canadian Academy for the History of Pharmacy, 1967), 74.

22 Garnet R. Paterson, 'Canadian Pharmacy, 1906–1956', *Canadian Pharmaceutical Journal* 89 (1956): 71–4.

23 Paul Soucy, 'The Proprietary or Patent Medicine Act of Canada', *Food, Drug and Cosmetic Law Journal* 8, no. 11 (1953): 706.

24 D.R. Kennedy, *One Hundred Years of Pharmacy Legislation* (Ottawa: Canadian Academy of History of Pharmacy, 1969), 33–6.

25 Proprietary or Patent Medicine Act, R.S.C. 1952, c. P-220.

26 Raison, *Brief History of Pharmacy in Canada*, 61.

27 W.A., 'Pharmacy in British Guiana', *Chemist and Druggist* 2 (September 1922): 335.

28 "The BP Addendum', *The Lancet* 157, no. 4039 (1901): 267–8.

29 Harkishan Singh, *Pharmacopoeias and Formularies* (Delhi: Vallabh Prakashan, 1994), 89.

30 Edmund White and John Humphrey, *Pharmacopedia: A Commentary on the British Pharmacopoeia 1898* (London: Henry Kimpton, 1901), xx, 535–63.

31 William Chattaway, *Digest of Researches and Criticisms Bearing on the Revision of the British Pharmacopoeia 1898* (London: General Medical Council, 1904).

32 Ibid., iii.

33 Ibid., 29–40.

34 Ernst W. Stieb, *Drug Adulteration: Detection and Control in Nineteenth Century Britain* (Madison: University of Wisconsin Press, 1966), 255.

Notes to pages 182–5   309

35 Anthony C. Cartwright, *The British Pharmacopoeia, 1864 to 2014: Medicines, International Standards, and the State* (Farnham, UK: Ashgate, 2015), 43.

36 *The British Pharmaceutical Codex: An Imperial Dispensatory for the Use of Medical Practitioners and Pharmacists* (London: Pharmaceutical Society of Great Britain, 1907).

37 Stuart Anderson and Virginia Berridge, 'Drug Misuse and the Community Pharmacist: An Historical Overview', in *Drug Misuse and Community Pharmacy*, ed. Janie Sheridan and John Strang (London: Taylor and Francis, 2003), 17–35.

38 For drug regulation and its impact on pharmacy practice after 1900 see Stuart Anderson, 'From Bespoke to Off-the-Peg: Community Pharmacists and the Retailing of Medicines in Great Britain, 1900 to 1970', in *From Physick to Pharmacology: Five Hundred Years of British Drug Retailing*, ed. Louise Hill Curth (Aldershot, UK: Ashgate, 2006), 105–42.

39 T.D. Whittet, 'Drug Control in Britain: From World War I to the Medicines Bill of 1968', in *Safeguarding the Public: Historical Aspects of Medicinal Drug Control*, ed. John B. Blake (Baltimore: Johns Hopkins University Press, 1970), 27–37.

40 'Physiological Testing', *Analytical Notes* 4 (1910): 2–3.

41 Stieb, *Drug Adulteration*, 99; C.G. Moor, *Suggested Standards of Purity for Foods and Drugs* (London: Bailliere, Tindall and Cox, 1902), 128.

42 E.M. Holmes, 'Is Physiological Standardization Necessary?', *Pharmaceutical Journal* 22 (1906): 127; William Kirby, 'Standardization', *Pharmaceutical Journal* 22 (1906): 200.

43 'Physiological Standards and Tests', *Pharmaceutical Journal* 22 (1906): 56.

44 For more on medicine stamp duty see Chantal Stebbings, *Tax, Medicines and the Law: From Quackery to Pharmacy* (Cambridge: Cambridge University Press, 2018).

45 Stebbings, *Tax, Medicines and the Law*, 126.

46 Ibid., 73.

47 *Precedents and Instructions 1904*, IR 78/60, 123, The National Archives, Kew.

48 Stebbings, *Tax, Medicines and the Law*, 179.

49 Ibid., 178.

50 Ibid., 207–8.

51 *Board of Customs and Excise and Predecessor, Medicine Stamp Duties 1936–39*, CUST 118/391, 68, The National Archives, Kew.

52 White and Humphrey, *Pharmacopedia*, 535–63.

53 *Report of the Sub-committee on the British Pharmacopoeia of the Committee*

310 Notes to pages 185–9

of Civil Research, Cmd 3101 (London: His Majesty's Stationery Office, 1928), 17 (hereafter cited as Macmillan Report).

54 Macmillan Report, 17.

55 *International Agreement Respecting the Unification of the Pharmacopoeial Formulas for Potent Drugs. Signed at Brussels, 29 November 1906*, Cd 3392 (London: His Majesty's Stationery Office, 1907).

56 Home Department, Government of India, Medical-A, November 1904, nos 87–8, National Archives of India, New Delhi.

57 Singh, *Pharmacopoeias and Formularies*, 70.

58 Home Department, Government of India, Medical-A, January (1905), nos 128–30, National Archives of India, New Delhi.

59 Nandini Bhattacharya, *Disparate Remedies: Making Medicines in Modern India* (Montreal and Kingston: McGill-Queen's University Press, 2023), 73–96.

60 Cartwright, *The British Pharmacopoeia*, 40.

61 *International Agreement Respecting the Unification of the Pharmacopoeial Formulas for Potent Drugs*.

62 Macmillan Report, 18.

63 Ibid., 19.

64 Ibid.

65 Ibid.

66 Cartwright, *British Pharmacopoeia*, 40.

67 *British Pharmacopoeia 1914* (London: General Medical Council, 1914), xxi.

68 Ibid., ix.

69 Singh, *Pharmacopoeias and Formularies*, 72.

70 *British Pharmacopoeia 1914*, xxiii–xxv.

71 Ibid., xxiii.

72 Stieb, *Drug Adulteration*, 37.

73 Ibid., 529–30; *British Pharmacopoeia 1914*, appendix 7.

74 *British Pharmacopoeia 1914*, 275–6.

75 Ibid., 71.

76 'The New Pharmacopoeia', *Chemist and Druggist* 84, no. 1796 (1914): 66.

77 'Some Pharmacopoeia Reflections', *Chemist and Druggist* 85, no. 1815 (1914): 47–8.

78 Review in *The Scotsman* cited in *Chemist and Druggist* 86, no. 1827 (1915): 118.

79 *Hong Kong Government Gazette*, 26 March 1915, 166.

80 Ibid.

81 Ibid., 168.

Notes to pages 189–93

82 Anuradha Roy, 'Growth and Development of the Chemical Industry in Bengal, 1900–47" (PhD diss., Jadavpur University [Kolkata], 1994), 58.

83 Kumar, 'Indian Drug Industry', 362.

84 Roy, 'Growth and Development of Chemical Industry', 61.

85 Bhattacharya, *Disparate Remedies*, 96–108.

86 "German Specialities', *Chemist and Druggist* 85, no. 1822 (1914): 88

87 Roy Church and E.M. Tansey, *Burroughs Wellcome & Co.: Knowledge, Trust, Profit, and the Transformation of the British Pharmaceutical Industry, 1880–1940* (Lancaster, UK: Crucible Books, 2007), 255–6.

88 Ibid., 257.

89 Ibid., 361–3.

90 'Aspirin Tablets', *Chemist and Druggist* 90, no. 2021 (1918): 43.

91 'Bayer Company Purchased by an American Firms', *American Druggist and Pharmaceutical Record* 67, no. 1 (1919): 58–60.

92 Church and Tansey, *Burroughs Wellcome & Co.*, 364.

93 Ibid., 278.

94 Stanley Chapman, *Jesse Boot of Boots the Chemists: A Study in Business History* (London: Hodder and Stoughton, 1974), 96–7.

95 'The Manufacture of Adalin', *Chemist and Druggist* 89, no. 1931 (1917): 106; 'The Flavine Patent', *Chemist and Druggist* 89, no. 1947 (1917): 430.

96 'BP 1914: Alteration and Amendment', *London Gazette*, 27 July 1917, 7678.

97 'BP 1914: Alteration and Amendment', *London Gazette*, 29 March 1918, 3954.

98 'Australian Aspirin Is Granted License', *Melbourne Herald*, 17 September 1915, 2.

99 R. Grenville Smith and Alexander Barrie, *Aspro: How a Family Business Grew Up* (Melbourne: Nicholas International, 1976), 5–6.

100 Ibid.

101 Haines, *Pharmacy in Australia*, 197.

102 Cited in Mike Ryan, *History of Organised Pharmacy in South Africa* (Cape Town: Society for History of Pharmacy in South Africa, 1986), 66.

103 H.L. Karnovsky, 'I Remember', in *Souvenir Programme* (Lynnwood: Pharmaceutical Society of South Africa, 1946).

104 Ryan, *History of Organised Pharmacy*, 66.

105 Macmillan Report, 20.

106 Cartwright, *British Pharmacopoeia*, 55.

107 'The British Pharmacopoeia', *British Medical Journal* 2, no. 1667 (1892): 1297.

108 'British Pharmaceutical Conference,' *British Medical Journal* 2, no. 2590 (1910): 475–7.

109 Cartwright, *British Pharmacopoeia*, 55.

110 'Duty on Patent or Proprietary Medicines,' *African Chemist and Druggist* 2, no. 13 (1923): 4.

111 Ryan, *History of Organized Pharmacy*, 79.

112 'Stamp Tax,' *African Chemist and Druggist* 2, no. 16 (1923): 14.

113 Ryan, *History of Organized Pharmacy*, 79–81.

114 Ibid., 78.

115 Ibid., 81.

116 George B. Griffinhagen, *Medicine Stamps Worldwide* (Greer, SC: American Topical Association, 1971), 79.

117 Dorothy W. Goyns, *Pharmacy in the Transvaal, 1894–1994* (Braamfontein: Pharmaceutical Society of South Africa, 1995), 38.

118 *Chemist and Druggist* 55 (1899): 694.

119 *Indian and Eastern Druggist* 9 (1928): 67.

120 Harkishan Singh, *Pharmacy Practice* (Delhi: Vallabh Prakashan, 2002), 120.

121 *Report of the Drugs Enquiry Committee 1930–31* (Calcutta: Government of India Central Publication Branch, 1931).

122 'An Outcome of Ottawa,' *Indian and Eastern Druggist* 13 (1932): 225.

123 Singh, *Pharmacy Practice*, 116.

124 Ibid., 118.

125 Bhattacharya, *Disparate Remedies*, 179–81.

126 Singh, *Pharmacy Practice*, 116.

127 P/11109, Government of Madras, Local/Municipal Public Health (*Asia, Pacific,* and African Collections), 1921, 1, cited in Bhattacharya, *Disparate Remedies*, 209.

128 V/27/850/41, 'Investigation of Indigenous Drugs,' Government of Madras, Local/Municipal Public Health (Asia, Pacific, and African Collections), 1921, 2.

129 'Indian Medicine,' *Chemist and Druggist* 95, no. 3 (1921): 52–3.

130 *Report of Drugs Enquiry Committee 1930–31.*

131 Ronald D. Mann, *Modern Drug Use: An Enquiry on Historical Principles* (Lancaster, UK: MTP Press, 1984), 544.

132 Ibid., 44.

133 Stieb, *Drug Adulteration*, 99–100.

Notes to pages 198–201

CHAPTER NINE

1 *Secret Remedies: What They Cost and What They Contain* (London: British Medical Association, 1909); *More Secret Remedies: What They Cost and What They Contain* (London: British Medical Association, 1912).

2 *Report from the Select Committee on Patent Medicines* (London: His Majesty's Stationery Office, 1914), para. 55.

3 Stuart Anderson and Virginia Berridge, 'Drug Misuse and the Community Pharmacist: An Historical Overview', in *Drug Misuse and Community Pharmacy*, ed. Janie Sheridan and John Strang (London: Taylor and Francis, 2003), 17–35.

4 PC8/1159, letter dated 15 October 1925, Medical School Teachers to Secretary, Medical Research Council, The National Archives (henceforth TNA), Kew.

5 Council Minutes, meeting 4 November 1925, Pharmaceutical Society of Great Britain, Royal Pharmaceutical Society Library (henceforth RPS Library).

6 Anthony C. Cartwright, *The British Pharmacopoeia, 1864 to 2014: Medicines, International Standards, and the State* (Farnham, UK: Ashgate, 2015), 351.

7 Council Minutes, meeting 2 December 1925, Pharmaceutical Society of Great Britain, RPS Library.

8 Cartwright, *British Pharmacopoeia*, 51.

9 Ibid., 51.

10 PC8/1159, 2 December 1925, letter William Glyn-Jones to Clerk of the Privy Council, TNA, Kew.

11 PC8/1159, 9 December 1925, letter William Glyn-Jones to Secretary, GMC, TNA, Kew.

12 Cartwright, *British Pharmacopoeia*, 52.

13 Council Minutes, meeting 3 March 1926, Pharmaceutical Society of Great Britain, RPS Library.

14 D.M. Dunlop and T.C. Denston, 'History and Development of the BP', *British Medical Journal* 2, no. 5107 (1958): 1251.

15 Cartwright, *British Pharmacopoeia*, 52.

16 Roy M. MacLeod and E. Kay Andrews, 'The Committee of Civil Research: Scientific Advice for Economic Development 1925–30', *Minerva* 7, no. 4 (1969): 680–705. The committee was replaced by the Economic Advisory Council in 1930.

17 *Report of the Sub-committee on the British Pharmacopoeia of the Committee of Civil Research*, Cmd 3101 (London: His Majesty's Stationery Office, 1928), 3 (hereafter cited as Macmillan Report).

18 Macmillan Report, 3.

19 Ibid., 57.

20 Cartwright, *British Pharmacopoeia*, 53.

21 Ibid., 53.

22 Ibid., 57.

23 Macmillan Report, 45.

24 Ibid.

25 Cartwright, *British Pharmacopoeia*, 53.

26 Macmillan Report, 35–6.

27 Ibid.

28 Ibid., 25.

29 Stuart Anderson, *Pharmacy and Professionalization in the British Empire, 1780–1970* (London: Palgrave Macmillan, 2021).

30 Macmillan Report, 25, para 58a.

31 Macmillan Report, 25, para 58a.

32 Macmillan Report, 27, para 58e.

33 James Bell, 'Minutes of Evidence', *Report from Select Committee on Sale of Food and Drugs Act (1875) Amendment Bill* (London: His Majesty's Stationery Office, 1879), 137–8.

34 Ernst W. Stieb, *Drug Adulteration: Detection and Control in Nineteenth Century Britain* (Madison: University of Wisconsin Press, 1966), 132–3.

35 Macmillan Report, 28.

36 Stieb, *Drug Adulteration*, 134.

37 The link between food and medicines in legislation continued until 1968 with passage of the Medicines Act. A 1938 Food and Drugs Act introduced penalties for misleading or false advertising.

38 Dominion Food and Drug Act, R.S.C. 1927, c. F-76, s. 4.

39 Pharmaceutical Act, S.M. 1924, c. P-164, s. 27 (Manitoba).

40 Pharmaceutical Act, c. P-164, s. 27.

41 Macmillan Report, 29.

42 MH55/2807, letter dated 14 November 1928 from Victoria state governor to secretary of state for Dominion affairs, TNA, Kew.

43 Macmillan Report, 30.

44 Ibid., 31.

45 Ibid.

46 Ibid., 32.

47 MH55/2808, letter dated 25 January 1926 to GMC from governor general of Canada, TNA, Kew.

48 Macmillan Report, 44.

49 Harkishan Singh, 'History of Drugs and Pharmacy Statutes', *Eastern Pharmacist* 42, no. 11 (November 1999): 31–7.

Notes to pages 209–18

50 Singh, 'History of Drugs and Pharmacy Statutes', 31–7.

51 Nandini Bhattacharya, *Disparate Remedies: Making Medicines in Modern India* (Montreal and Kingston: McGill-Queen's University Press, 2023), 74.

52 Ibid.

53 Macmillan Report, 13–16.

54 Ibid., 51–2.

55 Ibid., 52.

56 Bhattacharya, *Disparate Remedies*, 87.

57 Audrey M. Martin, *Pharmacy in Canada: Highlights of Its History from Early to Recent Times* (Vancouver: Pharmaceutical Association of British Columbia, 1955), 24.

58 Macmillan Report, 45.

59 Ibid., 46.

60 Ibid.

61 Ibid., 47.

62 Ibid.

63 Ibid., 48.

64 Ibid., 49.

65 Ibid.

66 Ibid., 49–50.

67 Ibid., 50.

68 Ibid.

69 MH55/2807, letter dated 14 January 1929, governor of Southern Rhodesia to Dominions Office, TNA, Kew.

70 Macmillan Report, 51.

71 Macmillan Report, 37, para. 97. In the summary of recommendations the new body was to be designated the Pharmacopoeia Commission (54, at para. 152(ii)).

72 Macmillan Report, 55.

73 Ibid., 56.

74 Ibid., 22; Frederick B. Power, *The International Conference for the Unification of the Formulae of Potent Medicaments* (Ann Arbor: University of Michigan, 1906).

75 Macmillan Report, 36.

CHAPTER TEN

1 W. David McIntyre, 'Dominion Status and the 1926 Declaration', in *A Guide to the Contemporary Commonwealth* (London: Palgrave Macmillan, 2001), 11–16.

2 John Darwin, 'A Third British Empire? The Dominion Idea in Imperial

316 Notes to pages 218–22

Politics', in *The Oxford History of the British Empire*, vol. 4, *The Twentieth Century*, ed. Judith M. Brown (Oxford: Oxford University Press, 1999), 69.

3 Judith M. Brown, 'India', in Brown, *The Twentieth Century*, 4:421.

4 Walter Sneader, *Drug Discovery: The Evolution of Modern Medicines* (London: Wiley, 1985); Mark Weatherall, *In Search of a Cure* (Oxford: Oxford University Press, 1990); Enrique Ravina, *The Evolution of Drug Discovery: From Traditional Medicines to Modern Drugs* (London: John Wiley & Sons, 2011).

5 Frederick Oliver, 'An Important Day for Pharmacy', *Pharmaceutical Historian* 26, no. 2 (1996): 15.

6 Anthony C. Cartwright, *The British Pharmacopoeia, 1864 to 2014: Medicines, International Standards, and the State* (Farnham, UK: Ashgate, 2015), 58.

7 Ibid., 60.

8 *British Pharmacopoeia 1932* (London: General Medical Council, 1932), xxix.

9 Audrey M. Martin, *Pharmacy in Canada: Highlights of Its History from Early to Recent Times* (Vancouver: Pharmaceutical Association of British Columbia, 1955), 24.

10 Editorial, 'The British Pharmacopoeia', *Indian and Eastern Druggist* 15, no. 4 (1934): 177.

11 Harkishan Singh, *Pharmacopoeias and Formularies* (Delhi: Vallabh Prakashan, 1994), 89.

12 Cartwright, *British Pharmacopoeia*, 61–2.

13 *British Pharmacopoeia 1932*, xxix.

14 *Chemist and Druggist*, 29 July 1933, 119.

15 Singh, *Pharmacopoeias and Formularies*, 89.

16 *British Pharmacopoeia 1932*, xvii.

17 *Chemist and Druggist*, 29 July 1933, 119.

18 *Chemist and Druggist*, 5 August 1933, 181.

19 Nandini Bhattacharya, *Disparate Remedies: Making Medicines in Modern India* (Montreal and Kingston: McGill-Queen's University Press, 2023), 75.

20 Stuart Anderson, *Pharmacy and Professionalization in the British Empire, 1780–1970* (London: Palgrave Macmillan, 2021), 217–47.

21 Singh, *Pharmacopoeias and Formularies*, 80; *Report of the Drugs Enquiry Committee 1930–31* (Calcutta: Government of India, 1931).

22 Singh, *Pharmacopoeias and Formularies*, 81.

23 Editorial, 'An Indian Pharmacopoeia', *Indian and Eastern Druggist* 13, no. 12 (1932): 249.

Notes to pages 222–5

24 Singh, *Pharmacopoeias and Formularies*, 94.

25 David Hooper, 'The Decline of Pharmaceutical Simples', *Pharmaceutical Journal and Pharmacist* 129 (1932): 326.

26 N.B. Dutta, 'Plea for an Indian Pharmacopoeia', *Indian Medical Record* 52 (1932): 97–101.

27 *Report of the Sub-committee on the British Pharmacopoeia of the Committee of Civil Research*, Cmd 3101 (London: His Majesty's Stationery Office, 1928), 55.

28 Cartwright, *British Pharmacopoeia*, 65.

29 Ibid.

30 Gregory Haines, *Pharmacy in Australia: The National Experience* (Deakin: Pharmaceutical Society of Australia, 1988), 284.

31 Cartwright, *British Pharmacopoeia*, 66.

32 Ibid.

33 Hugh N. Linstead, *Poisons Law* (London: Pharmaceutical Press, 1936), 54–5.

34 Linstead, *Poisons Law*, 1–18.

35 PC8/1260, letter, 18 April 1935, governor of Newfoundland to General Medical Council, National Archives (henceforth TNA), Kew.

36 P. Hamill, in *Favourite Recipes*, ed. Humphry Rolleston and Alan Moncrieff (London: Eyre and Spottiswoode, 1938), 11.

37 E. Lewis Lilley, in Rolleston and Moncrieff, *Favourite Recipes*, 209–11.

38 R. Mellon, 'Pharmacy in South Africa: Past and Present', *South African Pharmaceutical Journal* 1, no. 10 (1934): 16.

39 Mike Ryan, *History of Organised Pharmacy in South Africa* (Cape Town: Society for History of Pharmacy in South Africa, 1986), 95.

40 *South African Pharmaceutical Journal* 1, no. 10 (1934): 43.

41 Dorothy W. Goyns, *Pharmacy in the Transvaal, 1894–1994* (Braamfontein: Pharmaceutical Society of South Africa, 1995), 53.

42 Pratik Chakrabarti, *Medicine & Empire, 1600–1960* (Basingstoke, UK: Palgrave Macmillan, 2014), 192; Karen Flint, 'Competition, Race, and Professionalization: African Healers and White Medical Practitioners in Natal, South Africa in the Early Twentieth Century', *Social History of Medicine* 14, no. 2 (2001): 199–221.

43 Markku Hokkanen, 'Towards a Cultural History of Medicine(s) in Colonial Central Africa', in *Crossing Colonial Historiographies: Histories of Colonial and Indigenous Medicines in Transnational Perspectives*, ed. Anne Digby, Waltraud Ernst, and Projit B. Mukharji (Newcastle upon Tyne: Cambridge Scholars, 2010), 144.

44 Waltraud Ernst, *Plural Medicine, Tradition and Modernity, 1800–2000* (London: Routledge, 2002), 7–9.

45 Abena Dove Oseo-Asare, 'Bioprospecting and Resistance: Transforming Poisoned Arrows into Strophanthin Pills in Colonial Gold Coast, 1885–1922', *Social History of Medicine* 21, no. 2 (2008): 269–90.

46 'Synthetic Drugs', *British Medical Journal* 1, no. 3462 (1927): 888–9; J.M. Liebenau, 'Patents and the Chemical Industry', in *The Challenge of New Technology*, ed. J.M. Liebenau (Aldershot, UK: Gower, 1988), 135–50.

47 Roy Church and E.M. Tansey, *Burroughs Wellcome & Co.: Knowledge, Trust, Profit, and the Transformation of the British Pharmaceutical Industry, 1880–1940* (Lancaster, UK: Crucible Books, 2007), 319.

48 Cartwright, *British Pharmacopoeia*, 65.

49 Ibid., 66.

50 Ibid., 70.

51 For the impact of the Patent Act on drug discovery see Ronald D. Mann, *Modern Drug Use: An Enquiry on Historical Principles* (Lancaster, UK: MTP Press, 1984), 633.

52 MH55/2808, letter, 6 June 1938, Pharmaceutical Society of Ireland to GMC, TNA, Kew.

53 MH55/2808, letter, 18 March 1936, A.P. Beddard to Sir Henry Dale, TNA, Kew.

54 Keith Jeffery, 'The Second World War', in Brown, *The Twentieth Century*, 4:311.

55 Cartwright, *British Pharmacopoeia*, 68.

56 Ibid., 67.

57 Harold Davis, *Bentley's Textbook of Pharmaceutics*, 7th ed. (London: Bailliere, Tindall and Cox, 1961), 5.

58 Garnet R. Paterson, 'Canadian Pharmacy 1906–1956', *Canadian Pharmaceutical Journal* 89, no. 1 (1956): 71–4.

59 Jemma Houghton, '"Digging for Drugs": The Medicinal Plant Collection Scheme of the Second World War', *Pharmaceutical Historian* 52, no. 3 (2022): 65–74.

60 Laura Davies, *Fighting Fit: The Wartime Battle for Britain's Health* (London: Weidenfeld & Nicholson, 2016), 164; Judith Sumner, *Plants Go to War: A Botanical History of World War II* (Jefferson, NC: McFarland & Co., 2019), 191.

61 Davies, *Fighting Fit*, 159; 164; Ashley Jackson, '"Defend Lanka Your Home": War on the Home Front in Ceylon, 1939–1945', *War in History* 16, no. 2 (2009): 224.

62 Singh, *Pharmacopoeias and Formularies*, 93.

63 Minutes of the Drugs Technical Advisory Board, second meeting, 14 March 1944, Item 6, National Archives of India, New Delhi.

Notes to pages 230–3

64 Singh, *Pharmacopoeias and Formularies*, 94.

65 *Report of the Drugs Enquiry Committee 1930–31*.

66 Harkishan Singh, 'The Pharmacopoeia History of Colonial India', *Pharmaceutical Historian* 30, no. 2 (2000): 26–9.

67 Editorial, 'Post-War Development of Pharmacy in India', *Indian Journal of Pharmacy* 6, no. 1 (1944): 53–4; "The Indian Pharmaceutical List Committee', *Indian Pharmacist* 46, no. 1 (1945–46): 68–72, 78.

68 Singh, *Pharmacopoeias and Formularies*, 94.

69 *Pharmaceutical Journal* 158 (1947): 373–4; *Pharmaceutical Journal* 2 (1954): 172.

70 Singh, *Pharmacopoeias and Formularies*, 96.

71 Ibid.

72 'The Indian Pharmacopoeia Committee', *Indian Journal of Pharmacy* 10, no. 2 (1948): 117–18.

73 Editorial, 'Indian Pharmacopoeia Committee', *Indian Pharmacist* 4 (1948–49): 85–90. The *Pharmaceutical Journal* continued to take an interest. See also 'Pharmacopoeia of India', *Pharmaceutical Journal* 162, no. 4520 (1949): 13.

74 'The Indian Pharmacopoeia', *Pharmaceutical Journal* 173, no. 4751 (1954): 85.

75 Singh, *Pharmacopoeias and Formularies*, 103.

76 'The Indian Pharmaceutical List Committee', *Indian Pharmacist* 46, no. 1 (1945–46): 68–72, 78.

77 Cartwright, *British Pharmacopoeia*, 152–3.

78 Singh, *Pharmacopoeias and Formularies*, 101–18.

79 *Supplement 1960 to Pharmacopoeia of India* (Delhi: Government of India, 1960).

80 Singh, *Pharmacopoeias and Formularies*, 122.

81 Bhattacharya, *Disparate Remedies*, 96.

82 *British Pharmacopoeia 1948*, xxiv.

83 Cartwright, *British Pharmacopoeia*, 72.

84 *British Pharmacopoeia 1948*, v.

85 Ibid., xii–xiii.

86 Cartwright, *British Pharmacopoeia*, 73.

87 *British Pharmaceutical Codex 1973* (London: Pharmaceutical Society of Great Britain, 1973), ix.

88 *British Pharmacopoeia 1948*, 12.

89 Ibid., 69.

90 Ibid., 12.

91 Ibid., 835.

320 Notes to pages 233–6

92 CAB 128/8, Cabinet minutes (46) 108, Confidential Annex, 31 December 1946, cited by Wm Roger Louis, 'The Dissolution of the British Empire', in Brown, *The Twentieth Century*, 4:329. See also John Darwin, *Britain and Decolonization: The Retreat from Empire in the Post-war World* (London: Palgrave Macmillan, 1988).

93 Wm Roger Louis, 'The Dissolution of the British Empire', 329.

94 Louis, 329.

95 Andrew Egboh, *History of Pharmacy in Nigeria: A Guide and Survey of the Past and Present, 1887–1980* (Lagos: Pharmaceutical Society of Nigeria, 1982), 100.

96 John K. Crellin, *Newfoundland Drugstores: A History* (St John's: Flanker Press, 2013), 121–2.

97 *Addendum to British Pharmacopoeia 1948* (London: General Medical Council, 1951), xii.

98 Cartwright, *British Pharmacopoeia*, 75.

99 Ibid., 76.

100 *British Pharmacopoeia 1953*, xiv.

101 Ibid., xvii.

102 *British Pharmacopoeia 1948*, xxv.

103 *1951 Addendum to BP 1948*, xii; *British Pharmacopoeia 1953*, xvii.

104 American pharmaceutical companies establishing subsidiaries in Britain included Abbott, Lederle, Lilly, MSD, Pfizer, SKF, Upjohn, and Wyeth. See Leslie G. Matthews, *History of Pharmacy in Britain* (London: E. & S. Livingstone, 1962), 237.

105 Cartwright, *British Pharmacopoeia*, 79.

106 Teodor Canback, 'Pharmacopoeias and Formularies: BP 1958', *Journal of Pharmacy and Pharmacology* 9 (1958): 10.

107 Cartwright, *British Pharmacopoeia*, 80.

108 *British Pharmacopoeia 1953*, viii.

109 CO 859/1323, *Protocol for the Termination of the British Agreements for the Unification of Pharmacopoeial Formulae for Potent Drugs, 1957*, TNA, Kew.

110 Cartwright, *British Pharmacopoeia*, 77.

111 For other colonial responses see Cartwright, *British Pharmacopoeia*, 77–9.

112 Paul Cassar, 'Impact of British Pharmacy in Malta', *Pharmaceutical Historian* 8, no. 1 (1978): 3–4.

113 Patrick Chiu, 'Challenges and Opportunities for Western Pharmacy in Colonial Hong Kong, 1945–1984', *Pharmaceutical Historian* 50, no. 2 (2020): 49–50.

114 *Official Reports of Proceedings* (Hong Kong: Hong Kong Legislative Council, 16 July 1975), 900–3.

Notes to pages 237–42

115 Cartwright, *British Pharmacopoeia*, 80.

116 *British Pharmaceutical Codex 1973*, ix.

117 Lloyd C. Miller, 'The BP', *Journal of Pharmacy and Pharmacology* 15, no. 1 (1963): 766–8.

118 David Train, 'Pharmaceutical Standards', *Nature*, no. 4915 (1964): 118–19.

119 *British Pharmacopoeia 1968*, xix.

120 For the history and impact of the thalidomide disaster see Martin Johnson, Raymond Stokes, and Tobias Arndt, *The Thalidomide Catastrophe* (Exeter, UK: Onwards and Upwards, 2018); P. Knightley and H. Evans, *Suffer the Children: The Story of Thalidomide* (New York: Viking Press, 1979); Trent Stephens and Rock Brynner, *Dark Remedy: The Impact of Thalidomide and Its Revival as a Vital Medicine* (New York: Perseus Books, 2001).

121 Kenneth Robinson, 677 Parl. Deb. H.C. (5th ser.) (1963) col. 448.

122 Cartwright, *British Pharmacopoeia*, 90–1.

123 Ibid., 82.

124 *British Pharmacopoeia 1968*, xiv.

125 c816/02/01/1, Herbert S. Grainger, interviewed by Stuart Anderson, 17 May 1995, National Sound Archive, British Library.

126 Herbert S. Grainger, *An Apothecary's Tale: An Autobiography* (Hoddeston, UK: Noble Books, 2003), 226.

127 Ibid., 227.

CONCLUSION

1 'Notes', in *Drugs on the Page: Pharmacopoeias and Healing Knowledge in the Early Modern Atlantic World*, ed. Matthew James Crawford and Joseph M. Gabriel (Pittsburgh: University of Pittsburgh Press, 2019), 270.

2 Londa Schiebinger, 'Prospecting for Drugs: European Naturalists in the West Indies', in *Colonial Botany: Science, Commerce, and Politics in the Early Modern World*, ed. Londa Schiebinger and Claudia Swan (Philadelphia: University of Pennsylvania Press, 2005), 133.

3 Mark S.R. Jenner and Patrick Wallis, 'The Medical Marketplace', in *Medicine and the Market in England and Its Colonies, c.1450–c.1850*, edited by Mark S.R. Jenner and Patrick Wallis (London: Palgrave Macmillan, 2007), 15.

4 See Roy Porter and Mikulas Teich, eds, *Drugs and Narcotics in History* (Cambridge: Cambridge University Press, 1997).

Notes to pages 242–9

5 Nandini Bhattacharya, 'From Materia Medica to the Pharmacopoeia: Challenges of Writing the History of Drugs in India', *History Compass* 14, no. 4 (2016): 138.

6 Frances Watkins, Barbara Pendry, Olivia Corcoran, and Alberto Sanchez-Medina, 'Anglo-Saxon Pharmacopoeia Revisited: A Potential Treasure in Drug Discovery', *Drug Discovery Today* 16, nos 23–4 (2011): 1069–75.

7 Crawford and Gabriel, 'Introduction: Thinking with Pharmacopoeias', in *Drugs on the Page*, 11.

8 Pablo Gomez, 'The Power of the Unknown: Early Modern Pharmacopoeias and the Imagination of the Atlantic', in Crawford and Gabriel, *Drugs on the Page*, 268.

9 See for example Susan E. Bell and Anne E. Figert, 'Medicalization and Pharmaceuticalization at the Intersections: Looking Backward, Sideways, and Forward', *Social Science & Medicine* 75, no. 5 (2012): 775–83; Adele E. Clarke, Janet K. Shim, Laura Mamo, Jennifer Ruth Fosket, and Jennifer R. Fishman, 'Biomedicalization: Technoscientific Transformations of Health, Illness, and U.S. Biomedicine', *American Sociological Review* 68, no. 2 (2003): 161–94.

10 Stuart Anderson, *Pharmacy and Professionalization in the British Empire, 1780–1970* (London: Palgrave Macmillan, 2021), 69–97.

11 Bruno Bonnemain, 'Colonisation et pharmacie, 1830–1962: Une presence diversifiée de 130 ans des pharmaciens français', *Revue d'histoire de la pharmacie* 56, no. 359 (2008): 311–34.

12 Laurence Monnais, *The Colonial Life of Pharmaceuticals: Medicines and Modernity in Vietnam* (Cambridge: Cambridge University Press, 2019).

13 C.J.S. Thompson, *The Mystery and Art of the Apothecary* (London: John Lane, 1927), 280.

14 Gary B. Magee and Andre S. Thomson, *Empire and Globalisation: Networks of People, Goods and Capital in the British World, c. 1850–1914* (Cambridge: Cambridge University Press, 2010), 45–63.

15 Roy M. MacLeod, *Nature and Empire: Science and the Colonial Enterprise* (Chicago: University of Chicago Press, 2000), 10–15.

16 Mark Harrison, 'Science and the British Empire', *Isis* 96, no. 1 (2005): 63.

17 David Wade Chambers and Richard Gillespie, 'Locality in the History of Science: Colonial Science, Technoscience, and Indigenous Knowledge', *Osiris* 115 (2000): 221–40.

18 Claire Fowler, *Pharmacopoeia Londinensis 1618 and Its Descendants* (London: Royal College of Physician, 2018), 45.

19 George Urdang, 'Pharmacopoeias as Witnesses of World History', *Journal of the History of Medicine* 1, no. 1 (1946): 46–70.

Notes to pages 249–54

20 Fowler, *Pharmacopoeia Londinensis 1618*, 61.

21 Stuart Anderson, 'National Identities, Medical Politics, and Local Traditions: The Origins of the London, Edinburgh, and Dublin Pharmacopoeias, 1618–1807,' in Crawford and Gabriel, *Drugs on the Page*, 199–221.

22 Stuart Anderson, 'Pharmacy and Empire: The *British Pharmacopoeia* as an Instrument of Imperialism, 1864 to 1932,' *Pharmacy in History* 52, nos 3–4 (2010): 112–21.

23 George Urdang, 'The Development of Pharmacopoeias: A Review with Special Reference to the Pharmacopoeia Internationalis,' *Bulletin of the World Health Organisation* 4 (1951): 581.

24 Hugh N. Linstead, *Poisons Law* (London: Pharmaceutical Press, 1936), 2.

25 Derrick Dunlop, 'The Growth of Drug Regulation in the UK,' *Journal of the Royal Society of Medicine* 73, no. 6 (1980): 407.

26 Chantal Stebbings, *Tax, Medicines, and the Law: From Quackery to Pharmacy* (Cambridge: Cambridge University Press, 2018), 179–80.

27 *Regulatory Situation of Herbal Medicines: A Worldwide Review*, HO/TRM/98.1 (Geneva: World Health Organization, 1998).

28 Sandra Clair, 'The Challenges in Regulating Traditional Plant Medicines in the Era of Contemporary Evidence-Based Health Policy" (PhD diss., University of Canterbury, 2019).

29 For the early history of pharmaceutical texts see Paula de Vos, 'Pharmacopoeias and the Textual Tradition in Galenic Pharmacy,' in Crawford and Gabriel, *Drugs on the Page*, 19–44.

30 Robert Voeks, 'Disturbance Pharmacopoeias: Medicine and Myths from the Humid Tropics,' *Annals of the Association of American Geographers* 94, no. 4 (2004): 868–88.

31 Matthew James Crawford, 'An Imperial Pharmacopoeia?" in Crawford and Gabriel, *Drugs on the Page*, 77.

32 Orou G. Gaoue, Michael A. Coe, Matthew Bond, Georgia Hart, Barnabas C. Seyler, and Heather McMillen, 'Theories and Major Hypotheses in Ethnobotany,' *Economic Botany* 71, no. 3 (2017): 269–87.

33 Nélson Leal Alencar, Thiago Antonio de Sousa Araújo, Elba Lúcia Cavalcanti de Amorim, and Ulysses Paulino de Albuquerque, 'The Inclusion and Selection of Medicinal Plants in Traditional Pharmacopoeias: Evidence in Support of the Diversification Hypothesis,' *Economic Botany* 64, no. 1 (2010): 68–79.

34 See Reinaldo Farias Paiva de Lucena, Patricia Muniz de Medeiros, Elcida de Lima Araújo, Angelo Giuseppe Chaves Alves, and Ulysses Paulino de Albuquerque, 'The Ecological Apparency Hypothesis and the Impor-

tance of Useful Plants in Rural Communities from Northeastern Brazil,' *Journal of Environmental Management* 96, no. 1 (2012): 106–15.

35 Bhattacharya, 'From Materia Medica to Pharmacopoeia,' 131.

36 John V. Pickstone, *Ways of Knowing: A New History of Science, Technology and Medicine* (Manchester: Manchester University Press, 2000), 9.

37 Jonathan Simon, *Chemistry, Pharmacy and Revolution in France, 1777–1809* (Aldershot, UK: Ashgate, 2005), 170.

38 Ibid.

39 Freedom of Information Request, FOI 20/171 (Medicines and Healthcare Regulatory Authority, London, 12 May 2021).

40 *Pharmacy and Poisons Regulations L.N. 145 of 1978* (Hong Kong: Department of Health, Drug Registration and Import/Export Control Division, 2015), chap. 138, sec. 29.

41 Anthony C. Cartwright, *The British Pharmacopoeia, 1864 to 2014: Medicines, International Standards, and the State* (Farnham, UK: Ashgate, 2015), 135.

42 Roy Cunningham, *Consultation on the Future of the Two Volumes of the British Pharmacopoeia and the Companion Veterinary Volume* (London: Department of Health, 1999).

Index

acacia, 230

Accum, Frederick, 124

acetylsalicylic acid (aspirin), 189, 190, 192–3

acid, tests, 124; value, 55

aconite, 102

Aconitum heterophyllum, 143; *Aconitum napellus*, 169

Act of Union (1707), 94, 96

adulteration: definition of, 47; use of, 60, 124, 134, 206, 209

Adulteration Act (1860), 135

Adulteration of Food and Drugs Act (1872), 55

Agreement on the Unification of Pharmacopoeial Formulae for Potent Drugs (1930), 236

Ainslie, Whitelaw, 117, 138

Albania, 79

alchemists, 17

alcohol, 162

Algiers, 71

aloes, 230; and myrrh pills, 161

Alstonia scholaris, 143

amaranth, 230

ambergris, 91

America. *See* North American colonies; United States

American pharmacy, 128–9

American Revolutionary War, 21; American War of Independence, 104

analytical tests, 54, 189

Anglo-Sikh Wars, 119

Angola, 68

animal tests, 56

anis(e), 52

anthropology, 27–8; anthropologists, 255

anti-cholera vaccine, 220

antidotarium, 26

antidotus Matthioli, 101

antimony, 37, 87; organic antimonials, 220

anti-plague vaccine, 220

anti-pneumococcus serum, 220, 223

anti-venom serum, 220

apomorphine, 148

apothecaries, 18, 40, 50, 52–3, 60, 70, 73, 83, 86. *See also* Society of Apothecaries

Apothecaries Act (1815), 57, 106

326 Index

Apothecaries Hall, 10, 112
Apothecary, Wares, Drugs, and
  Stuffs Act (1540), 53
apparency hypothesis, 32, 254
arachis oil, 171, 173, 175, 188 192,
  221, 227
areca, 144
Aristolochia, 188, 231
Arnica flowers, dried, 173
arsenic, 50, 180, 185; tests, 187
Arsenic Act (1851), 57, 131
arsphenamine, 50, 189
aspirin. *See* acetylsalicylic acid
Assab Bay, 79
Assam, 115
Association of British Chemical
  Manufacturers, 235
Association of British Pharmaceuti-
  cal Industry, 235
Attfield, John, 55, 144, 146, 158,
  160–1, 185
atropine, 126, 190, 228
Auckland, 171
Augsburg Pharmacopòeia, 25, 26, 69,
  75, 89
Aushadh Kalpabali, 122
Australasian Journal of Pharmacy,
  169, 192
Australia, 21, 137, 151, 161, 169,
  192, 206, 207
Australian Pharmaceutical Formulary,
  178, 180
Australian wine, 208
Austria, 203
Ayurveda: medicine, 222; practi-
  tioners, 144, 173
Aztecs, 18

Bache, Franklin, 128
Baden Pharmacopoeia, 76

Bahamas, 234
Baker, Sir George, 101
Bald's Leechbook, 7
Balfour Declaration (1926), 218
balsam: of Copaiba, 134; of Peru, 8
Banks, Sir Joseph, 14
Barbados, 14, 137, 166
Barber, George, 146
barbitone, 187, 189
Basutoland, 167, 220
Battle of Buxar, 115
Battle of Plassey, 108, 115
Bavarian Pharmacopoeia, 76
bazaar medicines, 117, 121, 138,
  142, 177, 178, 196, 209, 247, 252
Bechuanaland Protectorate, 171
Beddard, Arthur, 219, 227
beeswax, white, 162
Belgian Congo, 81
Belgian pharmacopoeias, 69, 80–1
Belgium, 80, 203, 239
belladonna, 102, 221, 238
Bell, Jacob, 40, 130, 132
Bell, James, 205
Bengal: Presidency, 121; govern-
  ment, 134, 145
Bengal Dispensatory, 119–20
Bengal Pharmacopoeia, 128, 130, 137,
  210, 247
Benjamin. *See* benzoin
Bennett, R.R., 219
Bentley, Robert, 146
benzoin, 8, 91, 116
berberis, 187
Bergamo Pharmacopoeia, 87, 89
Berlin Conference (1884), 148, 152
Bermuda, 127, 166
betel, 187
Bevan, Joseph Gurney, 10; Bevan,
  Sylvanus, 110

Index

bezoar stone, 91

biological, medicines, 219, 220, 230; standards, 223; testing, 197, 203, 213, 221, 220

biomedicalization, 243

biomedicine, 17, 225, 230

bioprospecting, 17, 253

blood products, 235

boiling points, 125, 197

Bologna Pharmacopoeia, 87

Bombay: Presidency, 121, 145; government, 115, 116, 139, 153

Bombay Medical Union, 220

Boots (Nottingham), 223

botanical gardens, 12–13, 116, 159, 171

botanists, 14, 221

botany, 101, 105, 119, 134, 161

Brandenburg Dispensatory, 75

Brazil, 69

Breton, Peter, 122

British Disinfectant Manufacturers' Association, 235

British Guiana, 127, 166, 236

British Honduras, 166

British Medical Association, 58, 161

British Pharmaceutical Codex, 153, 182, 207, 224, 232

British Pharmaceutical Conference, 128, 193

British Pharmacopoeia Adopting Act (1898; Queensland), 208

British Pharmacopoeia Commission, 215, 219, 256

British Raj, 21, 128, 137

buchu, 125

bureaucratic regulation, 51, 176, 251

Burma, 164

Burroughs Wellcome, 189, 226

Burundi, 81

Butea: seeds, 187; gum, 188

Calcutta, 15, 116, 163; Calcutta Exhibition (1885), 146; government, 145; market, 122; medical college, 122; medical congress, 159

calumba, 102

camphor, 116, 196

Canada, 21, 137, 151, 164, 206; Canadian Committee on Pharmaceutical Standards, 220, 228; Canadian federation, 137; Canadian Medical Association, 210; Canadian Pharmaceutical Association, 180, 210; *Canadian Pharmaceutical Journal*, 137, 165; *Compendium of Canadian Formulary*, 180

Cannabis Indica, 135

cantharides, 70, 94

Cantonment Act (1924; India), 209

Cape Breton Island, 94

Cape Colony, 167; Colonial Medical Council, 167

Cape of Good Hope, 69, 115, 208

cardamom, 78, 91

Caribbean colonies, 71, 78, 99, 112

cascara, 228

cassia lignea, 8

castor oil, mixture, 192; seeds, 102

censors, 41, 54, 93, 107

Central Indigenous Drugs Committee, 159, 177, 186

Ceylon, 69, 168, 228

chalk, 134; mixture, 190

chamomile, 228

charcoal, 125

Chattaway, William, 181, 185

328 Index

chaulmoogra oil, 230

Chemical, medicines, 17, 128, 133, 134, 148, 218; nomenclature, 104; pharmacy, 102, 114; testing, 125, 134, 135, 148, 161, 187

chemistry, 14, 73, 105, 124, 134, 161; chemists, 133; corpuscular, 17

chemists and druggists, 131, 205; apprentices, 249

China, 196

China root, 8, 39

chloroform, 126, 134

Chopra, Sir Ram Nath, 222, 230

Christchurch, 171; botanic gardens, 171

Christison, Robert, 132

cinchona, 10, 13, 14, 15, 18, 70, 71

cinnamon, 78, 134

cloves, 14; clove oil, 134

cocaine, 15, 148, 161, 180, 182

cochineal, 94; production of, 116

Codex Medicamentarius, 180

Codex Medicamentarius, sive Pharmacopoeia Gallica, 74

Codice de la Cruz Badiano, 67

Codigo Pharmaceutico Lusitano, 67–8

cod liver oil, 126, 194, 227; emulsion of, 227

coffee, 242

Cohen, Lord, 239

colchicum, 102

College of Physicians (Dublin), 102–5

College of Physicians (Edinburgh), 96–9

College of Physicians (London), 53, 86–94

College of Physicians (Ontario), 207

College of Surgeons (Dublin), 104

Cologne, 69, 75, 90

Colonial Medical Service, 224

colonial pharmacopoeia, 115, 230, 248; colonial science, 15

Columba roots, 14

Columbian Exchange, 8, 84

Commission on Pharmacopoeial Revision (India), 220

Committee of Civil Research, 199, 201

Committees of Reference: in Botany 186; in Chemistry, 186; in Pharmacy, 161, 186, 193

Commonwealth Trade Descriptions Act (1906; Australia), 207

Company of Scotland Trading to Africa and the Indies, 95

Compendium of Canadian Formulary, 180

compounded medicines, 26, 30, 125

Concordia Aromatariorum, 65

Concordia Pharmacopolarum, 41, 65

constructive imperialism, 15

consumer sovereignty, 51, 140, 176, 251

convict pharmacopoeia, 113–14

Cook, James, 21

Cookworthy, William, 100

Corbyn, Thomas, 10, 110

coriander, 91

Corporation of Apothecaries (Ireland), 104

cortisone, 235

cotton, 78, 111, 116

cottonseed oil, 208, 227

Council of Europe, 239

counterfeit medicines, 47

Cranbrook, Viscount, 145

Crawford, F.J., 159, 163

creosote, 125–6

Cross, Viscount, 151
Culpeper, Nicholas, 17, 90, 93, 110
curare, 15
Curzon, Lord, 163
customs duties, 184, 195
Cyprus, 166

Daffy's Elixir, 110
Dale, Sir Henry, 227, 202
Dangerous Drugs Act (1920), 198–9
Dangerous Drugs Act (1930; India),
    222
Danish pharmacopoeia, 78–9
Danish West Indies, 79
Da Orta, Garcia, 25
Darien (Panama), 95
Darjeeling, 116
dates, 116
datura, 231
decolonization, 21, 197, 233
de Fourcroy, Antoine-Francois, 73
de la Cal y Bracho, Antonio, 67
de Laune, Gideon, 87
Delhi, 115
De Mayerne, Theodore, 87
Denmark, 78, 130. *See also* Danish
    pharmacopoeia; Danish West
    Indies
De Souza, Dr E.M., 164
Dey, Kanny Lall, 138, 156, 159
diamorphine, 189
digitalis, 148, 159, 228; compound
    pills, 225; powder, 221; tincture,
    105
digoxin, 184, 227
Diphtheria Antitoxin, 232
disintegration tests (tablets), 228
Dispensatorium Brandenburgicum, 76
Dispensatorium Coloniensis, 90
Dispensatorium Hafniense, 78

Dispensatorium Lippiacum, 75–6
dispensatory, 26, 103
disturbance pharmacopoeia, 254
diversification hypothesis, 30, 254
Dodoen, Rembert, 25
domestic remedies, 25, 48–9
Dominica, 236
Dominion Council of Health
    (Canada), 212
Dominion Food and Drug Act
    (1920; Canada), 206–7
Dominion pharmacopoeia, 151–3
dragon's blood, 8
Dr James's Powder, 102
drug cultivation, 189
drug regulation, 46, 73, 182, 198,
    224, 238; models of, 51
drug regulations: India, 140; Ire-
    land, 103
Drugs Act (India): of 1940, 144; of
    1944, 231
Drugs Enquiry Committee (1932;
    India), 195, 197, 222
Drugs Technical Advisory Board
    (India), 228
Dublin Pharmacopoeia, 45, 104–5
Du Bois, Jacques, 24
Dubosia, 228
Dufferin, Earl of, 151
Duncan, Andrew Jr, 14
Dunedin, 171
Dunlop, Professor Sir Derek, 235,
    252
Dutch East India Company, 69
Dutch East Indies, 69, 228
Dutch Guiana, 69
Dutch Pharmacopoeia, 70
Dutch West India Company, 69
Dutta, N.B., 222–3
Dutt, Shamachrun, 122

330 Index

Dymock, William, 138, 156

East India Company, 16, 38, 111, 140
economic botany, 13, 32; botanists, 222–3, 254
economic development, 256
Edinburgh New Dispensatory, 14
Edinburgh Pharmacopoeia, 96–9; use in North America, 110
Egypt, 228
English Civil War, 93
English Parliament, 103
ephedine, 227
Epsom salts, 193
ergot, 184, 221; ergotine, 148; ergotoxine, 226
Eritrea, 79
Ethiopia, 79
ethnobotany, 29, 34; ethnobotanists, 254, 255; historical, 34
ethnopharmacology, 29
ethno-pharmacopoeias, 30, 35, 253
European pharmacopoeia, 37, 39, 68, 239
exotic medicines, 7, 17, 228
Extra Pharmacopoeia, 136, 203. *See also* Martindale, William

Farmacopea per gli Stati Sardi, 80
Farmacopea Ufficiale del Regno d'Italia, 80
Farmacopoeia de D. Maria I, 68
Farmacopoeia Lusitana, 67
Farmacopoeia Mexicana, 67
Farmacopoeia Portuguesa, 68
Farrar, Frederick Willis, 153–4
Fayrer, Sir Joseph, 144–5, 149
fennel, 169
Fiji Islands, 171

Finland, 130
Food and Drugs Act (1875), 154, 205
Food and Drugs Act (1908; New Zealand), 209
Food and Drugs Act (1908; South Australia), 208
Food and Drug Acts (1913–14; Western Australia), 208
Formosa, 196
formulary, 26, 54, 73, 74; Australia, 178; Canada, 180; unofficial, 153
Fort St George, 115
foxglove, 102, 148
France, 80, 150, 187, 203, 239
fraud, 19, 40, 46, 86, 13
freezing point, 125
French Pharmacopoeia, 74–5, 180, 182

galenicals: definition of, 30; use of, 182, 184, 188
Galenic medicine, 87; pharmacy, 102, 114; principles, 16
gall apples, 70
Gambia, the, 220
garbling, 52; garblers, 52, 251
Garrod, Alfred, 132
gas gangrene antitoxin, 223
General Medical Council, 128, 131, 150, 251
Genoa treacle, 86
Gerarde, John, 25
German East Africa, 77
German Pharmacopoeia, 182
German South West Africa, 78
Germany, 80, 130, 187, 196, 203, 239
Ghana, 167. *See also* Gold Coast
Gibraltar, 166
ginger, Indian, 52, 220; tincture, strong, 161

Index

ginseng, 70
global: economy, 16; markets, 225; science, 16; trade, 10, 37
globalization, 7, 22
global pharmacopoeia, 36
glycerine (glycerol), 190, 192, 227
glyceryl trinitrate, 148
Glyn-Jones, Sir William, 200
Goa, 68
gold, 111
Gold Coast, 69, 111, 137, 225. *See also* Ghana
Good, John Mason, 40
Goodwin, James, 54
Government of Canada, 211
Government of India, 185, 189, 195, 210, 222
Government of Tasmania, 214
Granada, 166
Great Migration, 109
Greenish, Henry George, 185, 187, 193, 215, 219
Greenish, Thomas Edward, 152–3, 178, 179
Greenland, 78–9
Grindelia robusta, 169
Grocers' Company, 18, 86, 87
guaiac (guaicum), 8, 10, 35
Guatemala, 80
Gupta, Madhusudan, 122

hakims, 196
Hamilton, Lord, 163
Hampshire, Dr Charles, 219, 220
Hanbury, Daniel, 139, 146
Hartington, Marquis of, 145
Hartley, Sir Frank, 239
Hassall, Arthur Hill, 134
Heberden, William, 102
henbane, 102

herbal, 25, 30; medicine, 34, 36, 167, 253; remedies, 19, 33, 99
herbal pharmacopoeia, 28, 40
hexamine, 187, 193
Hills, Walter, 161
Holland, 203. *See also* Netherlands
Hollingsworth, R., 159, 163
honey, 40, 70, 125
Hong Kong, 158, 169, 188, 196, 236, 256
Hooper, David, 156, 164, 181, 222
Hyderabad (BMA branch), 210
hyoscine, 161, 228
hyoscyamus, 159, 228

iatrochemistry, 17
iatromechanics, 17, 98, 99
identity tests, 125
Imperial Economic Conference (1932), 195
imperializing pharmacopoeia, 83, 163, 166, 169, 171, 250
imperial pharmacopoeias: Britain, 63, 86, 107, 122, 143, 150, 163, 174, 181, 197, 211, 217, 233; France, 73, 74; Germany, 77; Spain, 64, 66, 67
incense, 40
Incorporation of Surgeons and Barbers (Edinburgh), 96
incunabula, 25
Indian and Colonial Addendum to the *BP*, 210, 221; *Government of India Edition* (1901), 174, 176
Indian Commission on Pharmacopoeial Revision, 230
Indian Medical Congress, 159
Indian Medical Council, 231
Indian Medical Department, 142

332   Index

Indian Medical Service, 115, 140, 145, 149

Indian Penal Code, 174

Indian Pharmaceutical Association, 231

Indian pharmacopoeia, 119, 121. *See also* Pharmacopoeia of India

Indian Pharmacopoeia Committee, 230

Indian Pharmacopoeial List, 229–30

Indian War of Independence, 21

Indigenous pharmacopoeias, 35, 253, 254, 255

indigo, 78, 116

Indochina, 71, 75

Indonesia, 71

inspection: of drugs, 54, 55; of premises, 85, 107, 209, 251

insular pharmacopoeia, 31

International Conference on the Unification of the Formulae of Powerful Medicaments (1902), 216

International Opium Convention (1912), 183

International Pharmacopoeia, 231, 236

iodine value, 55

ipecacuanha, 7, 10, 13, 14, 15, 35, 70, 134, 221, 228, 241

Ireland, 163, 215

Irish Free State, 215, 220, 227

Irish Parliament, 103, 105

Irish whisky, 94

iron, 55; compound mixture, 192; test for, 87

isinglass, 11

ispaghula, 143, 231

Italian Pharmacopoeia, 80

Italy, 80, 203, 239

Jabalpur Government Dispensary, 122

jalap, 8, 159, 241

Jamaica, 112, 127, 137, 166, 234

Jamestown, 109; weed, 8

Japan, 196, 228; pharmacopoeia, 75, 256

Johnston, Sir Harry, 167

kaolin, 161

Kashmir, 119

kava root, 171

Kemp, David Skinner, 164

Kenya, 228

Kimberley, Earl of, 148, 151, 156–7

King, George, 159

kino, 188; Botany Bay, 169

kola nut, 167

Koman, M.V., 196, 197

Korcula, 31

kousso, 166

labelling: containers, 195, 237; poisons, 252

Labuan, 169

Lagos, 167. *See also* Nigeria

laissez-faire policy, 206

lard, hog's, 162, 174

lead, 55

leeches, 94

lemon peel, dried, 162, 188

Libya, 79

limit tests, 148

Linacre, Thomas, 86

Linstead, Sir Hugh, 252

liquid paraffin, 161

lobelia, 230

London Pharmacopoeia, 85–6, 126, 132, 145, 166; Hindustani translation, 116

Index

Luxembourg, 80, 239
Lytton, Lord, 145

MacAlister, Donald Sir, 162, 200, 201, 219
Macmillan, Hugh Pattison, 202
Macmillan Report, 203, 217; publication, 223; remit, 201
Madagascar, 143, 167
Madras, 115, 143; botanic garden, 116; government, 145, 196; medical college, 158, 163; medical department, 39, 164
magnesia, manufacture of, 160
malaria, 29
Malaya, 228, 234
male fern, 166
Malta, 166, 236
Manitoba, 207
Martindale, William, 136, 146, 152, 161. See also *Extra Pharmacopoeia*
Martin, Sir James Ranald, 139
Massachusetts Bay Colony, 109
Materia Indica of Hindoostan, 117, 138
materia medica, 27, 91, 105, 119, 127, 128, 135, 241; India, 140, 142, 156, 196
Materia Medica Indica, 145–6
Materia Medica of Madras, 156
Mauritius, 28, 130, 169
Mayleigh, Thomas, 10
Medical Act (1858), 107, 128, 130
Medical Act (1862), 132
Medical Act (1915; Victoria), 208
Medical Act (1950), 235
Medical Act (1956), 237
Medical and Kindred Professions Ordinance (Malta), 236
Medical and Pharmacy Act Amend-

ment Act (1899; Cape Colony), 208
medical anthropology, 27–8
medical botany, 128
medicalization, 243
medical marketplace, 18, 23, 50, 242
medical philosophies, 87
medical reform, 40, 125
Medical Research Council, 199, 215, 227
medical sociology, 27, 28
medicines: efficacy, 38, 159, 174, 204, 213, 238; identity, 55, 60, 161, 163, 229; potency, 56, 60, 207; purity, 55, 60, 124, 148, 161, 163, 204, 207, 221, 229; quality, 19, 43, 60, 140, 161, 205, 207; safety, 38, 188, 236, 238; testing, 114
Medicines Act (1968), 57, 252
Medicines Commission, 219, 238, 251
Medicine Stamp Act (1802), 184
medicine stamp duty, 184, 194, 252
melon pumpkin seeds, 166, 173
melting point, 134, 197
menthol, 148
Merchandise Marks Act (1889; India), 174
mercury, 50, 53; thermometer, 102
metric system. *See* weights and measures
Mexico, 67
microscopy, 55, 134
migrant pharmacopoeias, 33
milk of sulphur, 53
Millington, Sir Thomas, 112
Monardes, Nicholas, 8
Montreal, 165
Montserrat, 165

Moreton Bay Penal Settlement, 113
Morocco, 40
morphine, 18, 105, 125–6, 148
Mouat, Frederick J., 122
'moving metropolis', 15
'multiple engagements', 246
mustard: oil, 47; paper, 161

Napoleonic Wars, 21, 108
narcotics, 61, 182 199; legislation, 62
narcotine, 105
Natal, 208, 209
National Formulary Committee, 224
National Institute for Medical Research, 227
nationalism, 21, 233; cultural, 12; Scottish, 94
national pharmacopoeia, 42, 74, 76, 81, 121, 136, 185, 194
National War Formulary, 227
natural, history, 14, 16; philosophy, 18
Nederlandsche Apoteek, 81
Neosalvarsan, 190
Netherlands, 80, 239, 245. *See also* Holland
networks, 246–7; botanical, 13, 116; industry, 235; Quaker, 10; scientific, 12, 128; trading, 61, 225
Newfoundland, 18, 165, 181, 215, 224
New Guinea, 171
'new imperialism', 152
New South Wales, 113, 169; New South Wales Pharmaceutical Society, 169
New Zealand, 21, 137, 151, 171,

179, 206, 209; New Zealand Pharmacy Board, 171
Nicobar Islands, 78–9
nicotinamide, 228
nicotine, 50
Nigeria, 137, 233. *See also* Lagos
Nine Years' War, 112
Nordic Pharmacopoeia Council, 237
North American colonies, 71, 165
Northern Rhodesia, 225
North-Western Provinces, 145
North-West Frontier Province, 119
Norway, 130, 203
Nova Scotia, 71; Nova Scotia Pharmaceutical Society, 151–2, 153
Nuevo Receptario. See *Receptario Florentino*; *Ricettario Fiorentino*
Nuremberg: *Dispensatory*, 24, 75; *Nuremberg Pharmacopoeia*, 54, 90
nux vomica, 221
Nyasaland, 225

occupational control, 51, 182, 251
Officina Medicamentorum, 66
olive oil, 171, 175, 188, 227
Ontario, 113, 175, 188, 227; College of Pharmacy, 180; College of Physicians and Surgeons, 180
opium, 10, 18, 35, 62, 105, 134, 174, 180, 182
Opium Act (1878; India), 174
Opium Ordinance (Transvaal), 62
Opium Wars, 61
optical rotation, 55, 182
Orange Free State, 195, 209
Orange River Colony, 208
orange tincture, 161
organoleptic tests, 54, 125

O'Shaughnessy, Sir William Brooke, 118, 139
Otago Pharmaceutical Association, 171

Pakistan, 233–4
Palestra pharmaceutica, 66, 114
Paracelsus, 18, 87; Paracelsian medicine, 87
Parisian Pharmacopoeia, 71
Paris, John Ayrton, 128
Park, Dr C.L., 212
Parliamentary Select Committee (1878–79), 205
Patea Domain Board, 171
Patent Act, 226
patent, letters, 232
patent medicines, 152–3, 180, 194, 195, 198, 224, 225, 252
Patiala Government, 222
Pemberton, Henry, 101
penicillin, 227–8
pepper, 8, 78
pepperers, 7, 52
Pereira, Jonathan, 127
Peru, 67
Peruvian bark, 12, 13
petroleum jelly, 179
pharmaceutical: anthropology, 28; chemistry, 119, 167; chemists, 73, 144; products, 30, 167
Pharmaceutical Act (1914; Manitoba), 207
Pharmaceutical Formulae, 184
pharmaceutical industry, 56, 76, 109, 151, 167, 184, 189–90, 195, 218
pharmaceuticalization, 243
Pharmaceutical Society of Great Britain: education, 57; founda-

tion, 18, 131; laboratory, 219; pharmacopoeia committee, 152; school, 106, 127; yearbook, 178
Pharmaceutical Society of Ireland, 215, 226
Pharmaceutical Society of Northern Ireland, 215
Pharmaceutical Society of Tasmania, 171
Pharmacia Antwerpiensis, 81
pharmacognosy, 77
Pharmacographia, 146
Pharmacographia Indica, 149, 156
pharmacology, 17, 77, 161; pharmacologists, 59, 77, 160, 255
Pharmacopedia, 181, 185
Pharmacopoea Austriaca, 80
Pharmacopoea Batava, 70, 81
Pharmacopoea Danica, 18–19
Pharmacopoea Germaniae, 76; *Pharmacopoea Germanica*, 76–7
Pharmacopoea Neerlandica, 70, 81
pharmacopoeia: definition, 22, 23, 41, 42; as expression of society, 31; and national identity, 124; universalization of, 35
Pharmacopoeia Act (1931; Ireland), 226
Pharmacopoeia Amstelredamensis, 69; *Pharmacopoeia Amstelredamensis Renovate*, 69–70
Pharmacopoeia Augustana, 25
Pharmacopoeia Belgica, 81; *Pharmacopoeia Belgica Nova*, 81
Pharmacopoeia Borussica, 76
Pharmacopoeia Britannica, 123
Pharmacopoeia Bruxellensis, 81
Pharmacopoeia Commission: origin, 215–19; membership, 235, 238; winding up, 239

336 Index

Pharmacopoeia Geral para o Reino e Dominios de Portugal, 67
Pharmacopoeia Harlemensis, 70
Pharmacopoeia Hispana, 66
Pharmacopoeia Matritensis, 64
Pharmacopoeia of India, 122, 182, 210, 230, 231, 247; supplement (1960), 231. *See also* Indian pharmacopoeia
Pharmacopoeia Ordinance (1958; Hong Kong), 236
Pharmacopoeia Portuguesa, 67–8
pharmacopoeia syphilitica, 37
pharmacy: by doctors, 19; practice, 34, 251; professionalisation, 6, 18, 40, 42, 244; regulation, 46, 252; separation from medicine, 42
Pharmacy Act (1852), 57, 130
Pharmacy Act (1871; Ontario), 137, 207
Pharmacy Act (1875; Ireland), 205
Pharmacy Act (1875; Quebec), 137
Pharmacy Act (1908), 182
Pharmacy Act (1908; New Zealand), 209
Pharmacy Act (1925; Northern Ireland), 205
Pharmacy Act (1948; India), 144
Pharmacy Act (1976; Nova Scotia), 137
Pharmacy and Poisons Act (1868), 57, 114
Pharmacy and Poisons Act (1933), 224
Pharmacy and Poisons Ordinance (1956; British Guiana), 236
Pharmacy and Poisons Regulations (1978; Hong Kong), 256
Pharmacy Council of India, 231
Pharmacy Ordinance (Nigeria), 233

Pharmacy Regulations (1921; New South Wales), 208
phenacetin, 155, 190, 193
phenylbutazone, 236
Phillips, Richard, 119, 125–6
physicians, relations with apothecaries, 53, 57, 86, 106
physiology, 105, 134; physiological testing, 184
Piper methysticum. See kava root
Pitcairn, Archibald, 99
Plantago ispaghula, 143
Plough Court, 110
Plymouth Colony, 109
podophyllum, Indian, 221
poisons: control, 45–6, 55; legislation, 52, 57; register, 182; regulation, 58, 85, 252; sale, 58, 209
Poisons Act (1919; India), 209
pomegranate bark, 166
poppies, syrup of, 166
Portugal, 82
Portuguese pharmacopoeias, 67–9
potash, manufacture, 160
Pouppée-Desportes, Jean-Baptiste René, 37
Powell, Richard, 25, 106, 123
Privy Council, 131–2, 153, 200
professionalization, pharmacy, 6, 18, 40, 42, 244
proprietary medicines, 153, 178–9, 183, 184, 211. *See also* patent medicines
Proprietary or Patent Medicine Act (1908; Canada), 180, 195
Prussia, 75
Pudina oil, 230
Pure Food Act (1908; New South Wales), 208

purity tests, 124, 135. *See also under* medicines

quack medicine, 184
Quain, Sir Richard, 136, 146, 160
Quaker, networks, 10
quassia, 102
Quebec, 137, 151; Quebec Act (1788), 113, 123
Queensland, 113, 162, 169, 208; pharmacy board, 214
quinine, 10, 18, 35, 105, 190, 241–2

Rangoon, 164
Ransom, Francis, 193
Receptario Florentino, 41, 86, 90. See also *Ricettario Fiorentino*
Redwood, Theophilus, 127, 136, 144, 146
refractive index, 55, 182
religious beliefs, 99, 174
rhubarb, 35, 53, 91, 230; compound pills, 125
riboflavin, 228
Ricettario Fiorentino, 24, 34. See also *Receptario Florentino*
Ripon, Marquis of, 145
Robinson, Kenneth, 238
Rose Case 1704, 57
Rowsell, Philip, 200
Royal African Company, 111
Royal Botanic Gardens, Kew, 14, 116
Royal College of Physicians (Dublin), 102–3
Royal College of Physicians (Edinburgh), 14, 97
Royal College of Physicians (London), 112, 125, 131
Royal College of Surgeons, 106

Royal Society, 125
Royle, John Forbes, 119, 138
rubber, 13
Russell, Patrick, 14
Russia: medicinal plants, 31–2; pharmacy in, 130
Rwanda, 81

Sale and Use of Poisons Act (1876; Victoria), 114
Sale of Food and Drugs Act (1875), 59
Sale of Food and Drugs Act (1887; New Zealand), 137
salicylates, 148, 160
salicylic acid, 148, 190
Salvarsan, 50, 189
Santo Tomas, 80
saponification value, 55
sarsaparilla, 8, 39, 91
sassafras, 8
scammony, 53, 134
scientification, 17, 73, 250
Scottish: colony, 94, 99; nationalism, 94, 97; Scottish Parliament, 95, 96, 98
Scramble for Africa, 21, 148
Sea Customs Act (1878; India), 174
Seidlitz Powders, 155
Select Committee on Patent Medicine (1914), 198
Senegal, 75
senna, 53, 91
sera, 56, 199
Serampore, 78–9
Serum Institute, Melbourne, 213
sesame oil, 175, 188, 192, 221, 227
Seven Years' War, 115
Seychelles, 169
shamans, 27

Sheriff, Moodeen, 143, 144, 156
sherry, 189, 206
Shillinglaw, Harry, 178
Sibbald, Robert, 97
Sibthorpe, C. (surgeon general), 164
Sierra Leone, 167, 220
silk, 69, 78
simples, meaning, 26, 30
Sindh, 115
Singapore, 168, 234
Sinhalese drugs, 168
sisal, 13
slavery, 21, 99, 111
Sloane, Sir Hans, 13, 100
social historians, 36, 37
social pharmacopoeias, 28
Society of Apothecaries: foundation, 18, 53, 87; medicine manufacture, 111, 112; medicine supply, 116, 125; reputation, 140; role in pharmacopoeia, 101, 106
soft colonial power, 249
Somalia, 79
South Africa, 21, 137, 151; Medical Association, 214; Pharmaceutical Association, 225; plant medicines, 167, 194, 206, 220, 225
South Australia, 169; Pharmaceutical Society, 179
South Carolina Act (1751), 111
Southern Rhodesia, 215, 225; Medical Council, 215
Spanish Pharmacopoeia, 65–7
Spanish War of Succession, 21
specific gravity, 124, 188, 220
spice, 69
spicers, 7
spikenard, 53
squill, 184

Squire, Peter, 126–7, 132, 135–6, 203
standardization, 59, 249
staphylococcus antitoxin, 223
starch, 125, 190
Statute of Westminster (1931), 218
St Christopher and Nevis, 171
St Croix, 78
steam baths, 136
sterilisation methods, 220, 227
Stevenson, Sir Archibald, 98
St Helena, 116, 167
stilboestrol, 228
St John, 78
St Lucia, 166
Storke, Samuel, 10
Stoughton's Elixir, 110
Straits of Magellan, 115
stramonium, 102, 115
strophanthin seeds, 148, 167, 221, 225
strophanthus, 167, 184
strychnine, 180
St Thomas, 78
St Vincent, 166
substandard medicines, 4, 48
substitution: of adulteration, 190; of drugs, 18, 83, 128; in India, 39, 156, 158, 177, 213, 216, 232, 248; of pharmacopoeia, 140; in Spain, 67; suggestions for, 163; suppression of, 159
Sudan, 228
suet: beef, 174; mutton, 174
sugar, 78, 99, 111, 116, 190, 227
sulphanilamide, 226, 227
sulphate of soda, manufacture of, 160
sulphur, 87, 91
sumbul root, 188
surgeons: colonial, 14, 113; collaboration with apothecaries, 18

surgical catgut, 235
Swaziland, 220
Sweden, 130, 203
Switzerland, 203, 239
Sydney, 15, 56, 114, 179

Tabasheer, 14
talc, as adulterant, 190
Tamil drugs, 168
tannic acid, 126
tansy seed, 52
Tanzania, 228
taraxacum, 159
Tariff Act (1894; India), 174
Tasmania (Van Diemen's Land),
    113, 127, 171, 214; Pharmaceuti-
    cal Society, 171
Tawell, John, 113
tea, 242
technology, 134, 160
technoscience, 61
thalidomide, 238
theophylline with ethylene
    diamine, 226
therapeutics, 161, 199, 204; botani-
    cal, 117; market, 222
Therapeutic Substances Act (1925),
    50, 199, 221
theriac, 91
theriaca Andromachi, 102
thermometer, 102
Thomson, Thomas, 128, 139
thymol, 148
thyroid, dried, 161
Tirard, Nestor, 160, 187, 194
tobacco, 8, 111, 242
Togo, 78
trade, 109; export, 110, 121; free,
    135, 149; names, 189; networks,
    225; re-export, 196; role in sub-
    stitution, 250. See also slavery

traditional pharmacopoeias, 29, 33,
    167, 243, 249
Tranquebar, 78–9
Trans-Jordan, 220
Transvaal: Pharmaceutical Society,
    192, 195; Pharmacy Board, 62,
    168
Treaty of Paris, 108
Treaty of Utrecht, 21
Trinidad and Tobago, 127, 165, 234
tropical climate, 143, 189
Turks and Caicos Islands, 166

Unani, 222; practitioners, 144, 196
Union Medical Council (South
    Africa), 214
Union of Crowns (1603), 94
Union Pharmacy Board (South
    Africa), 214
United States, 193, 196, 203. See also
    America
United States Pharmacopoeia, 111,
    165, 180, 182, 211, 223, 226, 232,
    235
universal pharmacopoeia, 35, 164

vaccines, 56, 199, 220, 232
Vaids, 196
Van Diemen's Land, 113. See also
    Tasmania
Victoria, 207, 208; BMA branch,
    169
Victoria Health Act (1915), 208
Victoria Pharmaceutical Society,
    178
Victoria Pharmacy Board, 114
Vietnam, 75, 244
Virginia Act (1736), 111
vitamin preparations, 223, 227,
    230

Index

Wakley, Thomas, 58
Warden, C.J.H., 149, 156, 159, 160
Waring, Edward John, 133–4, 138, 140
Warington, Robert, 136
Watson, Sir Thomas, 135
Watt, George, 146, 159, 160, 164
ways of knowing, 133, 61, 16
weights and measures, 94, 104, 127, 134, 135, 208; metric, 237; uniformity of, 228
Western Australia, 171
Western pharmacopoeia, 38, 121
wine, Australian, 208

wintergreen, oil of, 173
Winthrop, John, 109
Withering, William, 50
Woodward's Gripe Water, 194–5
World Health Organization, 236, 237, 253
wormseed, 52
wormwood, 40
Wurttenberg Pharmacopoeia, 75

Yearbook of Pharmacy, 153, 178

Zanzibar, 228
Zulu medicines, 168